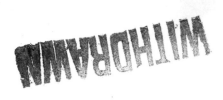

A History
of Psychiatry

Other Books by Edward Shorter

The Historian and the Computer: A Practical Guide

Work and Community in the West, editor

Strikes in France, 1830–1968 (co-author Charles Tilly)

The Making of the Modern Family

A History of Women's Bodies

Bedside Manners: The Troubled History of Doctors and Patients

The Health Century

From Paralysis to Fatigue: A History of Psychosomatic Illness in the Modern Era

From the Mind into the Body: The Cultural Origins of Psychosomatic Symptoms

A History of Psychiatry

From the Era of the Asylum to the Age of Prozac

Edward Shorter

John Wiley & Sons, Inc.

New York • Chichester • Brisbane • Toronto • Singapore • Weinheim

Copyright © 1997 by Edward Shorter
Published by John Wiley & Sons, Inc.

Library of Congress Cataloging-in-Publication Data:

Shorter, Edward.
    A history of psychiatry : from the era of the asylum to the age of
Prozac / by Edward Shorter.
        p.   cm.
    Includes bibliographical references.
    ISBN 0-471-15749-X (cloth : alk. paper). — ISBN 0-471-24531-3
(pbk. : alk. paper)
    1. Psychiatry—History. I. Title.
    [DNLM: 1. Psychiatry—history. 2. Psychoanalysis—history.
3. Psychotherapy—history. 4. Social Values. WM 11.1 S559h 1997]
RC438.S54 1997
616.89′009—dc20
DNLM/DLC
for Library of Congress   96-15292

This book is dedicated to my dear friends and fellow historians William Irvine and Michael Marrus: true comrades.

Preface

For historians of psychiatry who wrote 30 or 40 years ago—the last time anyone attempted an overview of the discipline—the story seemed relatively straightforward. First there were those wicked biological psychiatrists in the nineteenth century, then psychoanalysts and psychotherapists came along to defeat the biological zealots, establishing that mental illness resulted from unhappiness in childhood and stress in adult life. Freud's insights opened a new frontier in our understanding of mental illness and little more needed to be said.

Between the 1950s and the 1990s, a revolution took place in psychiatry. Old verities about unconscious conflicts as the cause of mental illness were pitched out and the spotlight of research turned on the brain itself. Psychoanalysis became, like Marxism, one of the dinosaur ideologies of the nineteenth century. Today, it is clear that when people experience a major mental illness, genetics and brain biology have as much to do with their problems as do stress and their early-childhood experiences. And even in the quotidian anxieties and mild depressions that are the lot of humankind, medications now can lift the symptoms, replacing hours of aimless chat. If there is one central intellectual reality at the end of the twentieth century, it is that the biological approach to psychiatry—treating mental illness as a genetically influenced disorder of brain chemistry—has been a smashing success. Freud's ideas, which dominated the history of psychiatry for the past half century, are now vanishing like the last snows of winter. The time has therefore come for a new look.

There is a place for a new history of psychiatry, a one-volume overview that will tell the basic story, highlight national differences, and point out how culture and psychiatry influence each other. A history is needed that will give the dramatic outlines of the story without sprawling into an encyclopedic country-by-country account. This volume takes on that task. I have not tried to tell it as intellectual history, as the arid succession of ideas and theories one after another, but rather as social history, recapturing the lives of some of the major players who now hover on the cusp of oblivion. It is a social history that identifies distinctive national contributions while not chronicling events in all places. And it is a social history that demonstrates how culture and commerce infiltrate what is often presented as a narrative of purely scientific triumphs.

Above all, I have tried to rescue the history of psychiatry from the sectarians who have made the subject a sandbox for their ideologies. To an extent unimaginable for other areas of the history of medicine, zealot-researchers have seized the history of psychiatry to illustrate how their pet bugaboos—be they capitalism, patriarchy, or psychiatry itself—have converted protest into illness, locking into asylums those who otherwise would be challenging the established order. Although these trendy notions have attained great currency among intellectuals, they are incorrect, in that they do not correspond to what actually happened. Psychiatry is, to be sure, the ultimate rulemaker of acceptable behavior through its ability to specify what counts as "crazy." Yet there is such a thing as mental illness. It has a reality independent of conventions of gender and class, and this reality can be mapped, understood, and treated in a systematic and scientific way. Just as one would not insist that Parkinsonism or multiple sclerosis are socially constructed, one may no longer argue that schizophrenia and depression are social constructs lacking a basis in flesh and blood. Yet how patients experience these conditions, and how society makes sense of them, are indeed subject to the influence of culture and convention.

The story I want to tell is straightforward. It begins in the newly therapeutic asylums of the late eighteenth century and ends in the quiet offices of private practitioners late in the twentieth. It commences with psychiatrists who believed that the brain was the basis of mental illness; it is then interrupted by half a century of divorcing brain from mind with the dominance of Freud's theories; and it concludes in our own time with the renewed triumph of views stressing the primacy of the brain.

The account the reader finds here is not unabashedly apologetic but rather semiapologetic. Once upon a time, real apologists of psychiatric history dominated the field, who argued that the rise of the asylum represented undiluted progress in the alleviation of human misery. Then in the 1960s, this judgment was completely overturned. The children of the 1960s insisted that psychiatrists and their institutions of brick and mortar had led us not into "progress"—a delusory notion at best, they scoffed—but into a historic nightmare of breathtaking proportions. Rather than alleviating madness, it was argued, the perpetrators of the "great confinement" had locked up people whose only offense was their poverty, their rebelliousness, or their unconventional manner of life. Indeed, the whole notion of mental illness appeared suspect to the activists of the 1960s, who preferred to use—always in mocking quotation marks—such bygone terms as madness or lunacy, the very ludicrousness of these phrases discrediting the proposition that mental disorder exists as a natural phenomenon. These detractors, I regret to say, now dominate the academic history of psychiatry, and the chapters that follow are intended to confront head-on their revisionism, which has become in its turn the new orthodoxy.

If mental illness is real, past efforts to relieve it do not automatically constitute a bourgeois plot. Nor are psychiatrists who point out this reality automatically guilty of self-serving efforts to boost their own professional influence. There are historians who detect professionalization and medicalization behind every turn in the history of psychiatry, meaning that doctors act not in the interest of their patients or of science, but to shore up their own sagging authority. Doctors, of course, wish to enhance their own influence and authority (as do the rest of us), but reducing the history of psychiatry to professional self-servingness ends up explaining little of a complex story.

The history of psychiatry is a minefield. Both the revisionists and neoapologists such as myself risk being blown up by uncharted pieces of evidence. The very richness of the sources makes it possible to demonstrate through selective quotation just about anything. But what counts is gaining a sense of the central tendency, the larger picture. After many years of studying the sources, I present the following chapters as being much closer to historical events than the revisionist version. Yet this is a young field of study, and many surprises may lie in store for us all.

I have several great debts to acknowledge. The last two chapters owe much to the generosity of David Healy, who shared with me the interviews he had conducted with important contemporary figures in psychiatry's history, and let me profit as well from the manuscript of his forthcoming book on the history of the antidepressants. Thomas Ban also very kindly read parts of the manuscript. Susan Bélanger helped with much of the library work. Any book addressing two hundred years of the history of world psychiatry will inevitably rely heavily on interlibrary loan services, and Roy D. Pearson of the Science and Medicine Library of the University of Toronto has done yeoman service here. Andrea Clark, the administrator of the History of Medicine Program at the University of Toronto, has been a great help to me throughout. Finally, it has been a great pleasure for me to work with Jo Ann Miller, my editor at John Wiley & Sons.

Contents

1

The Birth of Psychiatry

B efore the end of the eighteenth century, there was no such thing as psychiatry. Although individual doctors had occupied themselves with the care of the insane and had written manuals about it since the time of the ancient Greeks, psychiatry did not then exist as a discipline to which a group of physicians devoted themselves with a common sense of identity. Yet except for surgery, few other specialities had come to life either. The advent of medical specialism was a phenomenon of the nineteenth century.

Yet mental disorder as such had always been familiar. Having a partly biological and genetic basis, psychiatric illness is as old as the human condition. Although not all mental disturbances are buried in the integuments of our nervous system, some certainly are, arising from disorders of the chemistry of the brain itself. It follows then that human society has always known psychiatric illness, and has always had ways of coping with it.

A World without Psychiatry

What is it like to live in a world without psychiatry? In Ireland, it was like this: In 1817, a member of the House of Commons from an Irish district said, "There is nothing so shocking as madness in the cabin of the Irish peasant. . . . When a strong man or woman gets the complaint, the only way they have to manage is by making a hole in the floor of the cabin, not high enough for the person to stand up in, with a crib over it to prevent his getting up. This hole is about five feet deep, and they give this wretched being his food there, and there he generally dies."[1]

One may abandon immediately any romantic notion of the insane in past times as being permitted to gambol on the village green or ruminate idly in the shade of the oak tree. Before the middle of the nineteenth century, the people of villages and small towns had a horror of those who were different, an authoritarian intolerance of behavior that did not conform to rigidly drawn norms. Living in tightly organized face-to-face communities, the villagers of Europe attached great importance to inherited social roles, to customs preordained by tradition, and to daily lives dictated by the march of the seasons. Those who were forced by disorders of mind and mood to be different, to deviate from any of these rhythms, were dealt with in the most brutal and unfeeling manner. Consider, after all, the fate of those with major mental illnesses in the days of King Lear:

> Poor naked wretches, wheresoe'er you are,
> That bide the pelting of this pitiless storm,
> How shall your houseless heads and unfed sides,
> Your loop'd and window'd raggedness, defend you
> From seasons such as these?[2]

If turned out of their homes and villages, the mentally ill swelled the streams of beggars that wandered the roads of early modern Europe. Many of the "village idiots" were those who had suffered mental retardation or schizophrenia from birth trauma (protracted labor in the days of pelves narrowed by rickets). The "fool" with his staff was a standard iconographic image. Yet the picture of the insane as always having been with us requires nuancing. Outside of England, most people with mental disorders in past times had the right to be taken in and given poor relief in the place they were born. They could not be simply turned out.

So it was the family, not the community, that had to deal with them. Before the nineteenth century, looking after the insane was a family affair. And home care in the world we have lost was a horror story. Anton Müller, who in 1798 became chief of psychiatry at the Royal Julius Hospital in Würzburg, gave an account of some of the newly admitted patients. "A youth of sixteen, who for years had lain in a pigpen in the hut of his father, a shepherd, had so lost the use of his limbs and his mind that he would lap the food from his bowl with his mouth just like an animal." When admitted to the hospital, Müller's patients who had initially been in home care were routinely found to have "backs beaten blue, with bloody wounds." One man had been chained by his wife to the wall of their house for five years, losing the use of his legs. And when patients discharged from the Würzburg asylum were spotted in the village, the local youths would run after them shouting, "Looky looky, there goes the kooky."[3] These accounts are in every way typical of home treatment of the mentally ill during these years.

Such conditions persisted well into the nineteenth century. In the 1870s just prior to introducing an asylum, officials in the French-speaking Swiss canton of Fribourg conducted a census of the mentally ill. The investigators could scarcely believe their eyes. One-fifth of the 164 mental patients they identified had been under restraint at home, mostly in unheated rooms and stables, "narrow, dark, damp, stinking lockups." Two individuals detained in a stall were said to have "lain upon straw in their own feces, their faces covered with flies."[4] As Louis Caradec, a retired marine surgeon practicing in Brittany, commented in 1860 of the surrounding countryside, "In our rural areas, where people are still imbued with absurd prejudices, public opinion sees having madness in the family as shameful and will not send the person to an asylum. This is the principal reason that motivates our peasants to keep such poor afflicted individuals at home. If the insane person is peaceful, people generally let him run loose. But if he becomes raging or troublesome, he's chained down in a corner of the stable or in an isolated room, where his food is brought to him daily. . . . This happens quite frequently in the countryside, and often a number of years may pass before the authorities are informed of this crime [of sequestration]."[5]

In England, such patients, if not chained at home, might be fastened to a stake in a workhouse or poorhouse. Dr. William Perfect, who ran a small rest home in Westmalling, Kent, recalled being summoned in 1776 by the parish officers of Friendsbury to see "a maniacal man they had confined in their workhouse. . . . He was secured to the floor by means of a staple and an iron ring, which was fastened to a pair of fetters about his legs, and he was handcuffed." Was he integrated into the community? Through the bars of his windows, "continual visitors were pointing at, ridiculing and irritating the patient, who was thus made a spectacle of public sport . . . by several feats of dexterity, such as threading a needle with his toes."[6] So much for community care in this particular version of a supposedly gentle and caring "preindustrial society."

Conditions were scarcely better in the New World, as Dorothea Dix, the New England social reformer, discovered in the early 1840s when she rode about rural Massachusetts investigating local arrangements for "the insane poor."

3

At Lincoln she found, "One woman in a cage."

Medford: "One idiotic subject chained, and one in a close stall for 17 years."

Barnstable: "Four females in pens and stalls; two chained certainly, I think all."

Not all the mental patients in Massachusetts were confined at home. Some lay in the almshouses, as Dix found, "in wooden bunks filled with straw, always shut up." At Danvers, far before she reached the almshouse Dix could perceive "wild shouts, snatches of rude songs, imprecations, and obscene language" coming from a formerly respectable young woman who had been returned from a nearby hospital as "incurable." Now at Danvers, the woman stood beating upon the bars of her tiny uncleaned cage, "a foul spectacle. . . . the unwashed frame invested with fragments of unclean garments, the air so extremely offensive, though ventilation was afforded on all sides save one, that it was not possible to remain beyond a few moments without retreating for recovery to the outward air."[7]

These anecdotes do not represent the extreme or bizarre end of the spectrum; they are typical of the situation of those with a serious psychiatric illness in the years before the advent of the asylum. In a world without psychiatry, rather than being tolerated or indulged, the mentally ill were treated with a savage lack of feeling. Before the advent of the therapeutic asylum, there was no golden era, no idyllic refuge for those supposedly deviant from the values of capitalism. To maintain otherwise is a fantasy.[8]

Traditional Asylums

But since the Middle Ages, there have been asylums. The asylum is by no means an invention of the late eighteenth century. If we switch our view from villages and small towns to cities, the urban world has always had to confront the problem of homeless psychotic or demented individuals, and cities have organized institutions to accommodate them, sometimes within hospices for the sick, the criminal and vagrant, sometimes in jails and workhouses. Full-fledged asylums also existed. All of these institutions had solely custodial functions. Traditional society had no notion of delivering therapy to patients.

Among the oldest psychiatric hospitals in Europe was Bethlem, founded in the thirteenth century as the Priory of St. Mary of Bethlehem, which by 1403 housed six insane men among other denizens. In later centuries, the hospice was given over almost entirely to the insane, the name inevitably corrupting itself to Bethlem, or "Bedlam." In 1547, the City of London acquired custodianship of Bethlem, and it would remain a city-run asylum until 1948.[9] Recent scholarly accounts have mitigated somewhat the ghastly pictures of Bedlam that have come down to us from such sources as the eighth scene of William Hogarth's *The Rake's Progress*, drawn in 1733, showing the almost naked Rake lying manacled on the floor, his head shaved for lice, while a keeper or physician examines him. The private patients at Bethlem must have fared somewhat better because their families paid for their keep, yet the term "Bedlam" resonates as a synonym for chaotic madness.[10] By 1815, this most famous of all historic psychiatric hospitals had only 122 patients.[11] It therefore bulked little in the overall scene of care.

Although eighteenth-century England possessed seven other asylums or public charities, such as the Bethel in Norwich (founded in 1713),[12] it is likely that an equal if not greater number of patients were hospitalized in the private sector, in the numerous private "madhouses," or what would later be called "private nervous clinics," that dotted the landscape. Ranging in size from a handful of patients accommodated in a physician's home to facilities of four or five hundred, these private institutions offered custody, not therapy, for individuals too unmanageable for their own families at home. Conditions in the private madhouses were little superior to those in the public ones.[13] As John Haslam, the physician ("apothecary") of Bethlem, said of the private sector in 1809, "It is a painful recollection to recur to the number of interesting females I have seen, who, after having suffered a temporary disarrangement of mind, and undergone the brutal operation of spouting [forcing 'an entrance into the mouth through the barriers of the teeth'] in private receptacles for the insane, have been restored to their friends without a front tooth in either jaw."[14]

By 1826, when national statistics became available in England, only minimal numbers of individuals found themselves in either private or public asylums. Not quite five thousand insane people were confined in any form, 64 percent of them in the private sector, 36 percent in the public. Bethlem and St. Luke's together numbered only 500 patients, and a further 53 insane individuals were in jails—this in a country of 10 million people.[15] In England, it would be nonsense to speak, as the French philosopher Michel Foucault does, of any kind of "grand confinement."[16]

In contrast to the English tradition of private-sector custodialism, on the continent of Europe the public sector had always offered care. In France, through an administrative reorganization of 1656, Louis XIV established the two great Parisian hospices for the sick, the criminal, the homeless, and the insane—Bicêtre for men and the Salpêtrière for women—as part of a larger hospice program called the "general hospitals." These hôpitaux généraux were not hospitals but custodial institutions that attempted no pretense of therapy. Although both Bicêtre and the Salpêtrière came increasingly to house the insane, until the late nineteenth century they retained their character as hospices rather than psychiatric hospitals. Both retrospectively were known as scenes of horror, the inmates being regularly flogged, bound in chains, and subjected to stupefying hygienic conditions.

As part of the "general hospitals," the French government established hospices in several provincial cities as well. In none of these institutions was the number of psychiatric inmates ever very considerable, Bicêtre for example having in 1788 only 245 "insane" persons (including those with epilepsy and mental retardation).[17] By 1798, France had some 177 general hospitals, the great majority of beds given over to nonpsychiatric inmates of various kinds. Mental patients were also confined in a number of workhouses (dépôts de mendicité) and hospices ("hôpitaux," "hôtels dieux") scattered about the country.[18] At present, little is known about the exact mix of inmates, but the number of beggars, elderly people, and organically ill in these institutions seems to have been so high as to give them a decidedly nonpsychiatric stamp.[19] In France, Foucault's elect terrain with its almost thirty million people, it is absurd to insist on any kind of grand confinement. The number of psychiatric beds was minuscule in the context of these vast populations.

Central Europe, an assemblage of many small states, lacked the centralized government of France. Here, state, church, and local community divided the responsibility for psychiatric care in the form of asylums, almshouses, and jails. By the end of the eighteenth century, this form of care had fallen into a sad state. As Johann Reil, professor of medicine at Halle, depicted some of Germany's customary psychiatric lockups around the year 1800, "It is a remarkable sensation to come from the bustle of a big city into one of these madhouses." He found a whole "vaudeville" before his eyes as the insane in their delusions and hallucinations played out the roles of tyrant and slave, "fools who laugh without reason and fools who torture themselves without reason. Like criminals we lock these unfortunate creatures into mad-cages, into antiquated prisons, or put them next to the nesting holes of owls in desolate attics over the town gates or in the damp cellars of the jails, where the sympathetic gaze of a friend of mankind might never behold them; and we leave them there, gripped by chains, corrupting in their own filth."[20] Although several of these awful *"Tollhäuser"* (fools' houses) were founded in the Middle Ages, and a significant number cluster late in the eighteenth century, nowhere in Central Europe is there evidence of any "grand confinement" of the insane, supposedly touched off by the absolutist regimes of the seventeenth century.[21]

Foucault believed that psychiatry had been invented by the central state. But in statist Germany, psychiatry was a dead letter before the nineteenth century. As Würzburg's Müller later recalled, "Any physician of that time [the late eighteenth century] will know how little of importance medical students learned about mental illness, how much less one could pick up in practice, and just how greatly this discipline had been neglected." To be sure, the traditional physicians had always known of medications to give the insane for a supposed excess of "black bile" and the like. Yet here too, said Müller, "The use of hellebore, the art of the old doctors in healing the insane, seems to have been lost."[22]

The American colonies had little opportunity of experiencing a premodern madhouse phase. Although it was generally up to the colonial family to deal with "distracted persons," the town elders did occasionally construct little strong-houses for individual patients, such as the five-by-seven-foot house the town of Braintree, Massachusetts, helped Samuel Speere build in 1688 to confine his insane sister, Goodwife Witty. In 1701, the officials of Watertown, Massachusetts, ordered a "distracted child" to be placed in care, authorizing payments for its upkeep. When these arrangements collapsed the following year, the community authorized another resident to keep the child in a "little house . . . if he be distracted."[23] Thus confinement of some sort for mental illness dates far back in Colonial history.

As for colonial institutions, in 1729 the newly founded Boston almshouse created the first psychiatric ward by separating the insane from the other inhabitants.[24] Before 1800, there were only two hospitals in the United States, the Pennsylvania Hospital, established in 1752 at the instigation of the Religious Society of Friends, and the New York Hospital which opened in 1791. At some point, both institutions began admitting patients who were insane, the New York Hospital getting a separate psychiatric building in 1808 designated "Lunatic Asylum."[25] The first psychiatric hospital as such in the Colonies was founded in 1773 in Williamsburg, Virginia, "to make provision for the Support and Maintenance of Ideots, Lunatics, and other Persons of unsound Minds."[26]

Thus on both sides of the Atlantic, the history of psychiatry began as the history of the custodial asylum, institutions to confine raging individuals who were dangerous to themselves and a nuisance to others. It was the discovery that these institutions could have a therapeutic function that led to the birth of psychiatry as a discipline.

Heralding the Therapeutic Asylum

It was not the notion that madness was curable that changed at the end of the eighteenth century, for a kind of therapeutic self-confidence ran throughout traditional medicine with its bleeding, purging, and giving of emetics—all designed to cure. Rather, it was the notion that institutions themselves could be made curative, that confinement in them, rather than merely removing a nuisance from the vexed family or the aggrieved village elders, could make the patient better. This insight broke in an almost revolutionary way upon the scene.

Yet the eighteenth-century Enlightenment did flatter itself that through the use of reason it could much improve on the therapeutics of previous generations. The notion of curability was good Enlightenment thinking, part of a larger agenda of improvement through social, political, or medical engineering. If Revolutionary France could be given a constitution and the laws of market economics laid bare, so could illness be systematically treated through right-thinking therapeutic philosophies. Radiating from such centers as Edinburgh, a new therapeutic optimism engulfed the whole world of medicine in the second half of the eighteenth century, an optimism that psychiatry shared. A new generation of asylum physicians grew up filled with confidence in their ability to heal.

So diffuse was the spirit of change that it is difficult to identify a single individual as responsible for the new-style asylum. Germany's Johann Reil spoke of an international movement to help the plight of the insane. "The physicians of England, France, and Germany," he said in 1803, "are all stepping forward at once to improve the lot of the insane. . . . The cosmopolite sees joyously the untiring efforts of mankind to ensure the welfare of one's neighbor. The horrors of the prisons and the jails are over. . . . A bold race of men dares to take on this gigantic idea, an idea that dizzies the normal burgher, of wiping from the face of the earth one of the most devastating of pestilences."[27] Just imagine: Nothing less than eradicating insanity was what they had in mind, couched in the most delicious of Enlightenment rhetoric.

It is possible, however, to identify a handful of asylum physicians whose writings became beacons for the rest of the psychiatric world. In view of the great controversy surrounding this subject, one notes that the reform movement in psychiatry was truly international. There are scholars who associate the rise of psychiatry with various influences, some saying that capitalism was responsible, others the central state.[28] Yet the new therapeutic optimism of psychiatry originated in a wide variety of social and economic settings, making it unlikely that any single social force such as capitalism offers the answer. Enlightenment-style scientific thinking on the other hand spanned continents: Journals circulated widely, important books were soon translated, and individual physicians undertook trips abroad to learn what was happening elsewhere. It was this kind of scientific thinking, largely independent of social setting, that seems to have launched psychiatry.

The first psychiatrist to argue for the therapeutic benefits of institutionalizing patients was William Battie, the founding medical officer of St. Luke's Hospital in London, an asylum that opened in 1751. Battie, a distinguished figure, was owner of two large private madhouses and at one point president of the College of Physicians. The standard history of British psychiatry calls him "the leading 'mad-doctor' . . . of the day."[29] In 1758 at age 54, Battie wrote the *Treatise on Madness*, which specifically attributed therapeutic virtues to the asylum. He quoted an anonymous colleague to the effect that, "management did much more than

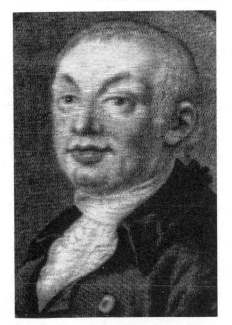

Vincenzio Chiarugi, late eighteenth-century Florentine psychiatrist who established one of the earliest therapeutic asylums (courtesy of Donatella Lippi).

medicine; and repeated experience has convinced me that confinement alone is oftentimes sufficient, but always so necessary that without it every method hitherto devised for the cure of madness would be ineffectual." Indeed it was a kind of isolation cure that Battie recommended, in which the patient was to receive no visits from friends (or spectators) and be attended not by his own servants but by the asylum orderlies.[30] This is the first influential statement of which I am aware on behalf of the asylum as a treatment center.

Battie went on to emphasize the curability of mental disorder: "Madness is . . . as manageable as many other distempers, which are equally dreadful and obstinate, and yet are not looked upon as incurable; such unhappy objects ought by no means to be abandoned, much less shut up in loathsome prisons as criminals or nuisances to the society."[31] Under the influence of psychoanalytically oriented history, such founders of modern psychiatry as Battie have been virtually forgotten.[32] Yet it was with Battie that the birth of psychiatry commenced.

The scene now shifts to Florence, Italy, where in 1785 a 26-year-old physician named Vincenzio Chiarugi, who had been employed in the overcrowded hospice of Santa Dorotea, proposed to the reformist Austrian Grand Duke Leopold, administrator of the province of Tuscany, that another hospital—the old Bonifazio—be renovated and that the psychiatric patients from Santa Dorotea be shifted there. In 1788, the Bonifazio mental hospital was opened and in the following year a handsomely printed set of regulations appeared—apparently Chiarugi's work—on how to maintain proper order in such an institution. In 1793 and 1794, Chiarugi then published his own three-volume work On Insanity, in which he made the case that asylums were not merely to segregate mental patients but to heal them. He outlined a scenario for doing so (the details of which I will discuss in the following section).[33] Chiarugi thus takes the credit for specifying the basics in running a therapeutic asylum.

Meanwhile in France, the Revolution was in progress. A month after Charlotte Corday's 1793 assassination of Marat, the Jacobin government asked a young physician named Philippe Pinel, then 38, to take over the operation of the Bicêtre hospice. Pinel was an example of the kind of self-made arriviste whom the Revolution had thrown into prominence. Born in 1745 in a village in the southwest of France, he was the eldest of seven children in a poorish medical family. He had studied mathematics at Toulouse, the regional university, and then went on to study medicine at Montpellier. Pinel went up to Paris as a kind of medical littérateur, writing and translating, attending salons, and—in the context of some as yet unclarified association with a private psychiatric clinic owned by

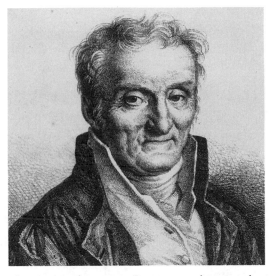

Philippe Pinel, early nineteenth-century Parisian psychiatrist who is considered the founder of modern psychiatry (courtesy of the Archives of the American Psychiatric Association).

the Belhomme family—developing a taste for the practical observation of patients (in contrast to the arid theorizing that then filled the medical texts).

After 1789, Pinel drifted into revolutionary circles, a man who, despite his lowly provincial origins and regional accent, possessed a political future. Imbued with Enlightenment psychology and a progressive social philosophy acquired in the salons during the 1780s, Pinel's head was filled with reformist ideals of both a humanitarian and a therapeutic nature.[34] His fame became guaranteed for having supposedly in 1793 directed the removal of chains from the madmen at Bicêtre (though it was hospital manager Jean-Baptiste Pussin who actually gave the orders). In 1795, Pinel abolished the chains at the Salpêtrière after becoming director of that institution.

Yet Pinel's name remains today a monument in the history of psychiatry not because of various purported freeings of the insane. Previous psychiatrists including Chiarugi had unchained their patients (also, Pinel replaced the chains with straitjackets). It was rather because of a textbook he published in 1801. On the basis of his experiences at Belhomme, Bicêtre, and the Salpêtrière, Pinel concluded that the asylum was a place where psychological therapy could be carried out, not explicit psychotherapy but using the experience of incarceration itself

11

in a healing manner. "The hope is well-justified," he said in 1801, "of returning to society individuals who seem to be hopeless. Our most assiduous and unflagging attention is required toward that numerous group of psychiatric patients who are convalescing or are lucid between episodes, a group that must be placed in the separate ward of the hospice . . . and subject to a kind of psychological treatment [*institution morale*] for the purpose of developing and strengthening their faculties of reason."[35] Although this was not the first statement of the asylum's therapeutic potential, it has been the historically most resonant. In most conventional histories of the subject, modern psychiatry begins with Pinel.

Pinel's 1801 text was vague on just how one organized life in an asylum to make it therapeutic, although we know that he himself was very endearing with the patients, that he calmed them with warm baths, and that he filled the idle hours with work and systematic activity.[36] It is in spelling out the therapeutic fine print that Pinel's pupil Jean-Etienne Esquirol enters the picture. Esquirol was born in Toulouse in 1772, the son of an influential family whom the Revolution had reduced to poverty. After

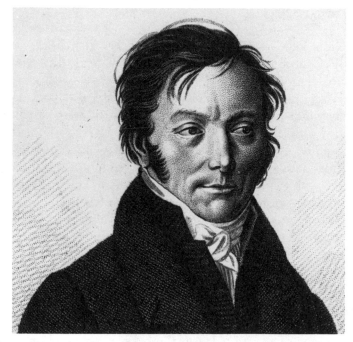

Jean-Etienne-Dominique Esquirol, early nineteenth-century Parisian psychiatrist who advocated what later would be called "social and community psychiatry" (courtesy of National Library of Medicine).

12

drifting about in search of a career, Esquirol migrated to Paris intent on medicine. In listening to lectures from hospital to hospital, Esquirol finally hit upon Pinel's at the Salpêtrière. A firm bond immediately formed between the two men. Almost at once, Esquirol, much like Carl Jung in his relationship to Sigmund Freud a century later, became known as the crown prince of reformed psychiatry. Esquirol began to make a name for himself with his 1802 doctoral thesis on the role of the "passions" in mental illness, and in 1811 he replaced the nonphysician Pussin as administrator of the psychiatric division of the Salpêtrière.[37]

It was Esquirol's plan to put the reforms of Pinel into practice. To help spread the word, in 1817 he began lecturing on psychiatry to the medical students. Eight years later, as he became chief physician of the large asylum in the Parisian suburb of Charenton, Esquirol already had a decade behind him of agitating for the cleanup of France's asylums, especially in the provinces.[38] Perhaps the most therapeutic notion of the Pinelian asylum, as put into operation by Esquirol, was that of the therapeutic community: patients and physicians living as community members in a psychiatric setting. In Esquirol's private nervous clinic across from the Salpêtrière (later moved to the suburb of Ivry), the patients would eat together at the same table with the Esquirol family.[39] Esquirol believed in the salutary effects of "isolation" from the outside world in the institution, and felt that removal from family and friends would contribute greatly to diverting the patient from the previously unhealthy passions that had ruled his or her life.[40]

The psychiatric current that Pinel and Esquirol originated would run throughout the Atlantic community in the nineteenth century, ending only when the pressure of sheer numbers swamped any notion of the asylum offering therapeutic benefit. Yet there were important international differences in the concept of the therapeutic asylum.

In Central Europe, the voice of Pinel was muted because Reil, the major authority on reform, happened not to care for the sage of Bicêtre and preferred Chiarugi instead.[41] Reil was one of those late-eighteenth-century Enlightenment polymaths. He made a name for himself in neuroanatomy and in internal medicine, only later turning his hand to psychiatry. Indeed, it is not clear that, except for his duties as physician at the Halle prison (whose population would have included some psychiatric cases), Reil ever had much contact with actual mental patients. But he had a lot of ideas and expressed them in *Rhapsodies on the Application of the Psychological Method of Cure in Mental Alienation*, a powerfully written but obscurely titled book that appeared in 1803 when Reil was 44.

Appalled by previous conditions in institutions, Reil asked in best Enlightenment style, "When it comes to saving others, where are the fruits of our famous culture, love for humankind, sense of community, supposed citizenship, and noble renunciation of self-interest?" He found before him a bleak psychiatric tableau. But here the "medical guild" can help, he said. "They have courage and energy, because everyone needs them. They are pupils of the large school of nature, a nature that refuses to keep us asunder as humans, and they react when they see this principle violated." (It was as though Reil and not Schiller had penned the "Ode to Joy.")

"What can doctors do about the problem of mental illness?" asked Reil. Institutions could help. Psychiatric hospitals, he said, were the one exception to the rule that sick people are better cared for at home. Family care of insanity was much less effective than institutional because "in family homes there are no baths, douches, open spaces and other adjuvants of therapy of which the physician disposes in public asylums." Given the scarcity of doctors interested in insanity, it made much more sense, he said, to concentrate the few available doctors in institutions rather than to disperse them in private family care. Thus, "As a rule public asylums must represent the basis of treating this kind of patient."[42]

There should be two kinds of institutions, for incurables and for curables. Reil dedicated an elaborate treatment regime to the latter, including both physical therapy and a psychotherapy that involved building theaters in asylums to stimulate patients' visual senses and making prostitutes available to male patients.[43] Much of this was merely Reil's fantasy—there were no actual plans to incorporate any of these features in asylum life. Yet it was a comprehensive program of institutional therapy that owed nothing to Pinel, only a few features to Chiarugi, and constituted a distinctively Central European strand in making psychiatry into a therapeutic profession.

Reil represents the latitudinarian stream in the history of German psychiatry. An authoritarian stream, however, arose at the same time in the figure of Ernst Horn, a 32-year-old army doctor who had gone into teaching and who became in 1806 the associate director of Berlin's Charité Hospital. In this capacity, he was charged with running the psychiatric service, established in 1798 after the penitentiary, the previous receptacle of psychiatric patients, had burned down. To understand the nature of Horn's proposals, bear in mind that the Charité was a military teaching hospital with an environment based on Prussian discipline. Yet in the context of the riotous disorder of the traditional asylum, such a strict regimen could generate favorable therapeutic results. Take, for example, the apparently trifling question of what patients were permitted to keep in their

14

rooms. When he arrived, Horn said, "Anybody could take into his room whatever he liked. Everybody wanted to build himself a little nest, without thinking that what was permitted the one must also be allowed the others, and so shortly the patient's entire room was overfilled in the extreme with things that caused untidyness. The sad consequences were not long in coming. I was forced to sacrifice the desires of the individual for the needs of the whole. The requests of the patients had to remain unheard, so that the community of patients would thrive better."[44]

It is true that when Horn arrived in 1806 he found chaos. Yet the order he imposed on this Goya-esque vista was not just tidy and appealing to the bureaucratic mind, it was therapeutic as well. He dictated a regimen of military drilling to the patients, inserted tight daily schedules to replace endless idleness, and installed a general sense of limits that helped give patients the feeling of being able to control their lives. "A lot of mentally ill people thanked him," commented Horn's biographer, "for their happy recovery."[45]

In the United States, European models held sway until the 1930s, which means that there were relatively few distinctive American psychiatric traditions—or few at least that were copied elsewhere. In talking about American "firsts" therefore, we must try to steer clear of the parochialism that has characterized much American writing on this subject.[46] Yet the American narrative is important, and it too begins with a founding figure.

The Philadelphia physician Benjamin Rush was officially acknowledged by the American Psychiatric Association in 1965 as the "father of American psychiatry."[47] Yet Rush, attending physician at the Pennsylvania Hospital, did little to serve as a beacon for the future. He was one with his European colleagues in seeing the brain as the basis of mental illness: "Persons who labour under the derangement, or want, of these faculties of the mind," he said in 1786, "are considered very properly as subjects of medicine; and there are many cases upon record that prove that their diseases have yielded to the healing art."[48] In his big psychiatry textbook, published in 1812, Rush stated coolly, "The cause of madness is seated primarily in the blood-vessels of the brain, and it depends upon the same kind of morbid and irregular actions that continues other arterial diseases."[49] This was garden-variety organicism and in no way distinctively American.

Rush's partisans have argued that his occasional musings on moral suasion anticipated later psychological therapies. Yet, psychological sensitivity is difficult to detect in his practice. As one visitor to the Pennsylvania Hospital in 1787 recounted of Rush's rounds, "We next took a view of the maniacs. Their cells were in the lower story, which is partly underground. These cells are about 10 feet square, and made as strong as a prison. . . . In each door is a hole, large enough to give them food, etc., which is closed with a little door secured with strong bolts." Most of the patients were lying upon straw. "Some of them were extremely fierce and raving, nearly or quite naked."[50] This was not the world of moral therapy and busy regimen, and it was quite at odds with the idyllic reforms of the Pennsylvania Hospital described in his textbook: "[The patients] now taste of the blessings of air, and light, and motion, in pleasant and shaded walks in summer. . . . They have recovered the human figure, and with it, their long forgotten relationship to their friends and the public."[51] As a founder of psychiatry therefore, Rush is a bit of a sham.

What do these many founders of modern psychiatry have in common? How about the Foucauldian notion that psychiatry was born in some kind of fiendish alliance between capitalism and the central state, enlisting psychiatrists in the larger game of confining deviant individuals in order to instill work discipline into an unmotivated traditional population? To be sure, Battie and Rush came from the stamping grounds of the nascent capitalist economy—Philadelphia and London—where they breathed the spirit of the marketplace. Yet Chiarugi's sleepy late-eighteenth-century Florence could scarcely have been less capitalistic, and it would be farcical to argue that Grand Duke Leopold was somehow extending the state-making writ of the Austrian monarchy to the Tuscan mental-health system.[52] Viennese moneyed interests had virtually no interest in Tuscany at this point and young Leopold (he was only 18 when his rule began in 1765) and his mother Maria Theresa counted more as traditional enlightened "despots" than as industry-backed state makers. Reil's Halle was at the time an economic backwater and unlikely to have suffused into Reil—the great friend of humankind—an urgency about encouraging industrial work discipline. The Foucauldian case would actually rise or fall with Pinel and Esquirol, themselves starkly different in class background and mind-set (Pinel a *philosophe*, Esquirol an early romantic). Aside from being close friends, what Pinel and Esquirol had in common was extensive experience with private clinics. Esquirol's thinking about therapy was certainly influenced by life at his own private clinic, though it is difficult to tell how Pinel's first five years in psychiatry at the Belhomme family's clinic affected him.

Why does it matter whether either man had cut his teeth in a private psychiatric clinic? Because the rise of the private clinic is anathema to the whole Foucauldian doctrine: By definition, these clinics arose from the private sector rather than the public. If the birth of psychiatry occurred mainly in private "madhouses," middle-class and aristocratic families voluntarily paying vast sums to rid themselves of manic relatives, what remains of the "grand confinement"?

Other scholarly accounts are scarcely more persuasive than Foucault's. Some have argued that "professionalization" was at work as psychiatrists sought to establish a self-serving hegemony over madness to boost their own wealth and power.[53] It is true that some private-sector physicians such as Battie did accumulate great fortunes. It is also true that in these years psychiatry did begin to constitute itself as a distinct discipline, claiming special intellectual and emotional qualities for its exercise. Yet this may be interpreted as a legitimate expression of therapeutic self-confidence rather than a power-grab.

These late-eighteenth-century psychiatrists believed that a new discipline was taking shape. Until the twentieth century, its practitioners would be called "alienists," one who treats "mental alienation." Reil enumerated the qualities making for a good psychiatrist: "Perspicacity, a talent for observation, intelligence, good will, persistence, patience, experience, an imposing physique, and a countenance that commands respect." He found these in short supply: "All those qualities required for the cure of the insane are so rare as to make the staffing of institutions difficult."[54] In 1808, Reil coined the term psychiatry, or "Psychiaterie," for the new discipline, which by 1816 he had shortened to "Psychiatrie."[55]

English writers too echoed this sentiment of psychiatry representing a special kind of discipline. As John Ferriar, chief physician of the asylum in Manchester, put it in 1810, plumbing the symptoms of madness required physicians better versed in Shakespeare than in the Greek medical writer Aretaeus. "From a want of that exquisite discernment in the traces of character, which rather qualifies a man for the composition of poetry or romance than for pathological discussion, some medical writers have limited their arrangement of mental disorders too narrowly," whereas others, Ferriar went on to say, had made the notion of insanity virtually coterminous with any "transitory excess of passion."[56] Thus for Ferriar, specializing in insanity required an understanding of culture and character.

In these years, "the concept of psychic medicine as science," as one of Reil's collaborators put it, was coming into being.[57] Psychiatrists were asserting a legitimate claim to guild status on the grounds that running an asylum in a therapeutic manner was an art and science as intricate as chemistry or anatomy.

Organizing the Therapeutic Asylum

The founders envisioned two aspects of life in an asylum as therapeutic—the setting itself with its orderly routines and communal spirit, and the doctor-patient relationship. A particular form of this relationship was often called "moral therapy." In both the setting and in moral therapy, the new asylum, as the founders conceived it, diverged from the traditional madhouse.

The eighteenth-century manuals said that madness came from excessive irritation of the nerves. Therefore a calmative setting was indicated. Battie sought to achieve in his asylum a kind of golden mean where, "Every unruly appetite must be checked, every fixed imagination must if possible be diverted." The patient's body and his quarters were to be kept clean, his diet light, "neither spirituous nor high seasoned." A "well timed variety of amusements" should neither be too long nor too diverting. The private nervous clinic should serve as a kind of rest home, in other words.[58]

If these late-eighteenth-century writers emphasized strengthening the patients' sense of self-control, it was not merely because they were creatures of a Methodist epoch that valued self-discipline but because self-control was therapeutic. Ferriar said that in "lunatic houses" the regimen should help the patient acquire the self-discipline that would permit him to "minister to himself." "A system of discipline, mild but exact, which makes the patient sensible of restraint without exciting pain or terror, is best suited to these complaints." The results were thought soon apparent. "It is owing to the sense of restraint that lunatics recover more quickly when they are removed from home," Ferriar said. The attention they received at home merely made the illness worse. "Among strangers, they find it necessary to exert their faculties, and the first tendency to regular thinking becomes the beginning of recovery." Thus the routine of the asylum should encourage limit-setting and focusing, encouraging in patients a sense of self-mastery. Above all, Ferriar stressed that "the management of hope and apprehension in the patient forms the most useful part of discipline. Small favours, the show of confidence, and apparent distinction accelerate recovery."[59]

How could one manage hope and apprehension in mental patients? How did one turn a "madhouse" into a "healing facility," as Reil put it? One might start by choosing an innocuous name, said Reil, a "Pension for Nervous Patients" perhaps, or a "Hospital for Psychological Healing." Situate it in a pleasant setting, midst brooks and lakes, hills and fields, with small villas clustered about the administration building. There should be no bars on the windows. Since the insane—Reil believed—tended to have a distinctive odor, the surfaces should be cleanable. The place would require baths, a "magic temple," and sites for "other exercises in attentiveness."[60] It would be decades before such temples to healing were actually constructed for the wealthy families of the great cities. Yet Reil's therapeutic vision was astonishingly prescient.

The therapeutic asylum in Central Europe was nothing if not orderly. At the Charité, Horn devised an hourly schedule for his patients, something unheard of at the time:

5–6 A.M. "Prompt arising, ablutions, and breakfast."

6–7 A.M. "Religious edification by reading out loud to the patients passages appropriate to their comprehension."

The day continued in this manner, with time slots for cutting wood, military exercises, drawing-and-painting class, geography lesson, and, between seven and eight-thirty (in good weather) in the evening, "bowling balls for little prizes."[61] Horn's timetable breathes the philosophy that orderly life is restorative.

Pinel urged structuring the day with work.[62] But it was his pupil Esquirol who, with his experiences in a private clinic, developed most fully in France the notion of the daily regimen itself as therapeutic. "The patient with mania, restrained by the harmony, order and rules of the house, will get his impulsiveness better in hand and yield less to eccentric acts." As Esquirol penned these lines in 1816, he might well have had Battie's advice of almost half a century previously in mind (though almost certainly he did not). Esquirol: "The calm that the psychiatric patients enjoy, far from the tumult and the noise, and the mental rest [*repos moral*] conferred by removal from their businesses and domestic problems, is very favorable to their recovery. Subject to an orderly life, to discipline, to a well calibrated regimen, they are obliged to reflect upon the change in their life. The necessity of adjusting [*se contentir*], of behaving well with strangers, of living together with their companions in suffering, are powerful allies in achieving restoration of their lost reason."[63]

There was a second sense in which the late-eighteenth-century asylum executed its historic break with the past: Physicians began using techniques related neither to the giving of medication nor to physical procedures. This was the advent of psychotherapy, the formal use of the doctor-patient relationship to restore patients. The special psychological relationship between psychiatrist and patients, sometimes called "moral therapy" after Pinel's 1801 phrase "le traitement moral" (a word which in this French context means "mental" not "moral"),[64] was actually not novel in principle. Informal psychological intervention is a technique with which physicians have always been familiar. Molière, the seventeenth-century French playwright, allows "Dr. Clitandre" to say in *L'Amour médecin*, "Sir, my remedies are different from those of the others. The others have emetics and bloodletting, medications and enemas. But I heal through words, through sounds, through letters, through talismans. . . . Because the mind has a firm hold upon the body, it is quite often through the mind that illness arises, and my habit has always been to heal the mind before proceeding to the body."[65] Reil was aware of a long train of physicians back to the Ancients preceding his own "psychological method of cure."[66] And in France after 1750, there had been a burst of writing on "la médecine de l'esprit."[67] As historian Roy Porter has demonstrated, the notion of moral management ran throughout psychological medicine in England during the eighteenth century.[68]

The late-eighteenth-century psychiatric writers tried to systematize these long-familiar techniques in the asylum, thus doing, in essence, formal psychotherapy. The first asylum physician to have experimented with moral therapy was Chiarugi at the Bonifazio asylum in Florence, who said in 1793 of treating depression, "It will be necessary in cases of true melancholia especially to promote and encourage *hope*, which is completely opposite to sadness and fear: this should be able to help change the physical and moral constitution of the person. . . . It has to be noted that this new feeling should be elicited in the most natural way so as not to cause resistance and spite in the melancholic patient."[69] Chiarugi can only be describing the physician's direct psychological intervention on the patient in the asylum.

Chiarugi's writing was largely unknown in England, where a whole generation of psychiatric writers in the first three decades of the nineteenth century preached the doctrine of "moral treatment" (see Chapter 2). The phrase was popularized in a private asylum founded in 1796 by William Tuke, a Quaker tea-merchant in York who wanted to improve the quality of care available to members of the local Quaker community with mental disorders. Although the York "Retreat" possessed a medical superintendent, the policies of care and gentleness for which it became famous were devised largely by laypersons. As Samuel Tuke, William's grandson, and also a merchant, wrote in an account of the Retreat published in 1813, "The judicious kindness of others appears generally to excite the gratitude and affection of the patient." This kindness offered a therapeutic grip on the patients, a hold by which to pull themselves back to wellness, Tuke believed.[70] Although the book seems naive in its starry-eyed conviction in the power of the will in "mania" and "melancholia," the two categories into which all mental illnesses were then divided, it had an enormous impact and, though written by a layperson, may be considered one of the single most famous documents in the history of psychiatry.

Meanwhile in France, Pinel had apparently never heard of the Tuke family nor the York Retreat. What he had seen, however, was the spectacle of Madame Pussin, the wife of the administrator at Bicêtre, sometime in the period 1793 to 1795 doing her version of psychotherapy. "I was astonished at Bicêtre to see her approach the most furious maniacs, to calm them with words of consolation, and to get them to eat meals that they would obstinately have rejected from any other hand. One day an insane patient, reduced to danger of starvation from his stubborn refusal to eat, revolted against her and, in pushing away the food she was serving him, reviled her in the most outrageous terms. This quick-witted woman put herself in unison with his delusional notions; she jumped and danced about in front of him, talked back to him in kind, and succeeded in making him smile. Taking advantage of this opportune moment to get him to eat, she saved his life."[71] Pinel doubtlessly was exposed to other such happenstance encounters in human sympathy as well, but chance favors a prepared mind, as Louis Pasteur later said, and Pinel's mind was prepared, sensitized by the philosophical and psychological discussions of the Enlightenment philosophers. He quickly came to the conclusion that the key to "giving the patients hope again," to using the asylum therapeutically, lay in "gaining their confidence." Patients normally try to conceal from one what they're thinking, he said. Only by "taking on an air of bonhomie and a tone of extreme frankness can one penetrate into their most secret thoughts, clear up their anxieties, and deal with apparent contradictions by comparing their problems to those of others."[72]

Pinel's 1801 book had such authority that it immediately launched moral therapy. Its only competitor was Reil's own elaborate system of psychological curing, of only academic interest because he apparently reasoned it all out in an armchair.[73] What the English called moral therapy and the French "le traitement moral" thus became the gold standard of enlightened asylum administration. Although Haslam, the medical officer of Bedlam, mocked Pinel for his pretentious talk about having an imposing manner and thunderous voice, Haslam nonetheless bowed to the wisdom of "devot[ing] some time and attention to discover the character of the patient, and to ascertain wherein, and on what points, his insanity consists." To achieve patients' confidence, Haslam said, one needed merely "a mildness of manner and expression, an attention to their narrative, and seeming acquiescence in its truth."[74] Nowhere will one find a more succinct expression of the qualities desired of the physician in the doctor-patient relationship.

Was the discovery of moral therapy thus a stroke of genius on the part of a handful of great men? Or did it lie in the intrinsic logic of the situation in which asylum physicians found themselves late in the eighteenth century? Determined to cure or ameliorate their patients' distress, it was obvious to them that some kind of psychological approach was necessary in addition to enema-giving and bloodletting. Clearly, patients would thrive better in a milieu that stressed productive activity and edifying pastimes as opposed to rolling around in straw covered with their own feces. It could not have been more evident to these physicians that patients respond to the comfort of the spoken word and to the expression of concern on the doctor's part, all of which are the essential and ageold ingredients of the much ballyhooed moral therapy. What is astonishing is not that it was discovered, but that it was later lost so completely from view in asylum life.

Nervous Illness and Nonpsychiatrists

Just as the major mental illnesses have always been with us, the minor ones such as anxiety, neurotic depression, and obsessive-compulsive behavior have accompanied humankind as well, though they seem by no means minor to those afflicted with them. Since the eighteenth century, they have often been referred to as "nervous illnesses," more recently as "neurotic" or "psychoneurotic" disorders. And every era has had its vocabulary for psychoneurosis. The ancient Jews thought "love sickness" to be capable of reducing a man to a skeleton.[75] Later epochs would contribute such additions to nosology as "hysteria" in the sixteenth century and "nerves" in the eighteenth.[76] All these expressions were quite nonspecific and could envelop just about any symptom imaginable. Jacob Isenflamm, for example, professor of medicine at Erlangen, disserted in 1774 about how hysteria and hypochondria could end fatally.[77]

Yet the so-called nervous disorders did not belong to psychiatry. They were assigned to family medicine or one to of the organic specialities such as neurology. In our own time, nervous and neurotic disorders have passed from the ambit of organic medicine to that of psychological medicine, becoming today the bread-and-butter of practicing psychiatrists.

How were such complaints considered at the end of the eighteenth century, our point of departure?

Minor psychiatric illnesses fell heavily to the lot of spa doctors. Europeans have traditionally sought relief at such watering places as Bath in England, Rigi-Kaltbad in Switzerland, Wiesbaden in Germany, and Plombières in France. In theory, the waters of the spa were seen as calmative; in practice their main benefit was probably to induce bowel movements, thus gratifying individuals who suffered the discomfort of chronic constipation and pleasing physicians who deemed open bowels the highway to health. Although the spas had blossomed in the High Middle Ages, they experienced a great decline in the early modern period following the Thirty Years War, also following rising wood prices and an epidemic of syphilis.[78]

By 1800, the spas were at a historic low point, seedy remnants of their late medieval glory. Bath in England was becoming a magnet for the poor rather than the wealthy.[79] Yet even at their nadir, the spas were still visited by the middle and upper classes for illnesses for which no organic cause could be found (in the medicine of the day, a vast gamut). In Germany, the watering places at Doberan in Mecklenburg, Nenndorf near Hanover, and Töplitz in Bohemia were seen as especially favorable for nervous illnesses.[80] Augustus Bozzi-Granville, a Milanese physician who in 1813 had settled in London and had a large society practice that included the Archduke of Clarence, described numerous nervous illnesses he had witnessed during his tour of the spas of Germany in the 1830s. Wiesbaden, for example, he deemed perfect for the hypochondriac: "He is sombre, thoughtful, or absent, in the midst of a laughing world. Forever brooding over his fate, his disease absorbs the whole of his attention. He disdains even the most trifling conversation with his fellow-creatures, and flies from those ephemeral acquaintances which are so easily formed at watering-places, exactly because one cares little how soon after they are forgotten. . . . Such a character one meets at Wiesbaden, as I found it at Gastein [in Austria], at Carlsbad [in Bohemia], and again at Töplitz."[81]

"Granville" as he called himself in print after his mother's name, encountered even more pronouncedly neurotic companions at "Bad Deinach" (Teinach, in Württemberg), the acidulous waters of which were said to be good for gout and rheumatism, also "for the cure of insane patients . . . and several of that class of patients, including hypochondriacal and melancholic persons, were in the course of cure at the time I visited the springs."[82] Thus the spa-physicians at Wiesbaden and Bad

Teinach would have to be quite adept at psychiatry, although they would not call themselves psychiatrists, alienists, *Irrenärzte*, or any of the other contemporary terms denoting madness: Nobody who was believed frankly mad would be encouraged to seek relief at a spa (though many did in fact, representing a chronic problem for the administration of the watering places).

Nor was the relief of nervous illness at chic spas a Germany monopoly. In June 1693, Lady Berisford's 19-year-old daughter was brought to Bath for symptoms "that usually accompany the virgin disease." She had great weakness in her wrists, what Dr. Peirce perceived as facial discoloring (owing he thought to premature onset of menstruation at 12), little appetite, and "vapours and strange fits." Peirce restored her with seven weeks of bathing and drinking the waters. He believed that "giving her to a good husband" should prevent a relapse.[83]

Outside of the spas, wealthy nervous patients might land in the hands of society doctors. In London, that meant the members and fellows of the Royal College of Physicians, who after the 1860s, would cluster increasingly on Harley Street and nearby West End addresses. Yet already in the eighteenth century, a clear corpus of society nerve doctors was identifiable, catering to the neurotic illnesses of a patrician population that wished to steer wide of "madness." Perhaps the prototypical society nerve doctor was George Cheyne, who in his 1733 book on the "English malady" and in other works launched the whole notion of "nervous illness" as a malady afflicting the nerves themselves. Cheyne, a Scotsman born in 1671, had studied at Edinburgh, then come down to London around 1701 to open a society practice, winning custom by "frequenting the society of the younger gentry," as his biographer put it, "and of free livers with whom he became extremely popular." For years, Cheyne indulged in long evenings of tavern dinners, recruiting intimates from his circle as patients and in the process becoming very stout, short of breath and gouty. After his own health broke, he sought treatment at Bath and was so pleased with his new regimen that he began spending the winters there, summering in London. In this climate of upper-class hypochondriasis and valetudinarianism, Cheyne penned his notions about nervous diseases as not representing madness but physical disorders of the nerves themselves ("a bodily distemper . . . as the smallpox or a fever"[84]).

And the suffering these nerves could inflict! "Of all the miseries that afflict human life and relate principally to the body, in this valley of tears I think nervous disorders in their extreme and last degrees are the most deplorable and beyond all comparison the worst."[85] Of course, his readers adored this analysis of the true nature of their suffering: organic illness over which the mind had no control. "His reputation with the public was immense," we are told, "and he was intimate with the most eminent physicians and other persons of note in his time."[86] One may spool ahead two hundred years and see such names as Karl and William Menninger in lieu of Cheyne. Yet even though the Menninger brothers and Cheyne all specialized in the same type of patient, Cheyne was seen as having nothing to do with insanity while the Menningers were celebrated as psychiatrists.

Many society nerve doctors followed in Cheyne's footsteps. Charles Perry was a medical graduate of Oxford who, giving a clue to his own social set, dedicated his volumes on world travel to his friend the Earl of Sandwich. In 1755, Perry wrote an account of the "hysteric passion." Was it a psychiatric illness? Not at all, rather a "nervous disorder" caused by "errors and defects in our accretions and secretions." In Perry's view, "Many thousands (I believe I may say millions) of women are daily, more or less, under its scourge and dominion." He had seen evidence of this himself. "I have in the course of a long practice, and a pretty large circle of acquaintance, had a great many hysterical patients under my care and cognizance: indeed I have had pretty many very remarkable cases of that kind under my care and management within a few years last past. And these in general I have treated with uncommon success and effect."[87] Nor was he necessarily boasting. There is much evidence that these physicians with their spa therapies and placebo treatments were vastly successful in lifting from their patients the burden of neurotic illness.

Society nerve doctors arose during the eighteenth century in every country, outfitted with such diagnoses as hysteria, hypochondria, and spleen. In 1763, Pierre Pomme popularized in France "vapours," a disorder already well known to the English. Pomme, who had come up from Arles to become a big social success in Paris and serve as medical consultant to the king, evidently treated a *beau monde* suffering from depression, "fatigue, pain and a sense of dullness. Sadness, melancholy and discouragement empoison all of their amusements." Pomme believed that chicken soup and cold baths would work wonders for the disorder.[88]

In the public utterances of the society nerve doctors, nerves and madness were miles apart. Yet in practice, they were not so far apart at all. Doctors who specialize in "nerves" will of course end up seeing patients with major psychiatric disorders, because the patients' relatives demand the illusion of organicity and shun the stigma of madness. Thus a physician like Joseph Daquin, a consultant in the city of Chambéry (which then belonged to the Italian Duchy of Savoy), would attribute the problems of the wealthy women in his private practice to "vapours." In his medical topography of Chambéry, published in 1787, he said, "Nervous afflictions are not frequent in Chambéry, yet we see today a greater number than previously; they have even spread to women of the countryside nearby the city." These nervous vapors, arising as they did from the uterus, could "derange all the functions of the brain."[89] Associated with women who led "a soft and sedentary life," such vapors sound like fairly significant disorders, deranging the functions of the brain and whatnot. But were these women "insane," in the sense of being candidates for admission to an asylum? Not at all. Their families would keep them at home.

At the same time, Daquin was medical director of the local hospice, or Hôtel-Dieu, of Chambéry, and treated poor patients for insanity. Some of these Hôtel-Dieu patients must have had symptoms similar to those of his private patients. Yet Daquin did not let the two worlds overlap. The author's extensive description on the title page of his topography says nothing about the psychiatric service of the Hôtel-Dieu. In conveying his ideas to the public, Daquin kept nerves and madness quite separate and did not advertise that he functioned as a psychiatrist.[90]

Eighteenth-century alienists covered only a narrow segment of the broad spectrum of disorders that the term psychiatry embraces today. The rest of the spectrum was taken over by practitioners who shunned any public identification with madness and sailed under the flag of spa doctor or society nerve doctor. Yet all were present at the birth of psychiatry.

Toward a Biological Psychiatry

Psychiatry has always been torn between two visions of mental illness. One vision stresses the neurosciences, with their interest in brain chemistry, brain anatomy, and medication, seeing the origin of psychic distress in the biology of the cerebral cortex. The other vision stresses the psychosocial side of patients' lives, attributing their symptoms to social problems or past personal stresses to which people may adjust imperfectly. (Both visions, by the way, attach considerable importance to psychotherapy, and it would be inexact to claim it as the monopoly of either.) The neuroscience version is usually called biological psychiatry; the social-stress version makes great virtue of the "biopsychosocial" model of illness. Yet even though psychiatrists may share both perspectives, when it comes to treating individual patients, the perspectives themselves really are polar opposites, in that both cannot be true at the same time. Either one's depression is due to a biologically influenced imbalance in one's neurotransmitters, perhaps activated by stress, or it stems from some psychodynamic process in one's unconscious mind. It is thus of great importance which vision has the upper hand within psychiatry at any given moment.

This bifurcation of vision was present at the very beginning of the discipline's history. At the beginning, the biological version was predominant. With the sole exception of Esquirol and his romantic theories about the "passions," the psychiatrists of the founding generation believed that the cause of mental illness lay in the integuments of the brain and that psychiatry was in a sense reducible to neurology. (The two disciplines were considered the same.) In 1758, William Battie worked out a complicated explanation of mental illness based on the medical theories of Hermann Boerhaave, the clinician from Leyden whose turn-of-the-eighteenth-century writings stressed the pathology of "solids" as opposed to humors. Battie had the idea that muscular "spasms" led to "laxity" of the blood vessels of the brain, which in turn caused "obstruction" of the vessels and an ensuing "compression" of the nerves, together with the advent of delusive sensations. Thus there could literally be "weakness of the nerves," in Battie's view, giving rise to anxiety among other sensations.[91] That Battie possessed no empirical demonstration of the rightness of any of these theories troubled him not at all: "Madness, though a terrible and at present a very frequent calamity, is perhaps as little understood as any that ever afflicted mankind," he said. He called for research, given what he considered the uselessness of previous writing on the subject. But in the meantime, he could relieve the laxity of his patients' nervous fibers by giving them appropriate "medical care."[92] (Assafetida, a nauseating plant preparation, and musk would have been typical "antispasmodics" of his day.)

For Chiarugi, the nervous system represented without question the basis of mental illness: "Insanity can be defined as a chronic and permanent idiopathic affliction [of unknown cause] of the brain, the principal part of the nervous system."[93] He did autopsies on many of his patients, and because so many of them died of infectious illnesses (frequently acquired while in Chiarugi's asylum), he often found brain lesions.[94]

Benjamin Rush was convinced that "the cause of madness is seated in the blood vessels of the brain," and that mental illness had nothing specific about it, being merely "part of the unity of disease, particularly of fever, of which madness is a chronic form, affecting that part of the brain which is the seat of the mind."[95] Pinel spoke approvingly of German physician Johann Greding's efforts to find lesions in mental patients at autopsy, or as Pinel put it, "structural lesions or developmental anomalies that do seem to be characteristic." Yet Pinel criticized such researchers for their lack of control groups, suspecting that many of the

27

same brain changes would show up in normal individuals.[96] Pinel and Rush wrote so sketchily of this whole subject that neither could really be classed a forerunner of biological psychiatry.

Johann Reil is another matter, however. Reil was so dogmatic about brain biology as the cause of madness that he stands as the first medical writer to foreshadow biological psychiatry. Whereas Chiarugi had little notion of mechanisms, or how alterations in the structure and chemistry of the brain might produce madness, Reil was full of theories based on the notion of "irritability" (from the mid-eighteenth-century Swiss physiologist Albrecht von Haller and the Scottish physician John Brown). To cure mental illnesses, one had to reduce irritability in the substance of the brain itself. "As the overly irritable nerve fibers are calmed, the inert ones become excited. The normal proportion in the dynamic of the organ of the mind is reestablished and the prominent delusions vanish."[97] In addition to moral therapy, Reil had a whole arsenal of physical therapies to effect these imagined brain changes, such as the administration of warmth, or stroking the patient's body, as well as the red-hot irons and mustard plasters of the philosophy of counterirritation (vexing the skin to draw out the irritants lying below).[98]

Subsequent generations would abandon these particular mechanisms and embrace others, such as phrenology, which in their turn would be abandoned in the late nineteenth century for still other hypothesized mechanisms of how the brain produced madness. No matter. What is important is that these early psychiatrists had some gut sense of organicity in the afflictions of their patients: The suffering was just too intense, the hallucinations too bizarre, the patient's whole physical habitus too transformed for the brain not somehow to be implicated.

The psychiatrists of the founding generation also anticipated later biological psychiatry with their emphasis on heredity. Heredity figures among those circumstances that physicians have "always known about," because the major psychiatric illnesses tend to cluster in certain family trees, and a doctor with knowledge of his patients' relatives would immediately spot this clustering. So striking, for example, was the recurrence of melancholia and suicide within certain Zurich families between the sixteenth and eighteenth centuries that local scribes often commented on it. The Schmid family's tendency to melancholia was considered to be something "in their blood." In eighteenth-century Zurich, phrases like *malum hereditarium* were in current use.[99] Such generational clumping is not in and of itself evidence of genetic influence, for families may transmit patterns of sociability from generation to generation as well as genes. Yet this clustering nonetheless provided stuff for rumination.

Thus did William Battie ruminate about heredity as an "original," or primary, cause of madness, speaking of "whole families derived from Lunatic ancestors. . . . There is more reason to fear that, whenever this disorder is hereditary, it is original," he said in 1758.[100] Battie thus inserted himself into a long tradition of British thought on the inheritability of madness. As Haslam of Bedlam commented in 1809, "Where one of the parents have been insane, it is more than probable that the offsprings will be similarly affected."[101] He went on to offer examples of family trees from which madness fairly bulged. The first example: "R. G. His grandfather was mad, but there was no insanity in his grandmother's family. His father was occasionally melancholic, and once had a raving paroxysm. His mother's family was sane. His father's brother died insane. R. G. has a brother and five sisters; his brother has been confined in St. Luke's [asylum], and is occasionally in a low spirited state. All his sisters have been insane; with the three youngest the disease came on after delivery."[102]

Other of psychiatry's founders were equally heredity-conscious. Even though Pinel and Esquirol gave only a few lines to brain lesions, they went on for pages about heredity. "It would be difficult," Pinel said in introducing the section of his book on heredity, "not to concede a hereditary transmission of mania, when one recalls that everywhere some members of certain families are struck in several successive generations."[103] In Esquirol's view, 110 of 482 melancholic patients seen at the Salpêtrière early in the century had a hereditary "cause" for their disorder.[104] Of the 264 wealthy patients at his private asylum, 150 owed their problems, in his opinion, to their heredity. "Heredity is the commonest predisposing cause of madness," he concluded.[105] Reil wrote of the "predisposition" (*Anlage*) to mental illness.[106] Chiarugi flatly assigned the "mental mania" of a 26-year-old man whose father and mother had both been manic to his "hereditary predisposition."[107] There was absolutely no doubt in the minds of this founding generation of psychiatrists, and in the minds of virtually all of their medical contemporaries, that individuals with a history of mental illness in the family stood a greater chance of falling ill than did individuals from non-mentally-ill families. A genetic perspective was present at the birth of psychiatry.

Romantic Psychiatry

Opposed to this neuroscientific perspective featuring brain-biology and genetics is the psychosocial perspective, emphasizing problems in one's personal history and social surroundings. Even though this perspective was not present at the very birth of psychiatry, it came along quickly enough, as one would expect, given that the real world of illness would inevitably tug psychiatrists toward human distress as it had tugged them toward human biology. This latter group of writers who sought to place distress within the category of morals and passions was retrospectively dubbed "Romantic psychiatry." (At the time they were known as the "psychically oriented," *die Psychiker*.)

The perception of passion was partly a generational issue. Members of the founding generation such as Battie, following in the tradition of John Locke, situated madness in "false perception" and the "confusion of ideas" that would inevitably follow such perception.[108] The next generation of Romantic psychiatrists by contrast sought out passions bubbling uncontrollably from the human soul. This tension within psychiatry flowed generally from the tension between the Enlightenment of the eighteenth century as a social and intellectual movement stressing reason, and the Romantic movement of the late eighteenth and early nineteenth centuries stressing feeling and sentiment. Thus a small clutch of psychiatric writers in Germany steered the discussion from reason toward mood and passion. Their underlying premise was that social circumstances (regulating the temptation to sin), not biology, governed passion, and that strict adherence to moral precepts was required for the control of these passions.

Unlike their biologically oriented colleagues, the Romantic psychiatrists had little interest in heredity or brain pathology and preferred to spend long hours talking to their patients about their subjective experiences. Otto Braus, at the time a young psychiatry resident in the Charité hospital in Berlin, recalled the contrast between the elderly Romantic psychiatrist Karl Wilhelm Ideler, then head of the psychiatric service, and his brash young deputy-chief Karl Westphal, who was very biologically oriented. The anecdote must have been in the late 1850s: Just after Braus came onto the service he introduced himself to Westphal, who said, "You'll see at once that our good old Professor Ideler is still wandering around in the olden days and using prescriptions taken from the pharmacopoeia of mental therapies, just because he sees these illnesses as independent and not related to illnesses of the body. He tries to prove to the patients that they've been the victims of delusive thinking, what the delusions are, how they acquired them, and so forth. You're going to have to tolerate listening in on these discussions, which can be quite boring.

"But if you take a shine to this work, a field that's quite new for you, I'll gladly loan you my books. You can help me out by working together with me in the autopsies, both on the gross [non-microscopic] side and the microscopic side, because our only salvation in dealing with mental illness in the future is going to be not just the interview room, but also the autopsy table and the microscope."[109] This vignette is situated toward the end of the period, as Romantic psychiatry was on the wane and Westphal's star was rising as the future professor of psychiatry in Berlin. But in the beginning, the Romantics had two powerful young advocates.

One of the original Romantic psychiatrists, though he would have dreaded the term, was Esquirol, the first major specialist to espouse the notion of psychosocial causation of psychiatric illness. Esquirol was a transitional figure with one foot in the biological camp, given his loyalty to Pinel, and one foot in the psychosocial, given his interest in statistical analyses of how such matters as age, sex, and occupation influence psychiatric illness.[110] But Esquirol shunned the ponderous moralizing that characterized the German Romantic psychiatrists.

The main German figure associated with Romantic psychiatry, the Leipzig professor Johann Christian Heinroth, knew Esquirol and felt a close affinity with him.[111] Born in 1773, Heinroth had been caught up in the fundamentalist Protestant religious movement of the early nineteenth century called Pietism. He had studied medicine in Leipzig, his hometown, and in Vienna in the 1790s, and then because of a death in the family had turned to theology, finally however pulling himself together to earn an MD in 1805. After serving in the army against Napoleon, in 1811 Heinroth took up an academic career at Leipzig teaching psychiatry, and became in 1827 the professor for "psychological therapy" at that university, the first such professorship in Germany.

Heinroth came to psychosocial perspectives through an obsession with morality and sin. People's passions drive them to choose evil, he said, and that choice leads to a kind of inner corruption. Once corrupt, external events such as terror, vexation, or disappointment can precipitate a mental illness. In his *Textbook of Mental Hygiene*, published in 1823, Heinroth reviewed the gamut of circumstances that could affect one's psychic well-being: food, drink, sleep, exercise, air pollution and, finally, poor attention to the cleanliness of the skin. A sample: "The passions are like burning coals tossed into the dwelling of life, or serpents that spit poison into the vessels, or vultures that gnaw at the entrails. From the moment someone is seized by a passion, order ceases to prevail in the economy of his life." What protection was there against the passions? Freedom! "The world however gives us no freedom; it will never leave us free. Only God makes us free."[112] Hardly what one expects to find in a psychiatry textbook.

Throughout Heinroth's work rang a kind of sanctimonious pietizing that sat ill with contemporaries. Carl Carus, later court physician at

Dresden, had met Heinroth in a fall journey through Leipzig in 1817 and pityingly attributed the sterility of Heinroth's ideas to the sterility of his marriage.[113] Heinroth probably would have sunk into oblivion had not later critics of psychoanalysis likened Freud to the Romantic psychiatrists, enraging Freud and grabbing the interest of the historians of psychoanalysis.[114] Yet Heinroth was among the first of the Germans to follow the Esquirol school of linking life circumstances to mental disorders. And his distant successors, who cast off Heinroth's moralizing and turned to social problems as the source of mental distress, were by no means worthy of the contempt of posterity.

The other Romantic psychiatrists were too unimportant to merit attention in a general volume on the history of psychiatry. Suffice it to say that in psychiatry almost from birth on, the neuroscience wing found a counterweight in the psychosocial wing. Happily or unhappily, the counterbalance was so weak that biological psychiatry dominated the discipline throughout the nineteenth century, right up to the time of Emil Kraepelin.

2

The Asylum Era

The rise of the asylum is the story of good intentions gone bad. That the dreams of the early psychiatrists failed is unquestionable. By World War I, asylums had become vast warehouses for the chronically insane and demented. Yet whether the failure of the asylum lay in the nature of the enterprise itself is a matter of controversy. Some argue that the asylum failed because it was overwhelmed by the ever-rising numbers of psychiatric patients in the nineteenth century. Others maintain that many people admitted to the asylum had no psychiatric illness and were confined merely because they were social misfits and outcasts, inconvenient rather than ill. Through this historical debate, as through psychiatry itself, runs the cleft demarcating neuroscience from psychosocial understanding. The neuroscientific side of the story sees growing pathology; the psychosocial version sees a social universe increasingly intolerant of deviance.

This debate is one of the most exciting in the social history of medicine. At the very beginning, therefore, I want to make my own point of view clear. I side with the people who see the increasing numbers of psychiatric patients as the result of changing patterns of psychiatric disease. But there is a psychosocial component in addition. It concerns the redistribution of people who were already mentally ill to asylums. "Already mentally ill" must be emphasized, for some scholars argue that those being redistributed from family and almshouse to the asylum were merely deviant or intolerable, and not ill at all.

At the end of the story, the asylum fails. But this does not represent a failure of the biological paradigm as a model for diagnosing and treating patients. It represents the tragedy of individuals whose good therapeutic intentions were overpowered by events. Here I part completely with the social constructionists who claim that psychiatry's apparent good intentions were a sham, a pretense for gaining professional power. The history of the asylum era is the story of how progressive and humane aspirations became relentlessly and repeatedly disappointed. The many well-meant initiatives of asylum psychiatry, central in the legacy that psychiatry's past has lent to the present, were almost all doomed to failure under the pressure of numbers.

In 1800, only a handful of individuals were confined in asylums. Beds in even the most famous of historic asylums, such as Bedlam in London, Bicêtre in Paris, or the "fools' tower" (Narrenturm) in Vienna, numbered in the dozens or low hundreds. In the nineteenth century, these numbers exploded. By 1904, there were 150,000 patients in U.S. mental hospitals, corresponding to a rate of almost two for every thousand population.[1] By 1891, France had 108 asylums.[2] A few years later, the London region alone counted no fewer than 16 asylums, including such giants as the London County Asylum at Colney Hatch ("Nut Hatch") with 2,200 beds, and the Hanwell Asylum (where in the 1840s John Conolly had publicized the nonrestraint of patients) with 2,600 beds.[3] The index of Heinrich Laehr's directory of asylums for German-speaking Europe published in 1891 contained no fewer than 202 entries for public asylums and 200 more for the private sector, to say nothing of the numerous institutions for the alcoholic, the morphinists, the epileptics, and the mentally retarded.[4] In a century's time, the confining of patients with a psychiatric illness had passed from an unusual procedure, born of grave necessity and done only in cities, to society's first response in dealing with psychotic illness.

National Traditions

As the physical platform for the practice of psychiatry, these asylums are central to the history of the discipline. They were founded everywhere at approximately the same time, in countries vastly disparate in social structure and level of economic development. As psychiatry arose in the United States in the early nineteenth century, it was in a sprawling, decentralized land with a tradition of voluntarism in the provision of public services. There would be no national regulation of psychiatric care until after World War II. The geography of early American asylums reflects no logic more than a series of local and adventitious initiatives:

Spring Grove State Hospital in Catonsville, Maryland, founded in 1798; Eastern State Hospital in Lexington, Kentucky, in 1824; Manhattan State Hospital in New York City, in 1825, and so forth.[5] In Britain as well, voluntarism rather than state intervention was the rule. Despite a law of 1808 empowering the counties to raise asylums, the regulation of psychiatric institutions in Britain remained in local hands until the Lunacy Act of 1890.[6]

Traditions of health care on the continent of Europe, by contrast, were very different. In France, state medicine had established itself with the general hospitals of the seventeenth century, followed by the county medical officers of the eighteenth. The rule was that the nation's health was directed from Paris. Extreme centralization characterized every aspect of health care in France, psychiatry included, and the establishment of asylums in the nineteenth century would occur from the top down (not from the bottom up, as in the United States). In Germany, Austria, and Switzerland traditions of state medicine reached far back in time. The notion of central control of medical matters was embedded in such concepts as "medical police" popularized by the Badenese physician Johann Peter Frank in his four-volume work of that title published between 1779 and 1788. Medical police included psychiatry. It was Frank who, after moving to Vienna, ordered in 1795 that a garden be laid down about the *Narrenturm* so that the patients could stretch their legs.[7]

All this administering was done in Central Europe, as in France, from high to low, from central chancelleries down to the asylum doctors in small towns on the periphery. The difference between France and Germany, however, is that France was a single, central state and Germany before 1871 a confederation of 39 separate states, each having its own tradition of administrative centralization. Some of these states led in founding asylums, others lagged. Prussia, by far the largest (except for Austria), was an innovator. Yet Bavaria, with one of the continent's renowned medical schools in Munich, lagged. A host of smaller states such as Baden, Württemberg, and the several "Saxonies" had universities with brilliant and far-flung international reputations, and played roles in the history of psychiatry quite disproportionate to their size.

Germany became the world leader in psychiatry during the nineteenth century precisely because of this dispersal of academic talent into many separate universities, each nurtured by the dynastic ambition of its own little principality. Germany possessed some 20 separate universities in addition to two medical academies, each struggling for glory and competing in a lively race for scientific advancement against the others. In almost every one of these little lands, academic talent was hooked up to asylum administration. The ministries of interior and education simply decreed that it would happen. France by contrast had basically one university, the Sorbonne in Paris. And even though some of the provincial cities had faculties of their own, they were dim bulbs compared to the great concentration of academic talent in Paris, the only place that mattered. Even today, Parisians indifferently lump the rest of the country together as "la province"; then as now, if one wished to have an important scientific career, it could be only in the City of Light.

The proliferation of German states also made the asylum psychiatrists in the various states more competitive against one another. All were avid for state honors. The German states had a long tradition of recognizing deserving officials and professors with almost meaningless titles, such as *Geheimrat* in Prussia (privy counsellor) or *Hofrat* in Austria (court counsellor). Seeking to demonstrate their devotion to duty, these asylum directors were constantly trying to innovate, reform, and thus distinguish themselves. The narrative of reform would thus become heavily German, in contrast to France where it was pointless to seek distinction in some provincial nest.

Despite these national differences, psychiatrists began everywhere early in the century with the same high intentions. Virtually to an individual, they intended to implement the principles that the founding generation had enunciated of daily regimen and moral therapy to foster the cure of psychiatric illness. One may distinguish between isolated early initiatives that led nowhere, such as Chiarugi's in late-eighteenth-century Florence, and the launching of a sustained wave of therapeutic asylums.

Sustained was the German wave. The new-style asylums gathered momentum earliest in Central Europe where, in the first decade of the nineteenth century, ministerial officials decided to give Pinel's and Reil's ideas a try.[8] This occurred first in the Kingdom of Saxony as the government decided to separate the hospice patients from the criminals. The Saxon government sent a family doctor named Christian August Hayner to study with Pinel, then in 1806 appointed him chief physician of a hospice at Waldheim. Entirely typical of its day, the Waldheim facility mixed together "curable and incurable mental patients, epileptics, the physically handicapped of every description, orphaned children, and criminals of the most diverse kinds in a chaotic mish-mash."[9] Hayner wanted to separate them, in particular dividing the curable from the incurable insane. In 1808, the Saxon government asked him to investigate the possibility of doing so by converting the fortress at Sonnenstein into an asylum for the acutely ill; two years later Hayner produced a proposal.

36

This kind of separation seemed like a clever idea. But in fact, the notion of making progress by separating the fresh cases from the chronic was somewhat of a will-o'-the-wisp.[10] Patients tend naturally to remit from such illnesses as depression and mania and even in many cases from schizophrenia, in contrast to dementia from which they do not recover. So most of the psychotic patients were potentially "curable" in that they would sooner or later get better anyway.

In 1811, the government opened Sonnenstein. Yet to Hayner's dismay, it was not he who was chosen as director but another psychiatrist, the 34-year-old Ernst Pienitz. Pienitz too had done a French apprenticeship, traveling to Paris at the same time as Hayner to see Pinel and Esquirol. (When Pienitz married a Parisian, Hayner and Esquirol were witnesses.) Pienitz had also studied in Vienna under Johann Peter Frank, and at the *Narrenturm* he had accompanied the director on rounds. Pienitz thus reflected the same liberal, humanitarian spirit that ran through this whole generation of physicians.

Cure of mental illness was the number one task of the Sonnenstein asylum. It corresponded to all of the "therapeutic asylum" notions of the time, containing a billiard room, gardens, music rooms with three pianos for concerts once every two weeks, and reading rooms that contained serious books ("no silly French novels").[11] Pienitz relied extensively on baths, or hydrotherapy. He was at great pains to find trustworthy attendants who would not beat the patients. He would make rounds with a surgeon (and a cleric), trying to remedy, in an across-the-boards assault on human unreason, any complaint at all that he could get a purchase on.[12] Pienitz did his task well. The Sonnenstein became celebrated as the "rising sun" of the new psychiatry, and he was rewarded for his efforts by becoming later in life an honorary "Privy Medical Counsellor" (*Geheimer Medizinalrat*).[13]

There is one other interesting theme in the Sonnenstein story. As part of the new spirit starting to blow through the private sector, around 1811 while Pienitz was director at Sonnenstein, he started taking patients into his home. He then established in the nearby city of Pirna an exclusive private asylum of about 20 beds, the third such in Germany. In the years ahead, reforming psychiatrists all over the Atlantic community would use such private establishments as a kind of clinical home base.

Meanwhile in the Rhineland, part of Prussia, another of the pathbreaking asylums was opening its doors. Prussia possessed, just as the Kingdom of Saxony, the same kind of interventionist senior administrators who saw in psychiatry a means of health reform and were willing to back practitioners such as Hayner and Pienitz. As early as 1805, the bureaucrats supported the efforts of Johann Langermann to reform the asylum in

37

Bayreuth. At the conclusion of the Napoleonic wars, the bureaucrats then returned to this task in earnest. In 1817, Karl von Altenstein, the powerful Prussian minister of education, decided to enlist Langermann to help apply the Pinel-Reil reforms in Prussia as a whole. To start with, they decided to turn the old buildings of the former monastery at Siegburg, about two hours' coach ride from Bonn, into a model hospital for curable psychiatric patients. The ministry chose as chief physician a specialist in state medicine named Maximilian Jacobi.[14]

Jacobi, 45 in 1820, had been educated in the most progressive settings, including Edinburgh, and had already made a name for himself through his efforts to reorganize the Bavarian state medical service. Soured at state medicine, Jacobi decided to try his hand at psychiatry and came into contact with Altenstein. In 1820, Jacobi did a tour of eight German asylums, after which the ministry let him take over the planning of the model asylum at Siegburg, which opened in 1825.[15]

It was really Siegburg and not Sonnenstein that became the beacon of psychiatric reform in Central Europe. Jacobi, unlike Pienitz or Langermann, published widely. And he managed to bring to bear therapeutically more than baths and good intentions. Jacobi applied almost to the letter the prescriptions of the founding generation about the restorative nature of an orderly regimen and the psychological impact that the physician himself, as a model of decency and duty, should have on the patients. His 1834 book on the organization of the asylum was translated into a number of languages, and motivated physicians from far and wide to come to Siegburg to observe. Jacobi conceived the asylum as a "hospital organized for the exclusive treatment of those organic illnesses that are associated with mental illness." Like any hospital, it had to possess a medley of therapeutic interventions, going beyond medication to include "baths of all kinds, electricity, galvanism and so forth, the whole array of the relevant treatments that belong to psychiatric as well as to somatic therapeutics, to which must be added diet, healthy air, suitable temperature, and keeping patients physically active and busy."[16]

How did Jacobi actually proceed with patients? Here is Heinrich N., "a strapping big, powerful farmer," who around the age of 39 began having periodic attacks of psychosis that would remit after a few weeks, leaving him in full possession of his senses until the next attack. Jacobi treated him with the standard medical therapies of the day, bloodletting, laxatives, and the like. But Jacobi also spent a good deal of time on nonmedical measures, such as worrying about the patient's diet, talking with him to win his confidence, physically laying-on hands by taking his pulse, and negotiating with him. When Heinrich raged in an attack, smearing his feces, Jacobi threatened the straitjacket and isolation room. This "greatly embittered" the patient, "who finally declared that he would behave peacefully and keep clean if we would agree not to use restraints. We gave in to him, and he kept his word. A few days later, he was decidedly on the path to convalescence." Later Jacobi was chatting with Heinrich about what seemed a psychotic fear of being burned alive. "He gave the following explanation. Earlier when he was in an agitated state, people would chain him fast in the barn, with straw for his bed, and hang a lamp directly overhead. He had always been gripped by the fear that a spark might fall down and burn him up with his bed, a fear of burning alive that accompanied him continuously thereafter."[17] Although there are features in Jacobi's management reminiscent of the traditional asylum, with its restraints and efforts to adjust the humors and irritations supposedly causing the illness, this use of the doctor-patient relationship therapeutically was thoroughly reformist, employing persuasion and the orderliness of a daily schedule to effect what he hoped would be a cure.

Siegburg's golden era occurred under Jacobi, who died in office in 1858. (Three years earlier, he had become a *Geheimer Medizinalrat*.) Psychiatrist Karl Pelman, who became a superintendent elsewhere and once had been an assistant physician at Siegburg, reflected about those halcyon days in the history of German psychiatry: "One cannot begrudge it to an asylum director if his thoughts travel back involuntarily to the old and in this respect better days, as he sits for hours at his desk and answers questionnaires whose purpose and sense are never quite clear to him. . . . In all my time at Siegburg, I never had to give a forensic expertise and nobody had yet invented [psychiatric reports on] accidents. We had all kinds of time, and we had to dedicate a part of this time to the patients, something that today is impossible even with the best of will." Pelman remembered Siegburg as having almost the intimacy of family life: "The whole asylum really was a kind of family, and everybody shared in the ups and downs of the individuals. Even patients in the agitated ward would feel a kind of obligation to be calm and make less noise if there had been a tragic event in the lives of one of the doctors' families."[18] It was in this kind of spirit that the reformed asylum in Germany was launched.

In France, the wave of reformist asylums washed scarcely beyond Esquirol's Paris. Asylums in the French provinces remained desolate custodial institutions, barely a step up from jails with no progressive energy or thoughtful experimentation.[19] The difference between Germany and

France is striking. In decentralized Germany, where everything was "province," local centers of innovation such as Siegburg and Sonnenstein had sprung up, jewels in the crowns of petty rulers. By contrast in centralized France, where a single haughty city confronted a vast provincial desert, neither Esquirol himself nor the administrators of the Ministry of the Interior in Paris cared much for what was happening outside. As historian Jan Goldstein puts it, "Esquirol took as axiomatic that all expertise in France about the treatment of lunatics was to be found in Paris and that any improvement in treatment procedures must necessarily take the form of an exportation of that expertise from the Parisian center to the benighted periphery."[20]

Thus Esquirol was able to shape events within the capital until his death in 1840. Becoming chief physician in 1825 of the Charenton asylum, which accepted patients referred by the state as well as family-supported patients, Esquirol was soon able to give the institution a handsome international reputation. He erected clean new quarters for the female patients, to which he attributed a salutary influence in improving the cure rate. For the private patients, he arranged "a salon where they may give themselves to various sociable games, to music and to dance, among each other and members of staff." Patients also had billiards and a large garden in which to stroll about. The men might go out on day passes. ("The women never go out alone.") The nonpaying patients as well had special gardens and activities, the women sewing, the men practicing military drills. "Thus organized, the Charenton institution offers very favorable conditions for the treatment of the insane," said Esquirol. What precisely was so therapeutic at Charenton? "The pleasant locality, the dependability and progressive spirit [douceur] of the administration, the zeal of the physicians, the ample provisions of care, the general atmosphere of the place . . .": All had made mental illness at Charenton treatable, he claimed.[21]

Yet in France, mental illness became "treatable" in this sense only at Charenton. No further wave of douceur radiated out. Bureaucratic inertia and political resistance stymied all of Esquirol's efforts to export his reforms to the 86 departments. Although Esquirol did place several of his students in outlying asylums—Achille-Louis Foville, for example, at the Saint-Yon asylum in Rouen (from which institution the fateful doctrine of degeneration would later emanate)—provincial France remained far behind provincial Germany.

Finally in 1838, the French bureaucracy contrived a national law regulating the administration of asylums in Paris and the departments. The law focused mainly on mechanisms of admission to an asylum (making a preliminary court order unnecessary), and aimed at extending a network of asylum services across the country. Moral therapy was definitely not the focus of these reforms, attracting little attention even in parliamentary debates.[22] Half a century later, many areas of France were still without public asylums, patients ending up in run-down private asylums resembling warehouses.[23] On the whole, the entire mental health apparatus created by the law of 1838 offered but a minimum of care. As the rising tide of patients overwhelmed asylum services in every part of Western society, in France it must be said there was little to overwhelm.

Britain resembled Germany for its lack of centralization. The British state bore as a birthmark its almost complete uninvolvement in healthcare and in medical research, offering the English a government so lean as to limit its powers to collecting customs and policing the streets. For this lack of engagement in medical matters, the English would later pay a price in laboratory research. (Even though state power in Germany was fragmented, each of the small principalities possessed age-old directorial reflexes, the complete opposite of Britain.) Yet a crucial issue in the diffusion of new ideas in medicine and psychiatry is whether the center overwhelms the periphery. In France it did. In England and Germany it did not. The scurrying administrative and industrial towns of England and Germany offered a more permissive terrain than did the ossified ministerial bureaucracy of the French state, which was bound to find moral therapy, with its implications of liberty for the patients, a nuisance.

Among English alienists in the first three decades of the nineteenth century, the concepts of moral therapy and the therapeutic use of daily routine positively blossomed. As John Ferriar, a general physician who also oversaw the Lunatic Hospital in Manchester, wrote in the 1810 edition of his *Medical Histories*, "A system of mildness and conciliation is now generally adopted, which, if it does not always facilitate the cure, at least tends to soften the destiny of the sufferer."[24] The moral treatment of William Tuke had become an English watchword. In 1813, William Tuke's grandson Samuel published a widely read memoir on exactly how the therapy worked: "The desire of esteem is considered at the Retreat as operating in general still more powerfully [than fear of punishment]. This principle . . . is found to have great influence, even over the conduct of the insane." Learning to overcome one's "morbid properties" resulted in "strengthening [the patient's] mind and conducing to a salutary habit of self-restraint; an object which experience points out as of the greatest importance in the cure of insanity by moral means."[25] These were classic lines in the history of psychiatry, even though they were written by a layperson. News of the

York Retreat traveled all over the United Kingdom and the continent, a reminder of what could be done.

Other reformist impulses came to Britain from the Continent. Asylum-owner George Man Burrows, for example, seems to have drawn his psychiatric liberalism from Europe. In 1816, he retired from general practice, where he had become a prominent medical spokesperson, to open a small private asylum in Chelsea. The following year, he visited the Parisian psychiatrists, to return to England where in 1823 he founded a more substantial private psychiatric hospital in Clapham that Burrows called "the Retreat." Burrows was among the first to prefer the term "asylum" to "madhouse," and gave, in a textbook on mental illness published in 1828, an account of the standard techniques of gentle management as then widely practiced on the Continent. "If the moderns have any claims to preeminence in the cure of insanity," he declared, "it is certainly from studying those means which have been denominated moral." Among the guidelines Burrows enumerated, such as not trying to argue acutely ill patients out of their symptoms, he included therapeutic use of "the soothing voice of friendship to calm the agony which reminiscence often generates."[26] The soothing voice of friendship: how appropriate a therapeutic mode for upper-middle-class doctors to deal with the kind of upper-middle-class patients enrolled in Burrows's asylum. And yet such techniques were effective. The textbook was "by far the most complete and practical treatise on insanity that had then appeared in this country."[27]

The English psychiatrist who described the new approach in greatest detail has nearly passed from memory because subsequent generations of medical memorialists found him as a phrenologist—a believer in the doctrine of diagnosing mental illness from the bumps on the skull—something of an embarrassment. William Charles Ellis was the founding superintendent of two new county asylums—the West Riding of Yorkshire Lunatic Asylum at Wakefield (beginning in 1818) and the Middlesex County Lunatic Asylum in London (from 1831 to 1838). He emerged as the principal Continental-style innovator in England. Conceiving his institution as a large family in the manner of Esquirol and Jacobi, Ellis saw asylum therapy as applied humanitarianism. As he wrote in 1838, "The moral treatment is by far the most difficult part of the subject. In this the most essential ingredient is constant, never-tiring, watchful kindness: there are but few, even amongst the insane, who, if a particle of mind be left, are not to be won by affectionate attention." And it worked, he said. "In many cases, there will be the delight of witnessing the gradual return to reason and happiness."[28]

In imitation of Edward Parker Charlesworth who had initiated "the nonrestraint system" at the Lincoln Asylum in 1821, Ellis at Hanwell abolished the policy of restraining agitated patients. In the manner of Horn at the Charité, he and his wife introduced crafts and activities with which to fill the day. By 1837, three-quarters of the 612 patients at Hanwell were doing some kind of useful daily work.[29] Even Ellis's eccentric doctrine of phrenology became an extension of moral therapy, for in running his fingers over his patients' heads and talking to them, Ellis conducted a highly therapeutic laying on of hands, calming and comforting them in a manner that previous medical therapy, with its purgatives and bloodletting, had not accomplished.[30]

If the Hanwell asylum in London was the English epicenter of moral therapy and busy regimen, Dumfries was the Scottish. Casting about for ways to deploy the inheritance of her late husband in the relief of madness, Elizabeth Crichton of Dumfries happened upon William Alexander Francis Browne's book *What Asylums Were, Are and Ought to Be*, published in 1837.[31] Browne was then at the nearby asylum at Montrose in Scotland. He had studied under Esquirol at Charenton, and as head of Montrose in the 1830s became an early partisan of the abolition of physical restraints.[32] Browne was filled with the spirit of the curative asylum. "The whole secret of the new system," he wrote in 1837, "and of that moral treatment by which the number of cures has been doubled may be summed up in two words, kindness and occupation."[33] This was precisely what Mrs. Crichton was looking for. She sought Browne out at Montrose, then donated £100,000 for a 120-bed hospital, the Crichton Royal Institution, that incorporated these principles and accepted patients from all classes.[34] It opened in Dumfries in 1839 with Browne its first medical director.

Thus by 1839, the new wave of asylums had well established itself in Britain. Here as on the Continent the notion became implicit that the function of the asylum was to cure, that of the alienist to use all the techniques implicit in the doctor-patient relationship and in the management of time to alleviate illnesses caused at bottom by disorder of the brain.

America lay distant on the periphery and came last as the reform wave broke across the Atlantic community. As in Europe, the alienists who carried forward this first wave tended to be experienced physicians, animated by a vision as intense as that of Jacobi or Ellis. By 1811, it had become apparent to the members of the Society of Friends in Philadelphia that the insane ward of Pennsylvania Hospital, to whose foundation they had in 1752 contributed so materially, was growing too crowded. They therefore resolved to build a regular asylum on a patch of land they bought in nearby Frankford, Pennsylvania. In May 1817, this first incursion of the new wave in America opened for business. Its model was the Retreat in York, England. As a later annual report of the Frankford Retreat boasted, "This asylum was the first erection of that kind on this side of the Atlantic in which a chain was never used for the confinement of the patients." At Frankford, as under similar regimens all over Britain and the Continent, the rule was, "Come what may, the law of kindness must prevail."[35] Unlike the Retreat at York, that at Frankford had a resident physician, Charles Lukens, from the beginning.

Now a series of foundations ensued. Impressed by the asylum at Frankford, Doctors Eli Todd and Samuel Woodward decided to animate the state medical society of Connecticut to erect a similar institution, or Retreat, at Hartford. A number of individuals subscribed to this quintessentially Anglo-Saxon kind of voluntary institution, and in 1824 the Hartford Retreat, semipublic in nature but open to the poor from Hartford, began admitting patients. Todd, a Yale arts graduate who like most of the physicians of his day had learned his medicine as an apprentice, was most active in the subscription and was appointed superintendent. Woodward, also a Yale graduate who had apprenticed to his physician father, consulted at the Retreat and to the penitentiary in nearby Wethersfield. Thus it was Todd's philosophy that guided the Hartford Retreat. Todd made, he said, "the law of kindness the all-pervading power of the moral discipline of the Retreat and required unvaried gentleness and respect to be manifested towards the inmates of the institution by every member belonging to it."[36] The Hartford Retreat later became entirely private, underwent several name changes, and exists today in that city as an exclusive private nervous clinic called the Institute for Living.

Almost simultaneously, Massachusetts acquired an asylum. Around 1810, the merchant princes of Boston decided to build a voluntary general hospital. But as events became protracted, the asylum that was to have been part of that hospital opened independently in 1818, even before the hospital itself (the Massachusetts General Hospital began accepting patients only in 1821). In 1826, this psychiatric service was renamed the McLean Asylum after the gift of John McLean, a Boston merchant who left the institution a sum of money. The first superintendent of McLean was Rufus Wyman, a Harvard graduate who had apprenticed in medicine in Boston. Wyman had read Pinel and Tuke and became a strong advocate of "the system of moral management." In his first report in 1822, he described the benefits of occupation and diversion in the regimen of the asylum: "Amusements provided, as draughts, chess, backgammon, nine-pins, swinging, sawing wood, gardening . . . divert the attention from the unpleasant subject of thought and afford exercise both of body and mind." To procure for the patients some outdoor exercise, Wyman arranged in 1828 for the asylum's first carriage and pair of horses. He later boasted that "chains or strait jackets have never been used or provided in this asylum" and that no attendant was permitted to lay hand upon a patient. (In fact early patients at the McLean Asylum were restrained.)[37] Like the Hartford Retreat, the McLean Asylum later went private once public beds for psychiatric patients became available in Massachusetts.

At this point, the baton fashioned by the private sector passed to the public. The first public asylum of any kind had been founded in Williamsburg in 1773. The first to arise from the new wave of therapeutic management arrived some 60 years later at Worcester, Massachusetts, proposed to the legislature in 1830 by the educational reformer Horace Mann. In January 1833, Worcester opened for business, its superintendent Samuel Woodward having come up from Connecticut where he had been a consultant for the Hartford Retreat. (Only in the United States did reserves of experience accumulated in the private sector fuel the public.) Woodward was not exactly a beacon of therapeutic *douceur*, it must be said. He blistered his patients' skin with caustic compounds in the hopes of getting the poisonous humors to the surface. He locked them in the strong room when they misbehaved. Nonetheless at Worcester, he brought tranquillity and orderliness to the lives of the "raving lunatics." "Of forty persons who formerly divested themselves of clothing, even in the most inclement seasons of the year," wrote the hospital's trustees in 1833, "only eight do it now. Through all the galleries, there is far less susceptibility to excitement, more quietude, more civility and kindness exercised towards each other. The wailings of the despondent and the ravings of the frantic are disspelled."[38]

Now many American public asylums began to dispel the wailings of the despondent. A number of asylums having therapeutic rather than custodial intentions were established in the 1840s, ranging from Utica State Hospital (where Amariah Brigham, cofounder in 1848 of the organization that ultimately became the American Psychiatric Association, held forth), to an asylum in Milledgeville, Georgia, that initially possessed the noblest of therapeutic intentions. Its superintendent would personally release new patients from manacles as they were brought for admission. The Milledgeville asylum later became an 8,000-bed hellhole.[39]

Thus by the 1840s, therapeutic asylums had burst forth all over the Atlantic community. In Europe as well as the United States, these young psychiatrists smelled the scent of victory in the air. In their reformed institutions, they were about to conquer mental illness.

The Pressure of Numbers

The reformers were defeated not by the faulty nature of their concept but by the pressure of numbers. The therapeutic asylum bore within it the seeds of success, for people with major psychiatric illnesses are indeed helped by sheltering in places they believe to be safe, by efforts to help them organize their time and lives, and by medication. The early asylum attempted all of these, yet under the assumption that physicians and attendants would be able to spend time treating patients rather than simply warehousing them. What happened was the overwhelming of the therapeutic asylum by numbers. By 1900, any hope of achieving the early reformers' ideals had been dashed by the flood of inmates hurled against the gates.

In the United States, the first pessimistic note was struck in 1869 with the establishment of an asylum in New York State only for chronic patients: the Willard State Hospital, the first American institution to abandon any pretense of cure and discharge.[40] Under the pressure of numbers, there were many Willards: average annual admissions to the typical American asylum climbed from 31 in 1820 to 182 in 1870, the average number of patients per asylum rising from 57 to 473.[41] Already in the 1870s, observers were transfixed at the remorseless rise in numbers, the unceasing need for ever more asylums. Said one New York banker to a visiting English psychiatrist in 1875 about the continuing demands, "I don't know how it is. They have cost enough, but we never know how the money goes. There is always a tap leaking somewhere."[42] After the 1880s, most American public asylums would abandon any effort at therapy in what historian David Rothman has described as "the decline from rehabilitation to custodianship."[43]

In 1895, the young Swiss psychiatrist Adolf Meyer found himself at the famous Worcester Asylum—birthplace of public-sector therapy—as a research scientist supposedly without clinical responsibilities. There were four other physicians at Worcester attending 1,200 patients, with 600 new admissions a year. Meyer protested this extreme work load (300 patients per doctor) and soon obtained a doubling of the medical staff. "How do you keep the boys busy?" a medical visitor asked him.[44] In other words, the expectation of being therapeutic had clearly vanished from the job description of the typical American psychiatrist.

Psychiatrists in Germany were no less hammered by the pressure of numbers as the rate of confinement grew from one psychiatric inpatient for every 5,300 population in 1852 to one for every 500 in 1911.[45] German psychiatrists were no less bewildered than American at this re-morseless rise: As soon as one asylum was built, another was needed. "Thus the lack of beds has become the permanent preoccupation of al-most all mental-health authorities," said one doctor in 1911.[46] Another lamented, "It is unsettling how patients needing institutional care are in-creasing, and bears no relationship to the increase in population."[47] Of Upper Bavaria, one wag said in 1907 that, if things persisted at the present rate, in 222 years the entire population of the province would be in an in-sane asylum.[48]

By 1911, the 11 pavilions of the Sainte-Anne asylum in Paris, origi-nally designed in 1867 for 490 patients, housed 1,100. When Vaucluse asylum in nearby Epinay-sur-Orge opened in 1869, it was slated for 500 patients; by 1911 it had over 1,000. The same unanticipated overcrowd-ing held true for almost every asylum in the Paris region founded after 1867.[49] Meanwhile in the classic Parisian asylums, overcrowding had worsened conditions desperately. A visitor to Bicêtre in the 1880s de-scribed "this melancholy conglomerate of overcrowded rooms and damp courtyards."[50]

In England, asylum inmates had more than doubled from 1.6 per 1,000 population in 1859 to 3.7 per 1,000 in 1909. In 1827, the average asylum had housed 116 patients; in 1910, the number reached 1,072.[51] Just before World War I, the head of the visitors' committee of one of the county asy-lums in Staffordshire noted in the register, "Our numbers have increased out of all proportion to our accommodation. On Saturday last we had the largest number, 916 patients, that has ever been in this asylum. . . . We have 36 males sleeping without bedsteads. I have ordered 20 iron bed-steads at a cost of 30/3d. each."[52] Montagu Lomax, a family doctor sec-onded to help out in an asylum during World War I, later reflected how completely English asylums had abandoned any kind of therapeutic role. "Our asylums detain," he said, "but they certainly do not cure. Or if they cure, it is only by accident, so to speak, and in spite of the system, not as a result of it." He never had fewer than 350 to 400 patients under his care, a number that "was sometimes doubled or trebled, and it was simply impos-sible to give them all individual attention." Had the superintendent at least maintained the hope of therapy? "If remedial treatment and methods of attempted cure were considered part of a Medical Officer's duties, I can only say that, as far as I was concerned, I received no hint of the fact during the whole of my term of office." Lomax concluded that, "public asylums for the most part exist merely to confine, not to cure, the insane."[53] The former hopes of a Battie or an Ellis had been shattered by the press of bodies.

Why the Increase?

Why this increase in numbers of asylum patients occurred is highly controversial within the social history of psychiatry. Several distinct schools have emerged. Dominating the field for the past two decades have been scholars who doubt the very existence of psychiatric illness, believing it to be socially constructed. These writers have attempted to trivialize the illnesses of the inmates and to make the case that capitalist society was venging itself on the patients for their unwillingness to work, for a Bohemian lifestyle, or even for a revolt against male authority. Thus society's growing intolerance of deviance is said to have led to the confinement of ever greater numbers of "intolerable" individuals.[54] It is astonishing that this interpretation could have achieved such currency as there is virtually no evidence on its behalf.

Another group of researchers argues that, while psychiatric illness is indeed very real and not necessarily an artifact of labeling, its incidence probably does not change very much over time. Therefore social explanations must be sought for the great nineteenth-century lockup.[55] This model is a serious contender, yet it is weakened by these researchers' reluctance to decompose "madness" into its component parts and see what happens to each. Yet differentiating is essential. To write a history of psychiatry that did not distinguish among dementia, psychosis, and feeblemindedness would be like trying to write a history of noise that did not distinguish between that made by computers and by tanks. Some psychiatric illnesses may well remain historically constant, others do not. Speaking in an undifferentiated way about lunatics, the insane, the distracted, and so forth, renounces at the outset any effort to peer beneath the surface of labels. The search for social causes therefore begs the question, causes of what, exactly?

A third group of writers argues that psychiatric illness is real and that it can change in frequency depending on social circumstances that might affect mind and brain.[56] I belong to this school. In my view, it is essential to disaggregate "madness," and to examine the many different diseases and syndromes whose final common pathway is dysphoria, psychosis, or

48

dementia. The massive increase in the number of asylum patients during the nineteenth century seems to have had two components: a "redistribution effect" and a genuine increase in the rate of psychiatric illness. Understanding these requires penetrating the monolith of madness to see the people and their conditions underneath.

Some of the increase in asylum admissions was a result of redistributing the ill. During the nineteenth century, individuals with major psychiatric illnesses were increasingly shifted from the family or the poorhouse to the asylum. This redistribution had nothing to do with the overall rate of mental illness. It simply involved rearrangements in care.

In addition, however, some kinds of psychiatric illnesses increased in frequency. During the nineteenth century, several major components of "madness" were on the rise, in particular neurosyphilis, alcoholic psychosis, and apparently, though this is less certain, schizophrenia.

The historical evidence of the authenticity of both of these processes—the redistribution of psychiatric patients and their rising numbers—is so overwhelming that it may no longer be ignored on the grounds that it is ideologically inconvenient. Many of the psychiatric historians who came of age in the 1960s and 1970s have constituted a kind of lost generation in that they have chosen to pursue puffs of smoke, displaying no interest in the question of just what happens historically to make mind and brain go awry. If we wish to tell the history of psychiatry empathically, we must deal with the story of illness rather than arguing that it is a nonstory or that it is unknowable.

Redistribution of Illness

Consider the plight of the impecunious family with a mentally ill relative at home. We are in nineteenth-century Vienna. "If the poor have to retain their mentally ill relatives in their overcrowded homes for a considerable period of time," said Viennese psychiatry professor Julius Wagner-Jauregg in 1901, "many family members suffer from interruptions of their night's sleep, or become fearful or exasperated by the patient's behavior, or cannot afford appropriate medical attention because money is short. A crisis is created. These are the people who bear the brunt of the overfilling of the asylum."[57]

Looking after the mentally ill fell in the first instance to the family. It was the family that decided to keep an afflicted individual at home or to seek care. "For the entire period from 1843 to 1900," concludes one student of American asylum psychiatry, "families continued to dominate the commitment process."[58] Thus, for the number of asylum patients to rise, families would first have to decide to send them away.

But why was it during the nineteenth century that families reached this decision so often? Was it because there previously had been no asylums to send afflicted relatives to? Or was it because of some change in the dynamic of family life? Was it the push of the family or the pull of the asylum?

Consider the pull argument. It is perfectly true that in the absence of asylums, families would have to keep distracted relatives at home, or send them out on the high road. But that is true only of poor families. Rich families too have always been plagued with the problem of mental illness, and these families could always have afforded to purchase outside accommodation, should they have so desired. Some did dump afflicted relatives on the Church, but we know that mad relatives in upper-class families were most commonly retained at home. The mad princes of Renaissance Germany would be locked in their rooms, or in fortresses.[59] Andrew Boorde, a Montpellier MD and cleric, devoted the "madnesse" section of his *Breviary of Healthe* published in 1552 to the domestic management of the condition.[60] Before a certain time, these wealthy families showed no interest in private madhouses. There were virtually none in England before the eighteenth century, and none before the nineteenth century on the Continent of Europe.

How do we explain the changed willingness of the wealthy to send their relatives away? I think that it is related to changing patterns of sentiment in family life.[61] As the family started to consider itself increasingly an emotional unit, disruptive relatives at home began to seem more and more intolerable. Before the eighteenth century, the family was based more on ties of property and lineage than sentiment. It had little intimacy to disrupt and did not celebrate its unity about the dinner table or at other private moments, of which there were few. Late in the eighteenth century, however, the sentimental climate of family life began to change. Relations became much more intimate, the evening meal an occasion for celebrating the private sentiments of "the little family's togetherness," as the French put it, *la petite famille bien unie*. Insane relatives no longer fit into this picture of bliss.

Bruno Goergen, owner of a newly founded private psychiatric clinic in early-nineteenth-century Vienna, explained why wealthy families had started turning to him. There was something intrinsic in psychiatric illness, said Goergen, that made a patient misinterpret the "consoling words of his relatives, the handwringing and trembling of his fiancée, the tears and sighs of those who are close to him . . . as being quite different than what they in reality are. His inflamed imagination, his sensibilities now thoroughly inimical to any sense of harmony, lead him all too often to see his dear wife for a mixer of poison, his loving children as devils, his agreeable dwelling for a prison. He hears voices that otherwise no one hears, he sees forms that otherwise no one sees. . . . And in his confusion this man, who otherwise had only a heartful of love for his family, lends neither eye nor ear to their torment, a torment that in gestures and words speaks its name aloud to him."[62] One is hard put to find utterances of this power in either the medical or the lay literature of previous epochs. We are dealing here with a new style of family life, for which mental illness in a dear member is no longer possible to behold.

Statistics show that the greater the disruption, the more rapidly did the family disembarrass itself of ill relatives. Wilhelm Svetlin, owner of a private psychiatric clinic for the wealthy in late-nineteenth-century Vienna, asked families about the duration of the patient's illness before admission to clinic: For 56 patients who came in with melancholia, a third of the families (36 percent) had been willing to wait half a year and more before bringing the patient to the clinic; only 18 percent of the melancholic patients were admitted within a month of less of the onset of illness. For the 16 patients with paranoia, not a single family acted within three months. But of the 22 patients with mania, a disorder that drives its victims restlessly night and day, 68 percent were brought in less than a month after the onset of symptoms.[63] This means that in the 1870s and 1880s, two-thirds of the wealthy Viennese families with manic relatives were unable to endure the patient's whistling, clapping, singing, yelling, and breaking of furniture for more than a month.

The implication of this is that in the 1670s and the 1770s such families *were* able to tolerate mania. What had therefore changed was not the availability of institutional care, for in the seventeenth century these families could have afforded outside care had they so desired, but the climate of family sentiment itself. The presence of an ostentatiously alienated member was impossible to contemplate within the tight little emotional nucleus that family life had become. Thus one component of the rise in asylum admissions was lessened family willingness to tolerate mental illness. Psychiatric illnesses once treated in the family now became assigned to the asylum.

The same growing readiness to disembarrass probably applied to the demented elderly. Whereas once families were willing to tolerate the presence of a demented senior, by the end of the nineteenth century at the latest, families started seeking outside care. In 1908, one English medical writer noted an increase in asylum admissions "due to the drafting into asylums of harmless old people, the subjects of senile dementia more or less pronounced, who were formerly kept in workhouses or allowed to remain with relatives or friends willing to look after them . . ."[64] At a county asylum in Buckinghamshire, the percentage of people over age 60 at admission climbed from 18.7 percent in 1881 to 24.0 percent in 1911.[65] The same trend held true in the United States. The proportion of patients admitted for "senility" rose sharply at Utica State Hospital in the late 1870s.[66] Data for Warren State Hospital in Warren, Pennsylvania, begin only in 1916, when 14.8 percent of all patients had "mental diseases of the senium." Between 1946 and 1950 the figure was 26.4 percent.[67] Historian Gerald Grob concludes that in the twentieth century, American mental hospitals became increasingly a repository for the elderly.[68] These then are examples of redistribution of illness from the family outward.

Another kind of redistribution involved shipping people previously housed in prisons and workhouses to the asylum. In England, a law of 1874 made imperial funds available for the removal of local pauper lunatics to county asylums, causing a clear shifting of the burden of care.[69] Some writers have argued that these pauper lunatics were more pauper than lunatic: unwanted rather than insane individuals whom the communities were happy to send away.[70] Yet well-informed observers of the day believed that, for the most part, the paupers ending up in asylum had some major psychiatric problem. The annual report of Burntwood Asylum in Staffordshire in 1887, for example, lets us glimpse a superintendent filled with humanitarian enthusiasm, standing at the door of his institution welcoming the latest arrivals from the workhouses: "The admissions from the Workhouses of helpless chronic cases requiring much special care were not a few. Complaint is sometimes made that Asylums should be hampered with these cases; but, for my part, I rejoice to think that the means placed at our disposal for nursing and caring for such poor and afflicted sufferers are happily and beneficially employed in lightening the burden of their troubles."[71]

Not until we have a retrospective analysis of these pauper lunatics and other redistributed patients, case by case on the basis of their files, will we be able to say if the redistributed patients were psychiatrically ill or merely inconvenient. But strong anecdotal evidence suggests that the individuals thus dumped on asylums by their families and local communities had some serious mental problem, rather than being confined for challenging capitalism, the patriarchal order, and all the other clutter in the storechest of scholarly hobbyhorses that has come down to us from the 1960s.

Rising Rate of Psychiatric Illness

A second major component in the press of bodies was a genuine increase in the rate of mental illness during the nineteenth century. Between 1800 and 1900, the risk grew appreciably that the average person in his or her lifetime would be visited by a major psychiatric disorder. Let us take the various elements of this increased risk in order, from the least controversial to the most.

The psychiatric illness that most demonstrably increased in frequency during the nineteenth century was neurosyphilis. The syphilitic infiltration of the central nervous system is of capital importance in the history

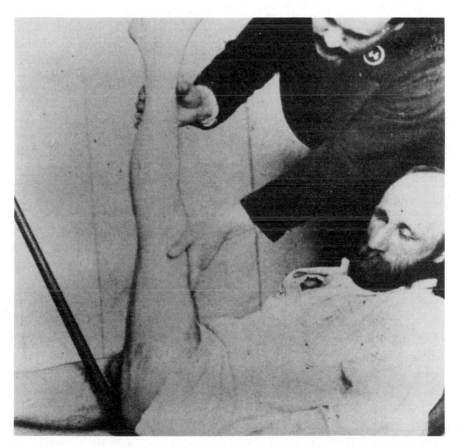

Patient with tabetic form of neurosyphilis in Colney Hatch asylum in London, c. 1900. Note hypotonia of joints, inability to raise eyelids ("ptosis").

Source: Psychiatry for the Poor by Richard Hunter and Ida Macalpine, 1974. London: Dawson. Courtesy of Dawson U. K. Ltd.

of psychiatry because it often announced itself clinically in the form of psychiatric symptoms. The end stages of neurosyphilis would be treated in public asylums and private clinics. It is the enormous rise in frequency of this disorder that explains part of the flood of patients into institutions. Once called "the disease of the century," neurosyphilis has been virtually forgotten today and is routinely ignored by historians of psychiatry, which explains why so much fantastical writing about "the social construction of illness" and the like has passed unchallenged. There was nothing socially constructed about neurosyphilis.[72]

Typically, a young medical student or businessman would have sex with a prostitute, in an era when "nice girls" were not available before marriage. He would experience the sore on his penis or perhaps the swollen lymph nodes of the groin that constitute evidence of primary syphilis. Then the signs of infection would go away, and the episode might pass from his mind. This partly explains why so many later victims in middle age would deny having had syphilis. Not only was it shameful, its first evidence—in an era when skin infections were daily affairs—often passed unnoticed.

But the spirochetes, the microorganisms that cause syphilis, would not leave the young man's bloodstream. Within a year, they might have invaded the meningeal lining of the brain and spinal cord though remaining clinically silent. Thus for many years, the young professionals and businessmen who were most at risk of the disease would walk about symptom-free. At this point, one of two things might happen. Either the body's immune system would overcome the disease so that it did in fact go away. Or, a decade now down the road, the infected individuals might start to become symptomatic, in the form, perhaps, of being unable to pronounce some kinds of phrases. In differentiating schizophrenia from neurosyphilis, the young doctor Lewis Thomas in Boston would ask patients to say, "God save the Commonwealth of Massachusetts."[73]

Or the early meningitis caused by the spirochetes might take the form of more frankly psychiatric symptoms, such as the grandiosity characteristic of mania. In one case, a distinguished Frankfurt chemistry professor suddenly interrupted his lecture and started to tell gossipy stories from the city. The previous day he had gone out and bought 10 automobiles and 100 wristwatches.[74] The sudden appearance of psychiatric symptoms of any kind in middle-aged businessmen and professionals made physicians of the day think immediately of neurosyphilis. But the symptom that most set clinicians' teeth on edge was the euphoria of spirochete-induced mania, for the patients always denied illness (they felt great!), and they had the capacity to bankrupt their families (as many did).

As the illness advanced, it might take one of two forms. If it affected primarily the spinal cord, it was known as tabes dorsalis (also locomotor ataxia), or wasting of the posterior part of the spinal cord. Tabes would cause lancinating pains to the abdomen as well as a high-stepping gait that patients described as "walking on cotton." (In the nineteenth century, it was not yet proven that such symptoms were the result of a primary syphilitic infection many years earlier, and so were not called neurosyphilis.) If the disease affected mainly the brain, psychiatric symptoms would be foremost, followed by dementia and paralysis. This form was known as general paralysis of the insane (GPI), dementia paralytica, or progressive paralysis, and was the kind most commonly encountered in the end stages in asylums; middle-class patients with tabes would be more inclined to seek relief at a spa.

Both forms of neurosyphilis were invariably fatal: Once a patient became symptomatic, he or she was finished. As Madame Maria Rivet, the operator of a private nervous clinic in Paris, said in the 1870s, "La paralysie générale . . . ne pardonne jamais" (General paralysis of the insane gives no mercy).[75] Early stages of the disease might appear in a variety of ways, and only physicians skillful at interpreting subtle changes in the pupils, eyelids, or reflexes would be able to spot it. But later stages, especially of GPI, were absolutely characteristic: There is no other disease in which primarily middle-aged men (it affected mainly males) suddenly become demented, then die paralyzed in the presence of terminal convulsions. Thus we may have some confidence that the reported statistics of the time give us a fair indication of the true level of neurosyphilis.

Neurosyphilis is not one of the age-old diseases like melancholia. It seems to have been largely unknown before the last quarter of the eighteenth century. Why this should be so is a mystery, since syphilis has been documented in Europe since the Middle Ages. Yet it was only in the 1780s and after that physicians began reporting the first cases involving the central nervous system.[76] Or what sounds like the first cases at least, for the diagnostic terms "tabes dorsalis" and "progressive paralysis" were coined only in the nineteenth century. Thus William Perfect, author of a psychiatry textbook of 1787, describes a patient whom a colleague told him about: a middle-aged man, "intemperately passionate, and misanthropic to the greatest degree; in this manner his insanity began to appear: he next drew upon his banker for sums immensely beyond what his account would afford, and, when disappointed in this respect, he became sullen, and immediately made out drafts for enormous sums upon houses with which he had not the least connexion." He began to think that he was the Lord Chancellor, King of Spain, and Duke of Bavaria. Thus far the man had shown the standard symptoms of mania. But then he became demented, something that does not happen in mania, and as Perfect's medical friend gave the most recent news, the patient had "gradually dwindled into a total decay as he approached to the verge of idiotism."[77] This sounds like an early case of progressive paralysis.

Almost simultaneously in Florence, Vincenzio Chiarugi was reporting patients who must certainly have had neurosyphilis, such as the 40-year-old soldier, his pupils immobile and unequal (a sign of a brain lesion), who proceeded to become demented, then "completely lost the movement of his lower extremities," dying in bed "of advanced atrophy." Chiarugi also reported a 37-year-old accountant who underwent an attack of mania, then became demented, dying "of a slow marasmus [wasting], having first become almost totally paraplegic."[78]

Within two decades of these early reports, experienced alienists were recounting as common this combination of paralysis and insanity. Said John Haslam, a physician at Bedlam, in 1809, "A course of debauchery long persisted in would probably terminate in paralysis. . . . Paralysis frequently induces derangement of mind." He believed the problem to be on the upswing: "Paralytic affections are a much more frequent cause of insanity than has been commonly supposed, and they are also a very common effect of madness; more maniacs die of hemiplegia [one-sided paralysis] and apoplexy [fits] than from any other disease."[79] Hence derived the connection between extramarital intercourse and madness that led contemporaries, by association, to warn against the spilling of semen as such, a presumed cause of general paralysis. For their pains, they would be mocked as moralizers by future generations of historians.

By the Napoleonic years, in French asylums this combination of paralysis and dementia had become an everyday occurrence. Esquirol, for example, described the various demented patients he had seen at the Salpêtrière and in his private asylum, the great majority of the private patients and a slight majority of the public ones being under the age of 50. Of these 235 individuals, more than half, he said, "presented some symptoms of paralysis." He concluded that dementia complicated by paralysis was quite frequent and incurable, but noted no particular difference between men and women.[80]

That was in 1814. Years later, Esquirol had another go at the subject, realizing now that young and middle-aged patients who had become both demented and paralyzed were very common indeed. "Paralysis is commoner among insane males than females," he said. "Eighteen years ago, when I was in charge of the psychiatric division of Bicêtre . . . I was struck by the difference in comparing the insane and paralyzed male patients of Bicêtre hospice with the [far fewer] number of paralytic females at the Salpêtrière." Esquirol said that his student Achille-Louis Foville, now in charge of the St.-Yon asylum, had noticed this as well: A tenth of all patients at St.-Yon had paralysis: two-thirds of them male, one-third female. And this strange paralysis of the insane was much commoner, noted Esquirol, in the Paris region than in the south of France or in Italy, citing statistics from confreres to prove this point. Yet the paralysis could not have been such a mystery to Esquirol, for in 1826 his young colleague Antoine-Laurent Bayle had demonstrated that both the paralysis and the delusions of grandeur of these patients were a result of chronic inflammation of the meninges, the lining of the brain.[81] These were psychiatric symptoms driven by organic brain disease, though the cause of the disease was as yet unknown.

Esquirol's and Bayle's observations about progressive paralysis became world renowned. It is often forgotten that in Germany as well, the epidemic of neurosyphilis began its acceleration in the Napoleonic years. In 1814, Christian Friedrich Harless, then professor of medicine in Erlangen, referred to the spinal version of neurosyphilis as "an already long-familiar constitutional illness" known to be fatal once the first signs of paralysis had appeared.[82] Three decades later, the great Berlin neuropathologist Moritz Romberg observed that this disease had recently increased "following the great military campaigns of our era." He baptized it tabes dorsalis.[83]

As an epidemic of venereal disease spread across Europe and North America in the nineteenth century, the epidemic of neurosyphilis lagged by 10 to 15 years, which is the average interval between the original infection and the appearance of psychiatric symptoms. Large numbers of people were involved: Five to 20 percent of the population would have had syphilis on a lifetime basis.[84] Of those, as many as 6 percent would go on to develop neurosyphilis.[85] Six percent of millions is a lot of people. Not all of them would have been admitted to asylums: Some died at home out of sheer shame, others perished in chic watering places like Lamalou in the Pyrenees, or sought suicide with morphine. The asylum population therefore is merely the tip of the iceberg. The point is that the paretics and tabetics bulked large in the life of the nineteenth-century asylum.

Because neurosyphilis tended to be a middle-class affliction, it was well represented in the men's wards of the private nervous clinics: Of 111 male patients in the early 1860s at the private Pöpelwitz clinic near Breslau, 32 percent had general paralysis of the insane; of the 75 female patients, not a one.[86] Among the major psychiatric illnesses at a "sanitarium for nervous and mental diseases" in Kansas City, Missouri, between 1901 and 1907, "general paresis" ranked in frequency only behind depression and mania, and ahead of schizophrenia ("dementia praecox").[87] A dozen other studies from the private sector reflect a similar prominence of neurosyphilis among the major psychiatric disorders.

Neurosyphilis carved its path through the public asylums of the Atlantic community. Before 1850, none of the Jewish patients admitted to the Frankfurt City Asylum had neurosyphilis. By the years between 1871 and 1880, 21 percent did, coming mostly from the class of merchants and other such paying patients.[88] "When I entered the Toronto Asylum in 1853," said Joseph Workman, superintendent of the asylum until 1875, "there was not a single case [of GPI], as far as I could judge, in the institution, but it was not long before it began to make an appearance." In the 10 years from 1865 to 1875, 65 men and 7 women died of paresis. "It is a melancholy confession, but it is the truth, that the asylum records of paresis have been a pretty nearly correct statement of the number of cases of this disease admitted."[89] England's Montagu Lomax said that patients with GPI "often form the majority of cases in the male hospital wards."[90] Thus did the tabetic, whose gait outside in the street heralded his arrival in the doctor's office, and the paretic, with his jumbled speech and irregular pupils, make their entry in the asylum.

What does all this mean for the social history of psychiatry as opposed to its biological history? Karl Edel's private psychiatric hospital in Berlin had, in fact, two wings: a luxurious one for private psychiatric patients from the upper orders, and an economy wing for public patients from the city of Berlin and surrounding area. In the late nineteenth century, neurosyphilis at the Edel clinic was very much a middle-class affair: 46 percent of the 976 men who passed through the private men's ward had neurosyphilis. There were many fewer paretics from the pauper class.

Of women at this clinic, 5 percent of the wealthy and 7 percent of the poor had neurosyphilis.

What is interesting in these statistics from the Edel clinic is what happened to patients after they were admitted with a diagnosis of paresis. Of the private patients, both male and female, around half were picked up by their families to die outside the asylum. The same is slightly less true for the working-class males: Only 30 percent of them were discharged by their families. Of greatest interest is the plight of the 22 working-class women admitted to the Edel clinic with this diagnosis: All died in the asylum. None were picked up.[91] This evidence suggests that the many scholars looking for social significance in the history of the asylum have been barking up the wrong tree: It is not the diagnoses, which tend to represent biological brain events, that are socially constructed but the experiences of the patients with these disorders. It is pointless to claim that psychiatric illness represents merely "labeling," or social efforts to make deviants conform, when we have these thousands of patients unable to move their legs, with bedsores discharging pints of pus because their attendants do not shift them often enough. Yet in these poor women, cast by their families into the outer darkness because they have a shameful illness, we have a real story, one alas largely untold.

Another cause of the tremendous rise of asylum admissions was insanity related to alcohol. Drinking large amounts of alcohol can affect the nervous system in various ways: The drug itself can cause hallucinations. Withdrawal from alcohol may produce psychosis, fits, and delirium tremens. And the chronic overconsumption of alcohol may cause a drinker to skimp on other calorie sources, producing a chronic psychosis and memory loss named after Sergei Korsakoff, the Russian asylum doctor who first described it in 1887 (thiamine deficiency is the real cause). Meanwhile Karl Wernicke, a German psychiatry professor and asylum physician, was describing (in 1881) the acute form of the same problem, the mental confusion and staggering gait that may suddenly strike alcoholics. Liver disease from drinking may carry its own psychiatric morbidity. There are, in short, many reasons why a large increase in the amount of alcohol that a population consumes could lead to an upturn in asylum admissions, some short and self-limiting, others long-term.[92]

Drinking increased very substantially in what one historian has called "the golden age of inebriation."[93] In England, the consumption of spirits per person rose 57 percent between 1801 and 1901, from less than half a gallon per person a year to more than three-quarters.[94] While an average adult American drank only 1.8 gallons of absolute alcohol in 1845, the figure had climbed to 2.6 in 1910.[95] Between the end of the eighteenth century and the beginning of the twentieth in France, the total production of alcohol and beer climbed 14-fold: from 1,170,000 hectoliters in 1781 to 16,700,000 in 1913.[96] And in the mid-decades of the nineteenth century, the consumption of beer in Bavaria doubled.[97] Rising standards of living and the cheap production of alcohol from beet sugar were driving this increase, as the French peasant started drinking wine with meals daily and the German craftsman having a bottle of whatever lay ready at hand.

Rising consumption spilled over into the number of patients admitted to asylum with alcohol toxicity. In Prussia, for example, in 1875 there were fewer than 600 such cases, in 1900 some 1,300.[98] Karl Bonhoeffer, later an important figure in German academic psychiatry and in the 1890s a psychiatry resident in the industrial city of Breslau, said of those years, "At that time . . . the admission room was dominated by the numbers of alcoholic patients wandering about in delirium, dragging pieces of bedding with them. On every summer day there was at least one such delirium patient. . . . It is simply inconceivable to us today what percent of patients in the psychiatric institutions of the large cities had alcoholic delirium. . . ." In the late 1880s at the Charité Hospital in Berlin, 39 percent of all patients had delirium tremens, Bonhoeffer said.[99] Cities like Berlin and Breslau had alcoholism rates far in excess of the population as a whole (given that, between 1875 and 1900, alcoholics were only 3 percent of all asylum patients in Prussia).[100] Nonetheless, compared with earlier times, such psychiatric illness was on the rise.

This increase was not just a German phenomenon. Among the 8,000-odd patients to pass through the forensic psychiatric service of the Parisian Prefecture of Police (the Infirmerie Spéciale) in the years from 1886 to 1888, alcoholism was the number one diagnosis (27 percent of all cases).[101] In the Parisian asylums, a third of the males were admitted because of drink (a tenth of the females). Valentin Magnan, the chief of the Sainte-Anne asylum, believed alcohol to be the main reason for the recent rise in admissions.[102]

In Britain, psychiatry was steeped in ethanol. Between 1874 and 1894, in the various wards of the Royal Edinburgh Asylum, alcoholics formed 15 to 20 percent of all male admissions (the female percentage was much lower).[103] Private clinics dedicated to drying out wealthy alcoholics sprang up all over, such as "Rivermere" for "inebriety and abuse of drugs" near Maldon in Essex, "an ideal private home for the treatment of ladies and gentlemen of the upper class." Or "Tower House" in Leicester, a "private high-class home for ladies," again for alcoholics and drug-abusers. The *Medical Directory* of the United Kingdom for 1908 carried ads for 24 such "homes."[104] It is evident that in the second half of the nineteenth century pathological drinking became a problem of considerable psychiatric proportions.

With neurosyphilis and alcoholism, the case is relatively straightforward. Both diseases increased in frequency with obvious consequences for admission to asylum. Yet these two conditions together represented overall only a fraction of all admissions (11 percent for Prussia as a whole in the period 1875–1900).[105] The vast bulk of asylum admissions consisted of patients receiving diagnoses that in retrospect are not transparent, "epileptic insanity," "hysterical madness," and the like. To peel back contemporary diagnostics from the underlying reality of illness, we need something more than these global diagnostic terms of former years: We need to make our own assessments of individual patients. Retrospective diagnosis on the basis of patients' charts is required, making a reassessment from the signs and symptoms reported in the file. Yet this kind of scholarship is very time-consuming, requires a knowledge both of context and of illness, and has only just begun. Therefore what I have to say about the third category of illness, schizophrenia, in which an evident increase in frequency occurred, is somewhat tentative. Yet I think there is enough evidence to justify the conjecture that the incidence of schizophrenia rose significantly during the nineteenth century.

It is now clear that schizophrenia is a genetically influenced disease of brain development, beginning perhaps in the uterus or in the trauma of childbirth as the child's brain does not grow properly, leaving the individual, often from the years of young adulthood on, unable to cope with normal human relationships, to deal with the usual stresses of life, or to organize his or her thoughts successfully (see pp. 268–270). The disease may also result in frank psychosis, meaning hallucinations, delusions, and illusions. Although what is called "schizophrenia" probably represents several different illness processes mixed together—some genetic, some not—there is no doubt that the disease is common, affecting perhaps one percent of the population. In the nineteenth century as well, much schizophrenia doubtlessly figured among the medley of psychotic disorders. But how much? And how does its frequency change over time?

The first descriptions of what is recognizable as schizophrenia appeared in 1809 by Pinel in France and Haslam in England. "Connected with the loss of memory," wrote Haslam, "there is a form of insanity which occurs in young persons": Individuals who previously were of "prompt capacity and lively disposition" start to become silent and incurious. "The sensibility appears to be considerably blunted; they do not bear the same affection towards their parents and relations." They become uninterested in their companions and unable to give any account of what they have just been reading, unable as well to put more than a sentence or two together on paper. Typical adolescent blues? "As their apathy increases they are negligent of their dress, and inattentive to personal cleanliness." They may become incontinent of urine and stool. "Thus in the interval between puberty and manhood," said Haslam, "I have painfully witnessed this hopeless and degrading change, which in a short time has transformed the most promising and vigorous intellect into a slavering and bloated idiot." Haslam described a young man who had amputated his own penis in a fit of fury. Yet after admission to Bedlam, the fellow appeared to recover. Haslam was mistrustful. "There was something in the reserve of his manner and peculiarity of his look which persuaded me he was not well, although no incoherence could be detected in his conversation." The patient appeared to Haslam to be walking rather lamely and on occasion sat with his shoes off rubbing his feet. He told Haslam that his feet were blistered yet declined to show them to the doctor. One day, again after seeing the patient rubbing his feet, Haslam insisted upon examining them: "They were quite free from any disorder. He now told me, with some embarrassment . . . that the boards on which he walked (the second story) were heated by subterraneous fires, under the direction of invisible and malicious agents, whose intentions, he was well convinced, were to consume him by degrees."[106]

The same kind of patients presented themselves across the Channel as well. In the context of "idiotism" among the young, Pinel reported a young sculptor, 28, "previously exhausted by the excesses of intemperance or the pleasures of love," who remained locked in a fixed position, "almost always immobile and taciturn. Sometimes he would give a kind of idiotic and stupid laugh, but there was no expression on the features of his face, and no memory of his previous life. Yet his appetite was never lacking, and even the approach of food would set his jaw to masticating."[107] It is impossible to say if either of these young patients of Haslam and Pinel had the disease that would later be described as schizophrenia. Yet if we find a large number of individuals affected with similar symptoms, it is not unreasonable to conclude that some of them had schizophrenia.

Haslam and Pinel attuned psychiatry to an apparently new kind of illness, one presenting itself as psychosis in young adults and progressing to chronic insanity. Such illness was called "dementia" in the language of the day but it did not in fact entail a loss of intelligence, rather chronic delusions and hallucinations accompanied by disorganized thinking. Descriptions of this kind of presentation are virtually absent from the medical literature before 1800. They become steadily more frequent thereafter.

Historian Edward Hare has called attention to a substantial increase in the number of patients reporting auditory hallucinations—voices speaking to or about them—during the nineteenth century. On the basis of such evidence, Hare launched the "recency hypothesis": schizophrenia as a recent disease rather than an age-old accompaniment of the human condition like depression.[108] His answer to the quarrel about whether the rate of insanity increased during the nineteenth century was an emphatic yes: "The condition we now call schizophrenia . . . was most likely to have been the main cause of the increased admissions."[109]

There are really three groups of players here. Hare's recency hypothesis has been attacked from two directions, by scholars who believe there is no such thing as psychiatric illness, and by a completely opposing camp insisting that schizophrenia has always been with us. It was, according to the antipsychiatry scholars, the madness-making environment of the late-nineteenth century asylum itself that converted individuals whose initial problems may have been mild into "chronic" cases that doctors labeled insanity.[110] According to this interpretation, these patients probably had no disorder at the time of admission and were just victims of labeling and medicalization.

A second group of scholars argues that schizophrenia is "probably very old," not a new disease at all, and that clear descriptions of it may be glimmed in the patchy premodern medical literature.[111] Thus what changes is merely the exactness and density of the medical literature, and not the phenomenon of disease as it exists in the real world.

A third group advocates the recency hypothesis. Represented by Hare and by some researchers who have undertaken retrospective diagnosis of individual asylum patients' charts, this school argues that schizophrenia is new and that it increased during the nineteenth century.

This three-cornered debate has stimulated a good deal of research. The stakes are high because the debate is really asking, do the origins of psychiatry lie in the manufacture of illness for reasons of professional gain, or do they lie in caring for a flood of patients afflicted with historically new diseases? Although it is still not possible to resolve the debate definitively, subsequent research has tended to support the recency hypothesis rather than those who argue for the social manufacture of madness.

Relying on nursing notes to diagnose patients retrospectively, one scholar found that descriptions of schizophrenic symptoms were rare in 1790 at the Pennsylvania Hospital in Philadelphia, and that on the basis of similar evidence they had become common by 1823 at Bethlem Royal Hospital. "This lends some more weight," he concluded, "to the evidence presented elsewhere for the recency hypothesis."[112]

In the retrospective diagnosis of individual patients' charts, several historians have documented the presence of frank psychotic symptoms that certainly sound like schizophrenia in a number of nineteenth-century private clinics and public asylums. Among children admitted to Bethlem after 1830, the incidence of auditory hallucinations and delusions suggestive of schizophrenia seems to have been on the rise.[113] Of 118 patients admitted to the York Retreat between 1880 and 1884, 31 percent displayed the delusions and hallucinations that would retrospectively qualify them for a diagnosis of schizophrenia. The authors, finding no evidence to support the contention that Victorian physicians "confused insanity with immorality or other forms of nonconformist behavior," concluded that most of the patients admitted to the Retreat in these years were "severely disturbed mentally."[114] Still other studies based on retrospective diagnosis have reached similar conclusions about the prevalence of schizophrenia in the nineteenth-century asylum.[115]

Nineteenth-century physicians who themselves believed insanity in young people to be increasing were probably not so wrong after all. Karl Kahlbaum, psychiatrist and owner of a private nervous clinic in the German town of Görlitz, was among the first to describe chronic madness in the young as a distinctive clinical entity, which he called "hebephrenia" (see p. 104). He observed in 1884, "It must be the experience of all psychiatric institutions that the number of youthful patients has recently undergone a considerable increase."[116]

Maria Rivet, daughter of the distinguished Paris psychiatrist Alexandre Brierre de Boismont, was not a physician, but she had grown up around psychiatric patients. She also ran the family's clinic, a classy establishment in the St.-Mandé quarter. Writing in 1875, she had the definite sentiment that there was something bizarre and unusual about all these young women turning up with major mental illnesses. An example: "Mlle. N. had undertaken a program of study at university that exhausted her mind. Reading medical books also contributed to the commotion in her brain, and despite her youth she is now struck by dementia, whereas this incurable disease generally strikes only the elderly." Wherein lay Mlle. N.'s madness? Initially she believed herself to be Eve, the first woman, "and demonstrated to us in eloquent and evocative terms the splendors of the terrestrial paradise at the time of creation, at which she was present." Then she refused to eat eggs for fear of being changed into a chicken. "The she believed herself to be God, the sun being the work of her hand, and we had to forcefully prevent her from staring at it. She was outraged, and insulted us for having dared deny her all-power. 'I created the sun myself,' she said." A long train of other delusions followed. Mlle. N. wrote letters from time to time giving voice to these delusional ideas, "but in an almost incomprehensible style." Recently, Mlle. N. had tamed three of the geese in the clinic's garden, one of them picking familiarly in her pockets while the other two sat on her shoulders. "She is almost always seated on the lawn, addressing long tirades to these beasts who seem to listen to her."[117] There are virtually no such accounts in the medical and psychiatric literature before the last quarter of the eighteenth century. It is impossible to read of the private Rivet clinic without feeling that, in the world of psychiatric disease, a new entity had raised its head.

Dead End

By 1900, psychiatry had reached a dead end. Its practitioners were concentrated for the most part in asylums, and asylums had become mainly warehouses in which any hope of therapy was illusory. Psychiatrists themselves had a rather poor reputation among their medical colleagues as the dull and the second-rate, just a step, if that, above the spa-doctors and the homeopaths.

Bulging with chronic paretics, dements, and catatonic schizophrenics, the asylums had achieved a desolateness that would have made the earlier generation of reformers heartsick. William Alanson White, superintendent of St. Elizabeths Hospital in Washington, had trained at the Blackwell's Island asylum in New York. He recalled rowing over early one morning from Manhattan and landing at a pier close to the asylum. "I could look back a distance of a few hundred feet and see the building where the women patients were confined. My memory of that vision is a building in which each window was a glare of light, and I can hear now the sounds that issued therefrom which reminded me of a hive of bees. These disturbed women, as they were called, were obviously in a state of continuous noisy activity all night long. . . ." What could one do about those who were too noisy? White described the restraining sheets used in the 1890s at the Binghampton State Hospital on violent patients in the absence of other (then taboo) mechanical restraints. "A perfectly hellish contrivance, literally speaking, in hot weather; and I am sure I have seen at least one patient die from heat exhaustion as a result of it "[118] Such an institution, of course, would be awful for the patients, but it also would be demoralizing for the physicians who served there. A profession composed of practitioners who did this kind of thing for a living would not hold its head up.

Britain was no different. In the judgment of one elderly psychiatrist formerly at the Buckinghamshire County Pauper Lunatic Asylum, "Between 1860 and 1930, say, British asylums remained backwaters."[119] The alienists themselves lost much of their contact with medicine, the life of a superintendent resembling more that of a gentleman farmer, "invited to tennis parties at the Rectory, fishing and even riding to hounds," as Eliot Slater, staff psychiatrist in the 1930s at the Maudsley Hospital in London, later said.

"Life was not quite so pleasant for the patients," Slater continued. "Confined to locked wards with an enclosed court for exercise, patients whose stormy illness had blown itself out leaving only residual symptoms, would remain year after year, unoccupied, deprived of incentive or responsibility of self-determination, getting more and more fixed in the straitjacket of an unchanging daily routine."[120]

From the 1830s on, the British had prided themselves greatly on abolishing mechanical restraints. Yet in an exercise that Montagu Lomax called "straining out a gnat and swallowing a camel," the British relied on (supposedly illegal) isolation cells that humiliated the patients even more than tying them down. One evening Lomax was called back to the asylum because a paralytic patient had fallen out of bed and broken his leg. "As I went through one of the wards on my way to the hospital I passed a single room in which a refractory patient was 'secluded.' It was after 7 P.M., and no attendant was within call. The patient was beating on the door with his fists and feet, and was shrieking out curses and imprecations. "For God's sake let me out, doctor! for God's sake let me out! O Christ, they are killing me! for God's sake let me out!"

"As I came back, after setting the broken leg, the same horrible sounds greeted my ears. They would probably continue for hours, keeping everyone in the vicinity awake, and ultimately might necessitate my giving the man a hypodermic injection. My reflections were not pleasant."[121]

Toward 1900, German asylums were probably the best-run in the world, because the German states supported them liberally, and because asylum physicians in Central Europe still retained the drive to do scientific research, a talisman of better care. (Care was also boosted by the "Herr Geheimrat" phenomenon, physicians intent on honors, who wanted to demonstrate themselves to the Ministry as medically up to snuff: This was almost unknown elsewhere.) Yet even in this birthland of reform, psychiatric conditions were upsetting. As Emil Kraepelin, later the most prominent of the academic psychiatrists, arrived at his new job as assistant physician at the Munich City Asylum in 1878, he had a migraine. A Mecklenburger from the North, he didn't know Bavaria at all. And the superintendent had put him in charge of the men's back ward. Kraepelin's thoughts were not pleasant as he confronted these 150 "demented, unclean [fecal is meant], half-agitated and fully agitated patients," many of whom were incapable of work and would hang around the hallways and courtyards, "where they would run around, yell, get into fights with each other, collect rocks, smoke, and chatter. The tendency to violence was very widespread; there was scarcely a daily rounds in which someone didn't report a fight, window breaking or destroying tableware. Often enough I had to suture or bind up the wounds that arose in this way."

Most fearsome in Kraepelin's daily itinerary was Ward G, housing the most violent of the male patients. One patient, locked in an isolation room, had managed to shatter a fellow patient's skull with a scrub brush. Later, the same patient nearly throttled an incautious attendant, took his keys away, and escaped into the city. As the patient was on the point of hurling a passerby into the Isar, the river that runs through Munich, he was overpowered and returned to the asylum. "Nobody," said Kraepelin, "had noticed he was missing."[122] This was not what Jacobi had in mind.

Not only had asylums themselves sunk to a historic low point, the profession of psychiatry had as well. "Who becomes a psychiatrist?" asked German psychiatrist Werner Heinz in 1928, tongue in cheek: (1) "Applicants for county medical officer who are afraid of failing the special exam in psychiatry if they don't get some practical experience"; (2) Those who are "physically inadequate," having rheumatism or a heart problem, or who "otherwise are not up to the exertions of a rural practice, maybe not even an urban practice"; (3) Those who are "intellectually inadequate, who instinctually seek out an asylum because they will stand out less there, and it's these latter, believe me, who later become the *superintendents*."[123]

Early in 1908, the superintendent of the Rheinau asylum in Switzerland asked the young Dr. Karl Gehry to consider a post there. Gehry was torn. On the one hand, he could face the uncertainties of opening a private village practice. On the other hand, "There was abroad a deep mistrust of psychiatry." His teacher, the famous Carl Jung, had told him in Zurich that "psychiatry is a stepchild of medicine" because it is not classed among the natural sciences, not weighing or measuring anything. "And people simply didn't think that a psychiatrist could do much. He simply declared everyone to be more or less mentally ill." Nobody, continued Gehry, would find it striking if he became a surgeon, "because surgery could support a family and had status. Psychiatry banishes you to an asylum where you're mainly isolated. The psychiatrist has to treat people who don't think they need treatment so that every day he has to swallow all those insults. . . ."[124] Such, roughly, was the position of everyday psychiatry.

Thus by 1900, the status of psychiatrists themselves had reached a low point. What a contrast with the earlier arrogant refusal of psychiatrists to associate themselves with the boil-lancers and enema-givers who constituted the rest of medicine. In 1853, the newly founded American organization of asylum physicians had refused to associate with the American Medical Association.[125] But then this self-imposed isolation had started to chafe. Alienists squirmed as Philadelphia neurologist and society nerve-doctor Weir Mitchell, in 1894, delivered his historic rebuke: "I shall have frankly to reproach . . . many of those who still bear the absurd label of 'medical superintendents,'" he told them at their annual meeting. "Where are your annual reports of scientific study, of the psychology and pathology of your patients?" he asked them. "We commonly get as your contributions to science, odd little statements, reports of a case or two, a few useless pages of isolated post-mortem records, and these are sandwiched among incomprehensible statistics and farm balance-sheets." Treatment? A sham, declared Mitchell: "Whatever the gullible public might believe about therapy, we [neurologists] hold the reverse opinion, and think your hospitals are never to be used save as the last resource."[126] Few psychiatrists could have emerged from this meeting without asking themselves, Am I still a physician?

Scarcely, answered William Bullard, president of the American Neurological Association at its meeting in Boston in 1912. To be sure, psychiatrists had done wonderfully, he sneered, at "direct[ing] the building and heating of their buildings, the buying of coal and groceries, the making up of accounts even to minute details." The problem was that in so doing they had lost contact with the rest of medicine.[127] In 1933, White declared most asylum physicians to be simply "dead wood."[128]

"Anchored in the setting of chronic illness, distant from the mainstream of medicine," as one rueful psychiatrist put it many years later, asylum psychiatry had come to the end of the road.[129] To establish that there was such a thing as a science of the brain and mind, and that the use of this science could help make patients better, the torch had to pass to other hands.

CHAPTER

3

The First
Biological Psychiatry

F or two centuries, the predominant theme in psychiatry has been har-
nessing the neurosciences to therapeutics. In the asylum, nineteenth-
century psychiatry ran into a dead end in achieving this goal. But outside
the asylum as well, in what one might call "the first biological psychiatry,"
nineteenth-century alienists attempted to enlist the neurosciences in caring for patients. As with the asylum, this initial attempt to give psychiatry
a scientific basis came to a dead end. What began as a promising attempt
to limn the biological and genetic roots of psychiatric illness ended in the
specter of "degeneration," the notion that inherited mental illness worsened steadily over the generations. Yet the parallel to the story of the asylum is striking. In neither the asylum nor biological psychiatry did the
failure of the idea mean necessarily that the idea itself was faulty. Rather,
it was that after 1900 the whole paradigm for looking at illness changed.

Enter Ideas

The first biological psychiatry was a movement of ideas rather than an
exercise in bricks and mortar. It asked, How do the genetics and the
chemistry of the brain actually make people ill? What therapies might
succeed with such illnesses? The answers were not to be found in the
humdrum routine of asylum life but in research done in universities and
institutes. What made the first biological psychiatry distinctive from

69

previous humoral theories was not the belief that psychiatric illness possessed an underlying neural structure—physicians since the Ancients have believed that—but the desire to lay bare the relationship between mind and brain through systematic research. It is this systematic element that was new, doing experiments on humans and animals, testing drugs, and examining brains postmortem.

Research in psychiatry was part of a larger nineteenth-century current toward research in medicine in general. Doctors began to apply the clinical-pathological method: reasoning back and forth from findings at autopsy to the signs and symptoms the patient displayed before death. This cross-reasoning permitted researchers to identify distinctive diseases. If one were interested in lung disease, for example, one would attempt to link the gurglings and rattlings in the lungs of a living patient to the findings at autopsy: Different diseases, such as emphysema and pneumonia, clearly separable at autopsy, made different noises antemortem. Psychiatry in the nineteenth century too tried to attempt this clinical-pathological method, hoping to demonstrate the correctness of the biological approach rather than merely accept it on faith. Generally speaking, these efforts took place not in asylums but in universities.

Thus there are two narratives to keep track of, although they largely overlap. One is the research narrative: How did biological psychiatry press forward? The other is the teaching narrative: How did psychiatry in general become a university subject? Linking both of these narratives is the practical reality that the family doctor had to know something about psychiatric illness to deal with upset families and mentally ill patients. The whole subject had to be de-demonized for the average medical student, who arrived in class with the same preconceptions as the lay public. Family physicians had to learn that mental illness was a familiar aspect of medical experience, as opposed to a satanic curse visited on the unfortunate by dark powers. In their practices, they would encounter much in the way of mania and depression, panic disorders, and dementia, and the stakes were enormous in deciding who was sick, who needed to be treated at home, and who required institutional care.

Sensitizing family doctors meant that mental illness must be "medicalized," or drawn into the circle of medical experience. Medicalization in psychiatry occurred at the same time as other physicians medicalized diseases such as tuberculosis and nephritis. The underlying logic was the same: Just as family doctors had to know something of the lung to treat TB, they needed to be familiar with the brain and central nervous system to treat mental illness. "Is it not necessary," asked Parisian psychiatrist

Ernest Billod rhetorically in 1884, "for the physician to possess knowledge of the illness that is as complete as possible. . . . in the grave eventuality of placing a patient in an institution?" The consequences of making a mistake could be dreadful he pointed out, "stigmatizing" the family with insanity.[1] The doctor had to know what he was doing.

Therefore in the nineteenth century, university instruction in psychiatry became organized all across the Atlantic community. To teach medical students, first there had to be lectures, then departments of psychiatry—or "clinics" as they are called in Europe—with access to psychiatric beds, and ultimately big psychiatric research institutes. The first biological psychiatry was thus driven simultaneously by the demands of education and scientific curiosity.

Within the very first reformed asylums of the eighteenth century alienists had begun lecturing to medical students. In 1753, William Battie started lecturing in psychiatry at St. Luke's Hospital in London, the governors of which had permitted Battie to attract "more gentlemen of the faculty . . . to make this branch of physic their particular care and study."[2] In 1805, Vincenzio Chiarugi commenced lecturing at his asylum in Florence.[3]

These were interesting beginnings. But for the next hundred years teaching and research in psychiatry would be dominated by the Germans.

A German Century

Giving so much attention to one country, or one language, in an international history of psychiatry requires some justification. The warrant is that the Germans truly did dominate the field. In modern medicine, the great majority of eponyms, or things named after individuals, are named after Germans. As one opens a medical dictionary to "signs," pathological phenomena that the physician discovers in a patient, the page swims with German names: "Berger's sign," a deformation of the pupils in early neurosyphilis, named after the Austrian ophthamologist Emil Berger; Möbius's sign, the inability to keep the eyeballs converged in thyroid disease, named after the Leipzig psychiatrist Paul Julius Möbius (who assured himself notoriety in the history of medicine by writing in 1900 a book titled *The Physiological Feeble-Mindedness of Women*); and Westphal's sign, the loss of the knee-jerk reflex in nervous disease.[4] This German dominance was owing to the many state-supported universities and asylums at which, from 1800 on, research and teaching were proceeding apace.

There were two mechanisms for hooking teaching to research in the German university. One was the tradition of the doctoral dissertation, for all medical students had to produce a dissertation to get the MD degree (the French did too, but there were many more German students). Second was a postdoctoral research project called the "habilitation" required from PhDs and MDs aspiring to teach at universities. Unlike the dissertation, often a scientific puffball, the habilitation had to make a serious contribution to knowledge to be accepted. After the habilitation, one would first be a private docent, entitled to lecture, then an associate professor (*ausserordentlicher Professor*), then a full professor (*ordentlicher Professor*). In no other country were so many students and postgraduates harnessed in this manner to publication and research. This academic structure, plus ample funds from the ministry, guaranteed scientific preeminence to Germany until 1933.

In Central Europe, lecturing in psychiatry began with Johann Heinroth in 1811 in Leipzig. Why is Ernst Horn, appointed in 1806 associate director of the Charité Hospital in Berlin and having responsibility for the psychiatry unit in that institution, not mentioned in first place? Because his formal psychiatry teaching there did not begin until 1818; and only after Karl Wilhelm Ideler took over psychiatry at the Charité in 1832 did it become an autonomous department.[5] None of these early professors fit the later model of chair-holder simultaneously in charge of an academic department and a psychiatric hospital (or "clinic"). Heinroth had no access to psychiatric patients. Indeed, the discipline vanished from Leipzig with his death in 1843 (not to resume there again until the appointment of Paul Flechsig in 1877, a tunnel-visioned brain anatomist).[6] Before 1865, such sporadic initiatives were undertaken at other German universities as well, such as Würzburg (1834) and Munich (1861).

Such was the strength of asylum psychiatry over university teaching in those days that a powerful asylum man such as Christian F. W. Roller could cause the newly founded (1826) teaching department at Heidelberg to collapse, as in 1842 Roller transferred the Heidelberg patients to his own new asylum at Illenau.[7]

These early efforts usually failed to teach the medical students much about psychiatry because the lectures themselves were situated in asylums often far distant from the students' other classrooms. Demonstrating the patients to the students was frequently less than illuminating because the asylums housed mostly chronic cases whose symptoms all seemed more or less alike. And the asylum psychiatrists themselves were often too preoccupied with administration to show much interest in teaching.[8] In their rustic isolation, they were also cut off from medicine.

As one university psychiatrist later put it, "In no branch of medicine were there so many peculiar eccentrics as among the older alienists."[9]

What was needed was a department of psychiatry situated close to the other medical departments, one that could admit patients whose illnesses the professors wanted to demonstrate in lectures and that could make psychiatry a convincing part of medicine by belonging to a general hospital. This was achieved in Germany in 1865, when Wilhelm Griesinger, then 48, whose career had flitted back and forth from internal medicine to psychiatry, agreed to become the professor of psychiatry in Berlin at the Charité hospital. Not only was Griesinger to become the single most influential representative of the first biological psychiatry, he established the modern model of the department of psychiatry as dedicated to teaching and research rather than to custodialism. It was with Griesinger that university psychiatry triumphed over asylum psychiatry.

Born in 1817 in Stuttgart, Griesinger had studied medicine in nearby Tübingen, then in Zurich under Johann Schönlein, returning to Tübingen for his degree. Schönlein was the man most responsible for turning German medicine away from philosophical considerations about the nature of life and toward the natural sciences. This was a time when

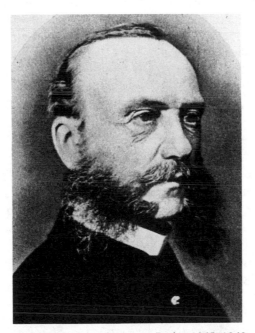

Wilhelm Griesinger, professor of psychiatry in Berlin 1865–1868, who is considered to be the founder of "the first biological psychiatry" (courtesy of National Library of Medicine).

questions were just starting to be asked about the biological substrate of illness in the tissues of the body, and the techniques of chemistry, physiology, and microscopy deployed to answer them. Under Schönlein, Griesinger came to understand that a physician should be trained as a scientist, studying patients through direct observation at the bedside rather than relying on thousand-year-old observations about humors.

Shortly after graduating from Tübingen in 1838, Griesinger spent two years as an assistant physician at the newly opened Winnenthal asylum near Stuttgart, which was then under the direction of a dynamic young psychiatrist named Albert Zeller, a member of the generation of reformers who had taken their inspiration from Jacobi at Siegburg. At the end of his Winnenthal stay, Griesinger permitted himself an astonishing piece of hubris for a 28-year-old doctor: He published in 1845 a textbook of psychiatry, which indeed achieved some recognition.[10]

At this point, Griesinger abandoned psychiatry, becoming an assistant physician at the internal medicine clinic in Tübingen. Then he moved on to such way stations as running the outpatient department at Kiel in North Germany, becoming the personal physician of the vice-regent of Cairo (relying on these experiences to publish a big book on infectious illnesses). Griesinger returned to Tübingen in 1854—at great remove from psychiatry—as the professor of medicine. Finally in 1860, he took on the professorship of internal medicine in Zurich, where he had begun almost 30 years previously as a medical student. It is actually remarkable that the bulk of the career of this the most famous German psychiatrist before Kraepelin should have been spent in quite another field.

Yet over his long trawl through internal medicine, Griesinger never fully lost sight of psychiatry, demonstrating psychiatric cases at his medicine clinic in Tübingen whenever he had the chance, or spontaneously organizing a course of lectures in psychiatry at the Zurich hospital. In 1861, Griesinger had returned to his textbook, completely revising it and bringing it out in a new edition, the text of which was in accordance with his current thinking about psychiatric illness as brain disease, or "nerve disease," as he put it. In contrast to the first edition, this second revised edition became a huge scholarly success and was perhaps the single most influential psychiatry textbook in the Western world until Kraepelin's big book in the 1890s (see p. 191).[11]

When Wilhelm Ideler, the Romantic psychiatrist who had been the previous holder of the psychiatry chair in Berlin, died in 1860, Griesinger was the obvious candidate to replace him. In 1865, Griesinger accepted the headship of psychiatry there. Although he would arrive to discover the psychiatric clinic at the Charité in complete disarray, he found the soil in

Berlin already well prepared for his notion that mental disease was brain disease. Berlin was rapidly rivaling Vienna as the world epicenter of medicine in those years, and Griesinger's old teacher Schönlein, for example, had been called to Berlin in 1840 as the professor of pathology and therapy, placing internal medicine there on a scientific footing that emphasized the physical examination of the patient in alliance with laboratory findings. The pathologist Rudolf Virchow, another great Berlin name, had often studied brains postmortem. (Psychiatrist Carl Wernicke later disparaged Virchow's brain sections, saying "This is the way you cut cheese."[12]) Thus in Berlin, Griesinger found a community of physicians accustomed to thinking of themselves as scientists and avid for leadership in the area of psychiatric illness.

Griesinger divided the Charité clinic into halves, one for "the usual nervous diseases," the other for "nervous disease with a primarily psychiatric presentation." Alternating between them by semester, he would hold three clinical lectures a week from 7 A.M. to 9 A.M. By the spring semester of 1867, 46 medical students were attending regularly (an impressive number, in view of the fact that psychiatry would not be on the exam), in addition to younger psychiatrists working in asylums, and a contingent of foreign physicians visiting Berlin. The medical students could also take individual patients out into the clinic's garden and practice testing their reflexes and looking at their eyeballs.[13]

The house staff (physicians in training) at the Charité experienced psychiatry not as it was practiced in an asylum but in a general hospital, for example, cross-covering other services. Robert Wollenberg, at the time a psychiatry resident, recalled being summoned full of fear and trembling to the obstetrical service in order to terminate a prolonged labor. Under the critical eyes of the staff midwives, he ended up performing a difficult maneuver called a "version." This meant reaching into the uterus, grasping the baby's feet and extracting it, an operation that would challenge any experienced obstetrician.[14] (Today's psychiatry residents, by contrast, tremble at the prospect of even doing an neurological exam.)

The Charité residents, as Griesinger told them, were there to learn how to diagnose. It was part of the new spirit that one had to watch an illness unfold for a while before one could determine its character, hence the notion of a short-stay urban asylum that would take on patients with few formalities (and little stigma), then either discharge them well or ship them off to a regular asylum.[15]

In 1867, Griesinger founded the flagship journal of the new neurologically oriented psychiatry, the *Archive for Psychiatry and Nervous Diseases*, which would overshadow the old *Journal of General Psychiatry* of the asylum doctors. The preface to the first issue of Griesinger's *Archive* contained one of those programmatic statements that in terms of historical resonance was comparable to Lenin's *What Is to Be Done?* "Psychiatry has undergone a transformation in its relationship to the rest of medicine," Griesinger said. "This transformation rests principally on the realization that patients with so-called 'mental illnesses' are really individuals with illnesses of the nerves and brain" (". . . dass die sogennanten 'Geisteskranken' Hirn- und Nerven-kranke Individuen sind"). Psychiatry must therefore "emerge from its closed-off status as a guild and become an integral part of general medicine accessible to all medical circles."[16] These are among the most portentous words ever uttered in the history of psychiatry. They inaugurated a new era of university psychiatry devoted to the study of brain and nervous tissue. In October 1868, a year after this first issue of the new *Archive* appeared, Griesinger died at age 51 of a ruptured appendix.[17]

Griesinger-style clinics now began appearing in a number of universities. Already in 1866, Ludwig Meyer, who as chief of the Hamburg asylum had made a name for himself by auctioning off the restraints used to bind patients, became head of a newly built university psychiatric clinic attached to an asylum in Göttingen. Meyer was co-editor of Griesinger's *Archive* and belonged to the inner circle of academic "nerve doctors" (*Nervenärzte*).[18] Further foundations followed. In 1872 in Munich, the brilliant student of brain structure Bernhard von Gudden transformed the psychiatric clinic there, which had been first opened in 1859, into a major research center. (Gudden died in 1886, dragged to the bottom of Lake Starnberg by his patient, the crazed Bavarian king Ludwig II.)[19] Carl Fürstner established a modest university clinic in Heidelberg in 1878 (the first asylum built within a university explicitly on Griesinger's lines).

Meanwhile in Austria, events unfolded in their own manner and in a way quite independent of Griesinger. In 1848, the 15-year-old Theodor Meynert moved with his family from Dresden, where he had been born, to Vienna, where his father was settling down to work as a journalist (Meynert's mother had originally been Viennese).[20] Meynert studied medicine in Vienna, having as a student the good fortune to be recognized as promising by the great pathologist Carl von Rokitansky. After graduating in 1861, Meynert specialized under Rokitansky in "the architecture and function of the brain and spinal cord." Thus there is no question of Meynert ever having been prepared as a psychiatrist. He was a neuropathologist and as such took a post as pathologist at the Vienna asylum. Yet from 1868 onward, Meynert also began lecturing in psychiatry. In 1870, the Austrian government appointed him associate professor of psychiatry, bringing him immediately into conflict with the older generation of humanitarian, psychologically oriented asylum clinicians. Meynert was a pupil of the Viennese school of natural science and of therapeutic nihilism, which maintained that the treatment of untreatable diseases is useless. He himself believed that he was in psychiatry in order to do research and not necessarily to cure patients. Indeed, he went on to do pioneer work in the microscopic structure of the brain and spinal cord, a challenging task involving discovering stains—carmine dye in Meynert's case—with which to visualize the various brain cells under the microscope, then differentiating layers (the cytoarchitecture) of the cerebral cortex and other specialized parts of the brain.[21] He worked on the fourth floor of his home, hunched over his microscope, hunting not just for structure but for pathological lesions in the neurons as well. And for this search, Meynert became an object of mockery among generations of the psychoanalytically oriented historians who came later, secure in the knowledge that Sigmund Freud, who had been a pupil of Meynert, had found the right way. That Meynert discovered little aside from the lesions of neurosyphilis did not necessarily mean that he was wrong, merely that he was searching with the wrong tools.

While Meynert's focus on the brain's frontal lobes would survive among subsequent generations as an object of humor, it was forgotten that Meynert, perhaps next to Griesinger the most famous representative of the first biological psychiatry of the nineteenth century, had forecast the second biological psychiatry of the twentieth. As Meynert wrote in 1890: "The study of human anatomy in its current form has passed from a solely descriptive science to something higher, to a form of knowledge that attempts to explain. . . . The more that psychiatry seeks, and finds, its scientific basis in a deep and finely grained understanding of the anatomical structure [of the brain], the more it elevates itself to the status of a science that deals with causes."[22] These were prophetic words.

Yet Meynert, like so many of his generation, had an Achilles heel when it came to patients. He basically had little interest in them, believing most to be beyond help. The Austrian physician and playwright Arthur Schnitzler, who trained for six months at Meynert's psychiatric clinic at the Vienna General Hospital, gave a sense of the man's clinical style: "[He] was a great scholar, a splendid diagnostician, but as a physician in the narrower sense, in his personal relations with the patients, . . . he did not win my admiration. As masterful as he may have been in the face of disease, in front of the sick person his behavior often seemed to me cool, uncertain, if not indeed anxious."[23] It probably was also unhelpful that Meynert was

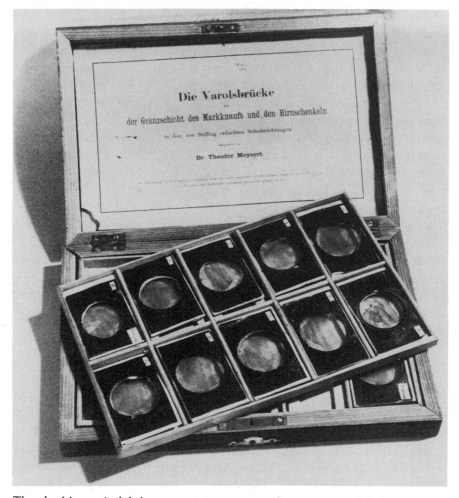

Theodor Meynert's slide box, containing sections of various parts of the brain. Meynert tried to find under the microscope the physical causes of mental illness (courtesy Institut für Geschichte der Medizin, Vienna).

a chronic alcoholic.[24] Malicious tongues claimed Meynert's only connection with psychiatry was that he had gone through a delirium tremens.

Nonetheless, Meynert was a pioneering figure. In 1868, he called for a fundamental reorientation of psychiatry—quite independently of Griesinger who was making the same demand in Berlin—away from preoccupation with labeling symptoms and toward understanding the underlying anatomical origins of psychiatric illness.[25] Meynert's work was the beginning of the last phase in the development of the first biological psychiatry: concentration on anatomy.

In the 1880s and after, an absolute craze for studying psychiatry with the microscope took possession of the German, Austrian, and Swiss universities. It is generally agreed that this craze led to a dead end, and that the first biological psychiatry died because it detached itself too completely from patients and their world. Yet misguided or not, these researchers were trying to achieve something more than merely mapping the architecture of the grey and white matter of the cerebral cortex. Following the model of neurosyphilis, they were trying to identify specific lesions in patients whose illnesses seemed to be primarily psychiatric rather than neurological. In other words they considered themselves at this point to be psychiatrists rather than neurologists (neurology in many places was a branch of internal medicine). The leaders in this field were almost all students of Meynert.

Two giants in the study of neuroanatomy and cerebral localization opened university clinics in the 1880s: Paul Flechsig in Leipzig in 1882 and Eduard Hitzig in Halle in 1885. Flechsig laid down the basic map of what regions of the cerebral cortex are responsible for what functions ("cerebral localization"), and Hitzig established that the brain responds to electrical stimulation. Both men had immense achievements.[26] Both were also terrible clinicians.

Here biological psychiatry in Germany showed the same shadow side as in Austria. Believing psychiatric diseases to be incurable, many of

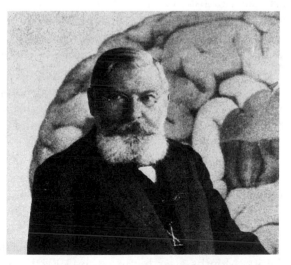

Paul Flechsig, professor of psychiatry at Leipzig 1877–1921, who pioneered the study of cerebral localization (but who was poor at dealing with patients) (courtesy of Museen der Stadt Wien).

these professors concentrated on research in the basic sciences and displayed little interest in clinical psychiatry. They had not gone into the discipline to make their patients better. Emil Kraepelin, who worked briefly as a resident under Flechsig until leaving in disgust, recalled Flechsig as being completely uninterested in learning about patients or their problems.[27] For Daniel Paul Schreber, a jurist who apparently had neurosyphilis and spent some time around 1884 in Flechsig's clinic, Flechsig was the "murderer of my soul."[28] (It was Schreber whom Freud in 1911 attempted retrospectively to psychoanalyze.[29]) Hitzig had the general reputation of being "intolerable." He knew little of psychiatry and, in one colleague's judgment, would never have lasted on the staff of a big psychiatric clinic had his scientific accomplishments not placed him in charge of one.[30] Accordingly, as research into brain anatomy and brain physiology accelerated, the first biological psychiatry became nihilistic about the possibilities of clinical care, seeking instead to become an annex of the basic medical sciences.

The first biological psychiatry slid to an end in the work of Carl Wernicke, narrowly balanced between "neuromythology" and brain anatomy. Wernicke, the most ambitious of the neurological psychiatrists, set out to establish that specific symptom complexes could be associated with specific areas of the brain. Here he had tremendous initial success, enshrining his name at the age of 24 in medical history. Having just graduated in 1870 from Breslau, he went to Vienna to work with Meynert. Wernicke established in 1874 that when a patient has a stroke in a specific part of the brain (the posterior perisylvian region), he or she will be unable to understand the spoken word and will be able to speak only in incomprehensible jargon. The area of the brain became known as Wernicke's area, and this particular aphasia became called "Wernicke's aphasia." This scientific windfall would stamp Wernicke's interests permanently. He spent the next years in Berlin attempting to identify other such areas, publishing between 1881 and 1883 a three-volume book on brain disease.[31]

At this point, Wernicke turned to a possibly more fanciful subject: whether psychiatric symptom-complexes existed that might be localized in certain areas of the brain. In 1885, he became professor of psychiatry at Breslau, spending almost all the rest of his days trying to match symptoms in patients to postulated brain abnormalities.[32] He developed thereby his own vocabulary for the accounting of psychiatric and neurological complaints. Months after his move in 1904 to the psychiatric clinic in Halle, he was mortally wounded when his bicycle was run over by a truck. Clinician to the last, as he lay dying he said reflectively, "I'm perishing of autopsychic disorientation."[33] Wernicke's vocabulary did not outlive him.

With Wernicke, the development in biological psychiatry that Karl Jaspers later characterized as "brain mythology" reached its end point.[34] Emil Kraepelin would shortly announce that the course of psychiatric illness offered the sharpest clue to its nature, rather than, as Wernicke believed, the kind of symptoms the patient had at any particular moment. Kraepelin espoused a longitudinal approach, Wernicke a cross-sectional. It was the historic victory of Kraepelin's views over Wernicke's that marked the end of the first biological psychiatry.

By 1911, Germany had 16 Griesinger-style university psychiatric clinics, 187 public asylums, and 225 private asylums, not to mention the many additional institutions in Austria and German-speaking Switzerland. By that year, Germany had almost 1,400 physicians specializing in psychiatry.[35] This pool of research energy was unmatched anywhere else in the world and explains the primacy of Central Europe in the science of mind and brain. But just as the particular development of the German states had given science policy a certain stamp, events in other countries would stamp the neurosciences there just as ineffably.

French Disasters

Unlike Germany, the history of university psychiatry in France is not synonymous with the biological approach, for Esquirol in particular had little interest in the integuments of the brain. What is intriguing about the French story is how politics destroyed virtually all efforts to launch university psychiatry of any kind—neuroscientific or psychosocial—before a government decree in 1877 finally created psychiatric clinics at the four main universities.

At some point before 1815, Pinel had offered a clinic in psychiatry for students at the Salpêtrière in addition to his university lectures in internal medicine and pathology. The clinic did not survive. In 1817, Esquirol began teaching a private course in psychiatry at the Salpêtrière. It was not an official course of the faculty, and not until 1821 did Antoine Royer-Collard begin offering the faculty's psychiatry lectures. They ceased a year later as the government abolished the entire School of Medicine in Paris for political reasons.[36] Therewith, formal teaching in psychiatry in Paris came to an end for the next half century.

France had gifted psychiatrists, many of whom made lasting contributions to the discipline. Yet their energies were never harnessed in the systematic manner of the German system with its 20-odd universities and armies of private-docents and professors.[37] The experience of the brilliant young Antoine-Laurent Bayle is instructive. In a doctoral thesis in medicine in 1822, Bayle attributed the psychiatric symptoms of neurosyphilis to a chronic inflammation of the meninges, thus making himself the first to discover a psychiatric disease with definite organicity, establishing that as the underlying disease worsens, the symptoms worsen as well.[38] What was the fate of this French Wernicke? Did he become the professor of psychiatry at Lyons (an analogous example to Wernicke's professorship at Breslau)? Hardly. Owing to political intrigues, Bayle never received even an asylum post to say nothing of a university professorship. Bayle was associated politically with Royer-Collard, under whom he had studied at Charenton. Royer-Collard had a falling out with the Pinel-Esquirol circle, and just after Royer-Collard died in November 1825, the members of this circle forced Bayle to take a position as assistant librarian in the Paris faculty of medicine. After returning to asylum psychiatry a few years later, his appetite for discovery presumably quenched, Bayle made no significant further contributions.[39]

Such maneuvers occurred regularly in France. Another victim was Josef Babinski, the gifted psychiatrist and discoverer of the reflex named after him (raking the sole of the foot will cause the big toe to turn up if brain disease, an upper-motor neuron lesion, is present). Political rivalries in the 1890s prevented Babinski from ever gaining an academic post.[40] A highly centralized system was permitted to shoot itself in the foot, so to speak, because everything was controlled from a single ministerial desk. And because opportunities in the provinces were so scant, there was no alternative venue to which people such as Bayle or Babinski could retreat, unlike the German psychiatry professors who regularly drifted from chair to chair. Wernicke, for example, had gone to Halle in 1904 after the Breslau city council interfered with the running of his service.

Thus in France, politics decreed that research in psychiatry would be situated in the asylum and not in the university. Of these asylum-based scholars, best known, or perhaps most notorious, was Bénédict-Auguste Morel, among the first to describe schizophrenia. It was Morel who launched the notion of "degeneration" on its fateful trajectory. Born into a family that became impoverished at the death of the father, Morel attended a religious boarding school in eastern France. Expelled from school, he came to Paris and became something of a penniless bohemian, toying with journalism and sharing a flat with the young Claude Bernard (who later became a famous physiologist but at the time, like Morel, was poverty-stricken). Both Morel and Bernard decided for medicine. In 1839,

Morel submitted a doctoral dissertation that touched among other things on insanity. Resolving to go further into psychiatry, he asked Bernard (then an interne at the Salpêtrière) to introduce him to Jean-Pierre Falret, psychiatrist and chief physician of the hospice. Thus Morel became involved in clinical psychiatry. In 1841, accompanying a patient on a voyage abroad, Morel chanced on an asylum for mentally retarded children run by Dr. Johann Jakob Guggenbühl at Abendberg, Switzerland. Guggenbühl specialized in children suffering from cretinism (later determined to be the result of iodine deficiency). The Abendberg visit hooked Morel's interest in the whole subject of mental retardation. Given the organicity of several forms of this condition such as Down syndrome, Morel would find it an easy step to organicist assumptions about psychiatry in general.

In 1848, Morel became staff physician at the Maréville asylum near Nancy, where he strode forth as a great reformer, releasing the patients from their fortresslike cells. Three years later, in 1851, he began teaching a course in psychiatry there. Although Morel's views might on occasion possess a romantic flavor, a result of his deep piety, there is no doubt that he was firmly within the biological tradition. "I believe that the brain is the organ of the soul," he declared.[41] By 1856, when Morel became chief physician of the St.-Yon asylum, he had acquired a kind of *idée fixe* about "degeneration" in its various forms, including mental retardation. Accordingly, Morel, the first major figure in France to have lectured in psychiatry since Esquirol and Royer-Collard, lined up on the biological side.[42]

To teach within the French university system, one has to pass a difficult examination called the *agrégation*. (Another reason why French psychiatry was behind: Young scientists spent all their time memorizing facts rather than doing research.) Morel did not become *agrégé*. But another of the comrades who hung about with Morel and Claude Bernard in their student days did pass the *agrégation*: Charles Lasègue.

It was Lasègue who rekindled the university teaching of psychiatry in Paris (as opposed to teaching non-academic courses in hospitals in the 1840s and after; several clinicians—such as Jules Baillarger at the Salpêtrière—offered hospital courses). Seven years younger than Morel, Lasègue had launched his career by the same route: He asked Claude Bernard to introduce him to Falret. Like Morel, Lasègue became captivated by psychiatry. Both men completed their MD dissertations at the age of 30. But rather than going off to some peripheral mental hospital as Morel did, upon graduation in 1846 Lasègue remained in Paris at the forensic clinic of the Prefecture of Police. He passed his *agrègation* in 1853 and became a staff physician in the Paris hospitals. Finally in 1862, he was given permission to teach a course in psychiatry at the faculty of medicine—yet without access to patients. Lasègue inaugurated the course on November 28 of that year in the Faculty's great, and only, lecture theater. He shifted further lectures to the Necker Hospital.

One might conclude that at last the genius of the French system had triumphed, that Lasègue, a truly talented man who had already made several original contributions to psychiatry (in 1873 he would describe anorexia nervosa for the first time as a distinct illness), had finally reached the point of Griesinger at the Charité in 1865 or Meynert in Vienna in 1870. But no. In 1867, five years after beginning his course, Lasègue became appointed professor of general pathology, not of psychiatry, for which there was as yet no chair. In 1869, Lasègue received the chair of clinical medicine at Pitié Hospital.[43] Few significant psychiatrists would train under him. Once again, the system had run into the sand.

Now psychiatry and nervous disease were becoming an embarrassment to the Ministry and to the Parliament, where there was great enthusiasm for such teaching. In 1875, two commissions recommended that a full chair in psychiatry ("maladies mentales") be created, and in 1877 a government decree determined that each of France's four medical faculties—the Sorbonne in Paris, and the faculties in Lyons, Nancy, and Marseille—would have teaching in psychiatry at the level of a full professorship. Here once again, the Ministry and Faculty defeated themselves. By this time, several distinguished psychiatrists in Paris were giving hospital-based lectures in psychiatry. Who should become the professor? After much political arm-twisting, Lasègue's candidate prevailed: an obscure 45-year-old psychiatrist named Benjamin Ball, born in Naples of an English father and a Swiss mother. Ball had little going for him save his powerful patron. At Lasègue's instigation, in the early 1870s Ball started to offer a complementary course of lectures in psychiatry at the Faculty. In 1879, he began lecturing at the Sainte-Anne asylum as the new chair-holder. But when the authorities created a chair for Ball at Sainte-Anne, they neglected to make him simultaneously medical director of the asylum. Intramural conflict at Sainte-Anne plagued Ball during his tenure in office. A disappointment to everyone, he died discouraged in 1893 at the age of 58.[44]

Following these negotiations is rewarding only because they illustrate why France remained a second-rate psychiatric power. Few stories, however, demonstrate so perfectly this inability to rise from mediocrity as the story of Jean-Martin Charcot, a man often hailed as a great psychiatrist though in fact he was an internist and pathologist, and understood almost nothing of major psychiatric illness. Born in 1825 of a working-class family, Charcot was a self-made man, a scholar and researcher who by the force of his own wit had pushed his way into a system dominated by upper-middle-class clinicians and bureaucrats. After jumping through the usual academic hoops, in 1862 Charcot became the chief physician of the Salpêtrière, a hospice that had its own medical service in addition to the psychiatric staff of which Charcot was not a member. In 1866, he began lecturing on chronic diseases at the Salpêtrière. Because the hospice, with its large population of aging (and mostly non-insane) women was a sort of treasure trove of pathology, Charcot became attracted to the study of neurological illness, just as Meynert had discovered the organic side of research in his association with Rokitansky. But Meynert at least taught on a psychiatric service, which Charcot never did. In the 1860s, Charcot made some fundamental discoveries in the area of neuropathology, linking anatomic changes to clinical symptoms in multiple sclerosis, for example, or describing ALS (amyotrophic lateral sclerosis, or "Lou Gehrig's disease"). These were major contributions and earned Charcot such a reputation that by the 1870s he was the best-known physician in France. In 1882, a chair in nervous disease was created specially for him.

In the early 1870s, Charcot became entangled in what would later constitute office-practice psychiatry, the undifferentiated mass of neurotic complaints that he termed "hysteria." Believing hysteria to be a real organic disease, transmitted genetically and associated with presumptive but unidentified changes in nervous tissue, Charcot elaborated a kind of air-castle of "iron laws of hysteria," a disease thought to follow its own rules. Thus it was that from the early 1870s until his death in 1893, Charcot poured most of his energy into hysteria, directing his many students toward it and forming, or deforming, an entire generation of researchers, many of whom were psychiatrists. He possessed titanic authority. All of Europe came to believe in Charcot's "hysteria," which willy-nilly had become the centerpiece of French psychiatry.

But after Charcot's death the whole edifice of Charcotian hysteria collapsed. The supposedly organic nervous disease called "grand hysteria" turned out to be nothing more than an artifact of suggestion, as did the presumed "stigmata" of hysteria, fixed physical signs such as supposed tunnel vision. An entire generation of physicians and patients had been gulled into believing, and reproducing in their illness behavior, the symptoms of a set of iron laws that never existed.[45] It was a complete disaster for French psychiatry, from which the French even by World War II had not fully recovered. (A Parisian symposium in 1925 on the centenary of Charcot's birth makes piteous reading.[46])

This history of misery was for the most part built into the French system. Only in France could a handful of chair-holders in Paris dominate the destiny of medical training in a country of almost 40 million people. When a system like the French produces a Pasteur, its extreme centralization has the potential to mobilize large amounts of talent. When it produces someone like Charcot, quite lacking in common sense and grandiosely sure of his own judgment, it harbors the potential for calamity.

One more calamity lay in the wings for French psychiatry in the nineteenth century. It took the form of Valentin Magnan, chief physician of the Sainte-Anne asylum.[47] Next to Morel, Magnan was perhaps the second most famous of France's biological psychiatrists. Born in 1835, he came up from Lyons where he had studied medicine to serve a prized internship in Paris, first at Bicêtre in 1864 under the organicist Victor Marcé and the hereditarian Prosper Lucas, then in 1865 for his second year of internship at the Salpêtrière. At the time, the Salpêtrière was a site of "prodigious activity"—as Magnan's biographer put it—in the area of neurology and organically oriented psychiatry.[48] Magnan involved himself fully in the research of such teachers as Jean-Pierre Falret. It was probably from Falret that Magnan derived his lust for classification that would later prove so fateful in the international isolation of French psychiatry.

Just after finishing his thesis in 1866, Magnan won a post in the admissions bureau of the Sainte-Anne asylum, which would open a year later. (The curious Parisian admissions system called for patients to be funneled from the forensic service of the Prefecture of Police to the Sainte-Anne admissions bureau, whence they would be distributed to the various asylums of the Paris region.) Here, Magnan stood in the midst of the great stream of psychiatric pathology coursing through the metropolis: In 1868 alone, he and his colleagues examined 2,600 patients. In that year, Magnan initiated at Sainte-Anne the kind of hospital-based lecture series then being attempted at other asylums and hospitals as well. (The course was shut down in 1873 by the authorities because of a public scandal over the demonstration of patients to students, resuming four years later.[49]) Passed over for the professorship in favor of Ball, Magnan remained at Sainte-Anne, the gray eminence of French psychiatry, until his retirement in 1912.

Among the patients passing through the admissions bureau, Magnan became particularly interested in the alcoholic, the epileptic, and those suffering nerve damage from the then popular drink absinthe (later banned as a neurotoxin). In short, Magnan singled out that class of patients whom Morel had identified as "degenerate," and in his writings Magnan would soon spread the doctrine of "degeneration" far and wide within Europe (see p. 181). That was one disservice to French psychiatry.

Magnan's other disservice was to elaborate, in imitation of Charcot, his own set of iron laws about the supposed evolution of psychotic illness, in which patients who began with fretfulness would end in dementia, the distinctively French "chronic delusional disorder with progressively downhill course" (*délire chronique à évolution systématique*). With the exception of neurosyphilis and Alzheimer's disease, no major psychiatric illness behaves in this manner, and the notion of carving out chronic delusional disorders as a privileged category makes little sense, for delusions are found in tandem with other symptoms in almost all psychotic illness. Yet Magnan's idiosyncratic approach to delusions stuck within French psychiatry and became a national tradition. It blocked the acceptance of schizophrenia, isolating France from the rest of the international community and stunting its growth behind a wall of nationalistic pride.[50]

Magnan represented the high-water mark in France of the first biological psychiatry. It was a version too permeated with his genetic reductionism to survive. After World War I, "mental hygiene" and other catchphrases of the psychosocial version of psychiatry would carry the day.

Anglo-Saxon Laggards

When in 1904 a young American psychiatry resident named Clarence Farrar visited London on a busman's holiday, he wanted quite naturally to tour the Bethlem Royal Hospital, most famous of all British psychiatric institutions. Staff physician William Stoddart, known as a "vast, portly figure arrayed in morning coat and top hat," came forward to show young Farrar around. The visitor asked his guide to characterize the state of English psychiatry. "Stoddart says English psychiatry is far behind that on the continent, that there exists in England no school of psychiatry," Farrar noted in his diary. "In Bethlem there is no pathologist and no pathology done except what Dr. Stoddart 'finds time' to do. In histological diagnosis, G.P. [general paralysis] is the only disease he thinks it possible to recognise. No psychology is done. It is considered to be much work with little result."[51] Farrar, who had just come from the great pathology laboratories of Heidelberg where such chiefs as Franz Nissl and Aloys Alzheimer bent over the microscope night and day to find the cause of psychosis and dementia, could scarcely believe the backward state of English psychiatry.

In England, where everything depended on private and charitable initiatives and nothing on public funds, research into biological psychiatry scarcely existed. "The following sketch," said surgeon Walter Rivington in his portrayal of medicine in the United Kingdom in 1879, "will show how widely different are the systems pursued in Paris and in London. In Paris 1 school of medicine, 1 staff of professors, 1 group of laboratories and museums, lecture theatre and dissecting-room. . . . responsibility to the State and centralisation are the main characteristics. In London, 11 schools, 11 staffs of professors and assistants, with 11 separate courses on each subject, 11 sets of offices and school buildings with their lecture theatres and laboratories. . . . Appointment of hospital staffs, without competition, by the lay authorities of the hospital through private influence or favour leavened by recommendation of future colleagues. . . ."[52] In this English system of extreme decentralization, no money could be found for laboratories or research institutes and little time spared from clinical duties for the microscope. Stoddart was in fact not untypical in his indifference to peeling back the mysteries of nature with laboratory research.

All this is not to say that British psychiatry was not biologically oriented. From the earliest days, British physicians had assigned a physical seat to mental illness. As Bedlam's John Haslam wrote in 1809, "From the preceding dissections of insane persons, it may be inferred that madness has always been connected with disease of the brain and its membranes."[53] From autopsies done at Hanwell, William Charles Ellis gained strength for his theories that "increased sanguineous action takes place on the commencement of insanity."[54] Yet while a somaticist theme ran throughout British psychiatry in the nineteenth century, it was sharply accented in the academic setting. Virtually without exception, the men who brought psychiatry to Britain's medical students were biologically oriented.

Since Battie's time, there had been sporadic lecturing on psychiatry in the London hospital medical schools. Yet a sustained course of academic lectures seems to have been first offered only in 1851 by David Skae, physician of the Royal Lunatic Asylum in Edinburgh. Organicist Skae proposed that types of insanity be classified on the basis of the bodily illness causing them, hence "mania of masturbation," "mania of pregnancy," and so forth, ending up with a list of 25: "Each may be described as *a disease* presenting a certain variety and kind of mental symptoms," he said.[55] In Dr. Skae's classroom at the Edinburgh Asylum in Morningside, disease thinking ran riot.

In London, it was William Sankey who in the 1860s at University College first began a course of psychiatry lectures. Sankey had been drawn to the subject of mental illness around the age of 40, having spent the first part of his career at the London Fever Hospital. Because many febrile illnesses cause delirium, the loss of orientation combined with psychotic symptoms, Sankey's interests in fever may have led him naturally toward psychiatry. A typical organicist, he did not doubt that melancholia possessed a morbid anatomy, though he was uncertain of its exact nature.[56] In 1854, he became the head of the female ward of the Middlesex County Asylum at Hanwell, leaving a decade later for a private clinic in the provinces, the Sandywell Park Lunatic Asylum in Gloucestershire. Around 1865, Sankey began as well to lecture on mental diseases at University College.[57]

Sankey got this post through the failed initiative of a young fellow of University College named Henry Maudsley. Maudsley, 30 at the time, had had a brilliant record as a medical student, graduating MB (medical bachelor, the British equivalent of the American MD) in 1856. At the surprising age of 24, he was appointed medical superintendent of the Manchester Royal Lunatic Hospital, coming down to London three years later to edit the flagship organ of British psychiatry, the *Journal of Mental Science*. In 1865, Maudsley proposed to University College that, as instruction in mental diseases was already available in Edinburgh, Paris, Vienna, and Berlin, a course be offered in London as well, because "every medical man has in his practice to deal with insanity as with any other disease; and it usually falls to him to deal with it at that early stage of the disease when there is always the best hope . . . of effecting a cure." The appointments committee of the College was convinced by his logic, but passed Maudsley over in favor of Sankey for the post.[58]

Maudsley had circumstances going for him other than his brilliance. In 1866 he had married the youngest daughter of the famous John Conolly, the alienist who in 1850 had widely publicized the virtue of abolishing restraints, as his predecessors had done at Hanwell and elsewhere.[59] With one swoop, Maudsley had now behind him the authority of his father-in-law (who died a month after the wedding). Maudsley also took over the lease of a small private nervous clinic, Lawn House, that Conolly had established in his own home in Hanwell, with quarters for eight patients, all wealthy females. Lawn House, plus Maudsley's consulting practice at his other residence in Hanover-square in London, became the basis of a considerable fortune.[60]

In 1869 Maudsley was appointed professor of medical jurisprudence, essentially a professorship in psychiatry, at University College Hospital. He went on to become the best-known psychiatrist of the Victorian era. He believed psychiatric illness to be a physical disorder of the body just as any other. "When a person is lunatic," he said in 1870, "he is . . . lunatic to his fingers' ends." For Maudsley as for Griesinger, mind disease was brain disease. "Mental disorders are neither more nor less than nervous diseases in which mental symptoms predominate."[61] In the context of Victorian psychiatry there was nothing at all daring or iconoclastic about these theories. Maudsley articulated what virtually every psychiatrist and medical man of the day believed, but he did so from a position of great authority, which gave him an opportunity to try and show that he was right.

In 1907, Maudsley offered £30,000 to the London County Council, the body that administered the asylums of the metropolis, for a new asylum on conditions that would have been familiar to Griesinger: that it accept only recently ill people, that it make provision for teaching and research, and that it be in the heart of the city near the medical schools. Completed in 1915, the new building was first used as a military hospital and only in 1923—four years after Maudsley's death—did it start to become the medical facility he had envisioned for "exact scientific research on the causes and pathology of mental diseases."[62] England, therefore, had to wait almost 60 years before getting its first university psychiatric clinic on the German model made famous by Griesinger in 1865.

The Achilles' heel, or genius if one prefers, of English psychiatry was that it was all clinical medicine and little science. The English were known as superb observers, clinical investigators, and examiners, but their clinical findings lacked the kind of anchor in the natural sciences at which the Germans were so gifted. Said a young Swiss medical student named Adolf Meyer after visiting London and Edinburgh in 1891, "One comes closest to the truth about English [sic] medicine in saying that it's conceived as the art of healing, to which science is subordinated. Practical matters receive priority everywhere. . . ."[63] It was not that the British were by nature more pragmatic or less inclined to rigor, merely that they were endowed with a system in which the teaching hospitals were dependent on charity. Government givers, as in Germany, had a penchant for science because its triumphs added to national prestige. Private givers, as in England, preferred to endow care because they were acting for humanitarian and dynastic reasons. Thus the kind of system that each country adopted made a big difference in the kind of psychiatry it produced.

To understand the backward state of American psychiatry at the turn of the century one must bear in mind the inferior condition of American medicine in general. "In 1900," writes historian Rosemary Stevens, "less than 10 percent of practicing physicians in the U.S.A. were graduates of genuine medical schools. About 20 percent had never attended medical school lectures. The majority were the products of apprenticeship or of the proprietary schools."[64] It cannot surprise us therefore that research and education in psychiatry in the United States got off to a slow start. In 1868, the year of Griesinger's manifesto, John Gray, the progressive superintendent at Utica State Hospital, persuaded the trustees to establish a pathology laboratory to make sections of the brain and spinal cord. Young Dr. Edward Hun of Albany, two years out of medical school at Columbia, was hired to do this work, and though we know little of his actual activity save that he left in 1873, we do know that he wrote on such topics as "the pulse of the insane" and "haematoma auris," or blood blisters within the ear sometimes called "insane ear" and thought characteristic of madness (in fact they were the result of asylum attendants clubbing the patients).[65] One cannot imagine a figure of such meager stature at a comparable post in Europe.

Hun was followed at Utica by John Deecke, a supposed scientific stalwart who cut a considerable figure in the eyes of visiting foreign physicians. When, for example, English psychiatrist John Bucknill came over in 1876, he found that "Dr. Theodore [sic] Deecke devotes his time exclusively to pathological investigations; and is engaged at the present time in producing photographs of cerebral and spinal sections of wonderful size and accuracy."[66] A scientific triumph, surely. Yet an observer closer to the scene tells us that Deecke, "who was a technician rather than a pathologist . . . could make sections but could not interpret them."[67] Deecke had never studied brain anatomy in medical school. The visiting British (unlike the eager young Dr. Farrar in London) did not discuss with Deecke what they were actually looking at. The "pathological laboratory" at Utica came to an end with Gray's death in 1886 and the entire episode left "the tradition of the histopathologist of the Utica State Hospital" as something of a joke among American psychiatrists.[68]

At this point, the story shifts to the young Adolf Meyer, who in 1891, had been visiting European asylums. Just after earning his MD at Zurich in 1892, Meyer migrated to the United States, to study neurology, he said.[69] Meyer was persuaded to make this ostensibly bizarre choice by a chance conversation in Berlin with an American neurobiologist who lauded the University of Chicago (perhaps Meyer believed possibilities for advancement were better in America than in Switzerland).[70] He landed in Chicago, which he found a scientific desert.[71] Then in 1893, Meyer was appointed staff pathologist at a mental hospital in Kankakee, Illinois, the Illinois Eastern Hospital for the Insane, which had opened its doors in 1879 as the first "noncongregate" asylum in the United

States, meaning that the patients lived in rows of little stone houses rather than in vast barracks.[72] Progressive though Kankakee was architecturally, at the time of Meyer's arrival the staff was "hopelessly sunk into routine and perfectly satisfied with it." Meyer began by offering a course in neurology to them, then saw that it was not hitting home. "When I realized this, I started with something in which the physicians were more closely interested every day. I began by having the new patients given an examination in the presence of the whole staff, quite unofficially, during an hour usually spent in recreation."[73] This was Meyer's hallmark: extensive history-taking, extensive investigation, extensive notetaking. If the British fetishized nonrestraint and the Germans the microscope, Meyer fetishized "the facts." From this point on, Meyer would move as a kind of Johnny Appleseed through the landscape of American psychiatry, dropping the seeds of what he always conceived as general "medicine" wherever he went (he tended to use the terms medicine and psychiatry synonymously).

In 1895, Meyer left Kankakee for the asylum at Worcester, Massachusetts, an institution created in 1833 by the original reform wave in American psychiatry but that, by the turn of the century, had become a warehouse of the mad. Meyer had come to Worcester almost through happenstance: At a convention of psychiatrists in 1895, he had been discussing with Edward Cowles, director of the McLean Hospital in Boston, the need for a pathology laboratory in the public sector at Worcester similar to the laboratory that Cowles had already established at McLean. The director of Worcester then wrote Meyer offering him the post, assuring him that he would be absolutely free to undertake whatever he wished in terms of research and training and not just be limited to autopsies. Meyer at this point was growing tired of autopsies anyway, beginning to interest himself in "the living patient."[74] Yet the psychiatry that he brought to Worcester was still a resolutely biological one. "The fundamental principle on which the psychiatry of today is built," he wrote in 1897, "is undoubtedly this biological conception of man." Exactly in line with his European preceptors, Meyer in his first decades in the United States saw the brain as the substrate of all mental activity: "We cannot conceive a disorder of the mind without a disorder of function of those cell mechanisms [of the brain]."[75]

After six years at Worcester, in 1901 Meyer was appointed director of the Pathological Institute in New York City, founded in 1895 to study brain sections from the state asylums. The Pathological Institute had drifted under its first director and now Meyer was called in to redirect it with the straightedge of German science.[76] In 1902, he relocated the

Institute to one of the buildings—a disused bakehouse—of the Manhattan State Hospital for the Insane on Ward's Island in New York.[77] Increasingly in these years, Meyer came to view the proper site for the study of psychiatry as the bedside rather than the "deadhouse." Yet his interests remained emphatically biological rather than psychosocial. For example, in 1903 he called the asylum physicians of all the state hospitals together to talk about his new agenda. "I sketched the general principles of pathology as adapted to psychiatry, the methods of the physical examination of the insane, and the most frequent issues and difficulties of general physical and neurological diagnosis, and some of the latest observations in these directions, such as one-sided apraxia [inability to carry out intentional movements] and one-sided delirium."[78]

When Meyer became professor of psychiatry at Johns Hopkins in 1910, he surveyed a landscape bereft of university science. Of the few laboratories approaching European standards, two he had created himself, at Kankakee and Worcester; several state hospitals had German-style laboratories, as for example Iowa and Minnesota; and the Government Hospital for the Insane (later St. Elizabeths Hospital) in Washington, opened in 1855, was building a scientific department. McLean Hospital probably approached the European model closest with its corps of physicians and small number of beds.[79] By the turn of the century, scarcely an American university was implicated in the systematic study of psychiatry, though many offered lecture courses.[80]

Characteristic of the development of psychiatry in the United States, therefore, was the separation of teaching and research, the opposite of the Continental model. This is why the founding of the Johns Hopkins Medical School in 1893 was of such significance: It promised to bring together science and the clinic, and Meyer's journey to Baltimore in 1910 would accomplish this for psychiatry. It was, ironically, Meyer's tenure at Hopkins that put an end to the first biological psychiatry in the United States.

Degeneration

Psychiatrists of the nineteenth century pioneered the modern understanding of the genetics and biology of neuroscience. But then they went one step further. They asserted that not only do the major mental illnesses have a heavy biological and genetic component, but that these illnesses get worse as they are passed from generation to generation, causing progressive degeneration within family trees and within the population as a whole. Here psychiatry stood on very risky ground, ground that in fact would crumble into catastrophe as these ideas were appropriated by politicians as an agenda for action.

There is some truth to the concept of degeneration, although the term rings infamously on late-twentieth-century ears tutored to its misuse in the Holocaust: Some diseases with a psychiatric and neurological presentation do become worse as they are passed on. The genes that cause these illnesses expand in size (called technically trinucleotide repeat mutations) as the illnesses descend the family tree. The number of DNA base pairs becomes larger. Examples are the "fragile-X" syndrome, the second commonest cause of mental retardation after Down's, and Huntington's disease, involving involuntary, jerky movements (chorea) and mental deterioration.[81] So there is something to the notion of deterioration across the generations for select illnesses. Yet by the end of the nineteenth century, the advocates of degeneration had expanded the concept to embrace much of psychiatry and anthropology. The idea of degeneration began to bolster such social policies as sterilization, euthanasia, and persecution of the Jews on the grounds that they were a "degenerate" people.

In 1857, Benedict-Augustin Morel launched the concept of degeneration on its historical trajectory. Shocked by the "incessant progression" in Europe of such evils as general paralysis of the insane, epilepsy, suicide, and crime, Morel was attempting to identify underlying "natural forces" shaping the destiny of the human condition. He was struck that many of his patients looked funny. Some of the patients with mental retardation ("the cretins"), for example, had goiters (a result of iodine deficiency). Asylum patients, generally speaking, seemed to Morel to have a "special cachet in their physiognomy." What was the matter with these people? It was not just that they were suffering from inheritable insanity, he thought. All psychiatrists of Morel's day believed mental illness to be directly inheritable. It was that "they recapitulate in their bodies the pathological organic characteristics of a number of previous generations," that they were on the receiving end of the combined weight of generations of madness. Borrowing a term current in the comparative zoology of his day, Morel decided to call this pathological momentum within a family tree "degeneration." And not only was it bad for the family, it was hurtful to society. Morel wrote, "The degenerate human being, if he is abandoned to himself, falls into a progressive degradation. He becomes . . . not only incapable of forming part of the chain of transmission of progress in human society, he is the greatest obstacle to this progress through his contact with the healthy portion of the population." Happily, "The span of his existence is limited as is that of all monstrosities."[82]

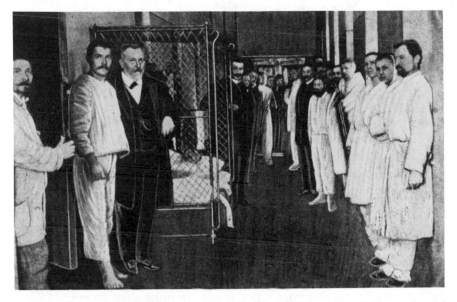

Richard von Krafft-Ebing, professor of psychiatry in Vienna 1892–1902, on clinical rounds at the Vienna General Hospital. He is identified with "degeneration" theory and with his study of sex life *Psychopathia Sexualis* (1886) (courtesy of Institut für Geschichte der Medizin, Vienna).

Thus Morelian degeneration was loosed upon the world. It might start as an acquired characteristic: alcoholism for example, or dissolution in the slums of the big cities. These vicious characteristics would then pass into the individual's seed and be transmitted via heredity, worsening with each generation. What began as maternal tuberculosis might end three or four generations later as dementia and sterility, he thought. This was truly a challenging agenda both for the social hygienists (clean up the slums and bars) and the healing professions, for if acquired characteristics could become inherited, action was required to remedy these evils. There was also another kind of action agenda. Morel believed, though he did not develop the point, that the degenerate should be sequestered.[83]

In every country, Morel had his signal advocates, representatives on mission to carry the doctrine of degeneration to the local psychiatric community. In Central Europe, it was Viennese psychiatry professor Richard von Krafft-Ebing, who is remembered by posterity mainly as the author of *Psychopathia Sexualis*, a kind of schoolboy's masturbatory compendium published in 1886 of what would later be called the alternative sexualities. Yet *Psychopathia Sexualis* merely gave Krafft-Ebing later notoriety. What lent him his initial authority were the big textbooks on forensic psychiatry and general psychiatry he wrote in the 1870s.

Born and educated in Germany, in the late 1860s Krafft-Ebing was a staff psychiatrist at the Illenau asylum in Baden when he first warned readers of Morelian degeneration as a cause of criminality.[84] Later he declared, "Madness, when it finally breaks out, represents only the last link in the psychopathic chain of constitutional heredity, or degenerate heredity."[85] This was good Morelian doctrine, and its amplification in Central Europe increased as Krafft-Ebing himself climbed. In 1874, he became director of the provincial asylum in Graz, Austria, and professor of psychiatry at the university there. Five years later he wrote a textbook that became the German bible of degeneration theory. A sample: "[In degenerates] it is specially frequent for sexual functioning to be abnormal, in so far as there is either no sexual drive at all, or it is abnormally strong, manifesting itself explosively and seeking satisfaction impulsively, or abnormally early, stirring already in early childhood and leading to masturbation. Or it may appear perversely, meaning that the kind of satisfaction is not oriented to reproduction."[86] By the time he wrote *Psychopathia Sexualis* in 1886, Krafft-Ebing, shortly to be summoned to a chair in Vienna, was seeing degeneration literally under the bed. The onanists, homosexuals, and premature ejaculators who paraded through its pages (later editions became even more colorful) were virtually without exception stamped as "degenerates."[87] The book remains a classic example of psychiatry run off the rails, of the misuse of scientific authority to demonize cultural preferences. As one colleague said of Krafft-Ebing, "He was a man who was gifted in literary terms, yet scientifically and critically he was incapable to the point of feeblemindedness."[88]

In France, Valentin Magnan became the main standard-bearer of degeneration after Morel's death in 1873. Magnan first warmed to the subject in his lectures at Sainte-Anne in 1882, producing a decade later a widely read summary of the subject. Coming as he did after Darwin, Magnan interpreted the degenerates as losers in an epochal battle for survival among the species. A society that did not wish to succumb in the "hereditary struggle for life" would trim its load of degeneration, he said in 1895 with his collaborator Maurice Paul Legrain.[89] "Degeneracy is more than an individual disease, it is a social menace: It is important to combat it with a rigorous form of social hygiene. One must not forget that the degenerate is often a dangerous individual against whom society should and must reserve the right to defend itself." Even better, the authors hinted ambiguously in the last sentence of their work that one might "cut off the problem at its roots."[90] Subsequent developments did not belie the ominousness of this promise.

Although it was Sankey who in 1857 introduced Morel's ideas to England, their primary apostle was Henry Maudsley.[91] As early as 1870, Maudsley suggested, with Morel, that his colleagues search for the stigmata of degeneracy in "malformations of the external ear . . . tics, grimaces, or other spasmodic movements of muscles of face, eyelids or lips . . . stammering and defects of pronunciation," as well as in eyes that possessed "a vacantly-abstracted, or half-fearful, half-suspicious, and distrustful look." "These marks are, I believe, the outward and visible signs of an inward and invisible peculiarity of cerebral organization."[92]

These teachings were absorbed by patients and physicians alike in late Victorian England.[93] How difficult it was, noted Samuel Strahan, senior medical officer of Berrywood Asylum in Northampton, to elicit a family history of mental illness from relatives who were all terrified at the specter of degeneration in the family tree. "We are all only too well acquainted with the manner in which these people, even in the poorer ranks of life, endeavour by every means to keep from us a knowledge of such family taint." The percentage of patients with family taint ranged in the statistics considerably. Yet in Strahan's view these statistics measured mainly "the amount of prevarication and untruth practised by the relatives of the insane." In reality the "inherited insane diathesis [tendency]" was to be found in "the majority of such cases," he said.[94] This is what most British alienists came to believe by the last two decades of the nineteenth century. At Brookwood asylum in Surrey, the percentage of patients in whom physicians whiffed a hereditary causation increased from 4 percent in 1870–1872 to 40 percent by 1890–1892.[95] Doubtless, many of these patients did have a positive family history but that is not the point. It is that many members of the psychiatric profession in England and elsewhere became convinced that a juggernaut of heredity born across the generations was bearing down on their patients, which is very different from noting that a genetic component may be present among many other circumstances in the unleashing of mental illness in a given individual.

Within psychiatry itself, the belief in degeneration in the sense of an inexorably gathering genetic fate, fell relatively quickly by the wayside. By the *belle époque*, degeneration had started to go out of style among alienists. Magnan died in 1916, an isolated and disbelieved old man.[96] Samuel Strahan, the social Darwinist, left medicine and went into law. Degeneration started to become an object of ridicule among physicians.

In a lampoon of 1911, Freud's collaborator Wilhelm Stekel makes the fictional Viennese coffeehouse "At the Sign of Degeneration" (*zur Degeneration*) a rendezvous for doctors.[97]

A new generation of psychiatrists began to assess these doctrines with a cool eye. As Oswald Bumke, then a 31-year-old private docent at the psychiatric clinic in Freiburg, said in 1908: "The great edifice that the doctrine of inheritability had once erected has been demolished in recent years piece by piece, and all that remains is bits of rubble." His greatest problem at the moment was dissuading general practitioners from putting down "hereditarily burdened" (*erblich belastet*) as the cause of psychosis in their patients. Heredity does play a role, he told his target audience of family doctors, but let's not exaggerate it.[98] Other nonbiological interpretations, such as Karl Jaspers' 1913 "phenomenology" (stressing empathy with patients' subjective symptoms[99]), were gaining pride of place. Thus by the beginning of World War I, degeneration was being discredited within psychiatry. In the years between the World Wars, those who continued to preach that mental illness accelerated across the generations like an express train were viewed as marginal, eccentric figures.

But the genie was out of the bottle. In the last quarter of the nineteenth century, degeneration passed from an object of discussion within the closed world of academic psychiatry to the boulevard press. In a demonstration that ideas have consequences (and that physicians must be very careful about the correctness of what they believe before they make announcements to the public), the public seized with horror on the concept of degeneration. The educated middle classes began believing implicitly that European society was doomed unless action was taken to stem the poisoning of the well of heredity.

Novelist Émile Zola, in his series on the fortunes of the Rougon and Macquart families, depicted vast social forces battling each other, driven by the iron laws of social Darwinism; the degenerate were destined to slide under. As soon as we learn in Zola's 1885 novel *Germinal* that young Étienne Lantier's mother was a Macquart, we know that his fate is sealed:

"You shouldn't drink," Catherine says to Étienne.
"Oh, don't worry, I know I shouldn't."
Étienne nodded his head; he hated liquor with the hatred of the last-born of a race of drunkards, the hatred of one who suffered so from a wild, alcohol-steeped inheritance that the least little drop was poison to him.

But Catherine has her own hereditary problems. As the wicked Chaval sets about to rape her, "She fell back on some old ropes and stopped resisting—submitting to the male, before her time, with that hereditary submission which made the girls of her race tumble in the open air while still in their childhood."[100] On and on it goes, the characters, all victims of degeneration, driven through life by their genes.

Part and parcel of European culture, the fateful notion of degeneration was picked up by the eugenists, by social-hygienists intent on combating mental retardation with sterilization, and by antidemocratic political forces with a deep hatred of "degenerate" groups such as homosexuals and Jews. Psychiatry's responsibility for all this is only a partial one. Academic psychiatrists in the 1920s were not generally associated with right-wing doctrines of racial hygiene, though there were exceptions to this, such as the Swiss psychiatrist Ernst Rüdin who after 1907 worked at the university psychiatric clinic in Munich, and the Freiburg professor Alfred Hoche who in 1920 coauthored a justification for euthanasia.[101] Academic medicine in Germany on the whole stood waist-deep in the Nazi sewer, and bears heavy responsibility for the disaster that followed. After 1933, degeneration became an official part of Nazi ideology. Hitler's machinery of death singled out Jews, people with mental retardation, and other supposedly biological degenerates for campaigns of destruction.[102]

The Nazi abuse of genetic concepts rendered any discussion of them inadmissible for many years after 1945. The notions of degeneration and inheritability became identical in the minds of the educated middle classes. Both were synonymous with Nazi evil. After World War II, any reference to the genetic transmission of psychiatric illness, whether as one factor among many or as inexorable degeneration, became taboo. The mere discussion of psychiatric genetics would, in civil middle-class dialogue, be ruled out of court for decades to come.

The End of the First Biological Psychiatry

The first biological psychiatry as a clinical approach died long before the Nazis. It was not necessarily discredited by research findings. That's not the way paradigms change within medicine. People simply lost interest in brain anatomy once a new way of looking at psychiatric illness appeared on the horizon. The new approach saw illness vertically rather than cross-sectionally: trying to understand the patient's problems of a given moment in the context of his or her lifetime history, in contrast to the biological approach of trying to correlate the symptoms of the moment with neurological findings and with brain findings postmortem.

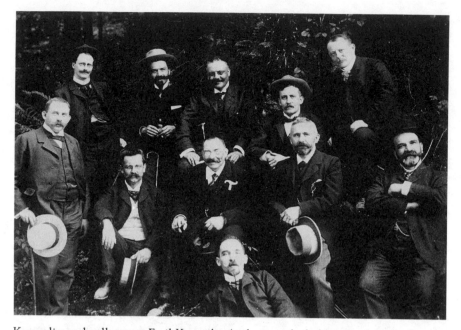

Kraepelin and colleagues. Emil Kraepelin (at lower right holding hat) and colleagues at a meeting of the Association of Southwest German Neurologists and Psychiatrists (Wanderversammlung der südwestdeutschen Neurologen und Irrenärzte), probably sometime between 1902 and 1904. Kraepelin was then professor of psychiatry at Heidelberg. From left to right in the top row are Albrecht Bethe (Strasbourg), and Aloys Alzheimer (Heidelberg). Franz Nissl (Heidelberg) seated to the left of Kraepelin cradling his characteristic walking stick in his arm. Robert Gaupp, Kraepelin's later opponent who was then at Heidelberg, is seated at lower left with hand on knee. The photograph was found in the papers of Dr. C. B. Farrar, courtesy of the estate. (Another copy of the photograph, with some incorrect identifying information, was published in the German edition of Emil Kraepelin's autobiography.)

Seminal in introducing this new vertical manner of looking at illness was Emil Kraepelin.

It is Kraepelin, not Freud, who is the central figure in the history of psychiatry. Freud was a neurologist who did not see patients with psychotic illness. His doctrine of psychoanalysis, based on intuitive leaps of fantasy, did not stand the test of time. By contrast, Kraepelin and his data cards provided the single most significant insight that the late nineteenth and early twentieth centuries had to offer into major psychiatric illness: that there are several principal types, that they have very different courses, and that their nature may be appreciated through the systematic study of large numbers of cases. Ironically, Kraepelin, in his impatience with hypothetical theories about the brain, brought the first biological psychiatry to an end.

The American Kraepelin was Adolf Meyer, who helped to terminate the first biological psychiatry in the United States. Although Meyer never became an international figure (his brief vogue in Britain notwithstanding), he was the most prominent American psychiatrist before World War II, and his distinctive style did much to shape and misshape the evolution of American psychiatry in general. One is therefore entitled to speak of Kraepelin and Meyer in the same breath, keeping in mind that the influence of the former was worldwide and enduring, and that of the latter evanescent and parochial—yet important in the American story.

Kraepelin's psychiatric career began in revolt against biological psychiatry.[103] Born in 1856 in North Germany, he earned his MD in 1878 at Würzburg, then went down to Munich to serve as a resident of the brain biologist Bernhard von Gudden. The clinic in Munich, founded in 1859, had figured among the early university psychiatric clinics, even before that of Griesinger. Gudden, the second chief of that clinic, belonged to the generation that believed the mysteries of psychiatry could be unfolded through the microscope. Many influential researchers, such as the Swiss August Forel, graduated from the Munich clinic.

As Kraepelin, a cool North German arrived in Munich, he became friendly with a young doctor from the Bavarian Palatinate named Franz Nissl, also a resident. But while Nissl, Gudden, and all the others were busy looking at brains through their microscopes, Kraepelin could not take part because he had an eye problem. Unlike the other Munichers, Kraepelin was also extremely interested in human psychology as a dimension of psychiatric illness. He had been keen on psychology since youth, and as a medical student avidly read the work of the experimental psychologist Wilhelm Wundt, who is considered the virtual founder of modern psychology. When Wundt established a psychological laboratory in 1879 at Leipzig, Kraepelin, the young psychiatrist, vowed to go there and study with him. Thus with Gudden's blessing, Kraepelin left Munich in 1882.

Kraepelin's attraction to psychology, and his repulsion at anatomically oriented psychiatry, were strengthened by his experiences in Leipzig. To earn his living, he had to work as an assistant with Paul Flechsig, whose only interest lay in the microscope and dissecting table. Kraepelin so hated Flechsig that he left his service after three months and plunged himself further into psychological studies with Wundt. In a story similar to that of Griesinger, who was young and inexperienced when he wrote a textbook, at 27 Kraepelin too attempted a textbook, a slim *Compendium* of no particular merit published in 1883.[104] He wrote it because he wanted to marry and needed the money.[105]

Kraepelin at this point was in almost the exact situation in which Freud found himself during these years: having to make a living because of a decision to marry. In 1884, Kraepelin became an asylum physician, just as Freud in 1886 entered private practice to earn a livelihood. But unlike Freud, luck struck early for Kraepelin. In 1886, he received a professorship of psychiatry at what was then Dorpat University, after World War I called Tartu University, in the Estonian city of the same name.

At Dorpat, Kraepelin started to become intrigued with the kind of observation that had failed to interest the Gudden school: What happened to patients at the end of the road? How did their illnesses turn out? Yet his inability to speak Estonian left him unable to investigate the subject systematically.

In 1890, Kraepelin left marginal Dorpat for a professorship of psychiatry at Heidelberg, a university clinic at the epicenter of German academic life. At Heidelberg, moreover, there was no pressure on psychiatrists to do neurology, which was treated in a separate clinic. Here Kraepelin came into his own. He could now combine his interest in patients' illness trajectories with the psychological approach he personally favored. He could also incorporate in the Heidelberg clinic the anatomical psychiatry he had learned at Munich and which was still de rigueur for the day. Kraepelin undertook two innovations in particular. He began keeping little cards on each of his patients, noting previous history and condition at discharge. Second, in imitation of the comprehensive Griesinger-style department of psychiatry, Kraepelin wanted to surround himself with the best researchers available.

The people Kraepelin brought to the university psychiatric clinic in Heidelberg read like an honor roll of turn-of-the-century German neuroscience. In 1895, he lured his old Munich chum Franz Nissl to Heidelberg from the Frankfurt city asylum, which was then—under the dynamic Emil Sioli—something of a research center and not just a city lockup. Nissl was by now a famous neurohistologist who had discovered stains that permitted the nuclei and other structures of nerve cells to be seen, making possible the division of the cerebral cortex into numerous local areas and cell layers.[106] A curious man with a blunt demeanor, a large birthmark on his face, and an absolute indifference to sartorial display, Nissl was also well known among insiders for his bizarre work habits, spending the time from seven in the evening until dawn at his lab bench.[107] Working alongside Nissl at the Frankfurt asylum was another gifted young neurohistologist named Aloys Alzheimer, discoverer in 1906 of the disease later named after him.[108] Alzheimer and Nissl were great friends and notorious workaholics, and Alzheimer too was known for sleeping during the day and working through the night at his microscope. Alzheimer followed his friend to the Heidelberg clinic in 1903. (The two were otherwise as unalike as cheese and chalk, Alzheimer an expansive family man, Nissl an obsessive-compulsive bachelor.) So on the organic side, the Heidelberg clinic had the two great students of the microscopic structure of the brain.

Although Kraepelin's interest in psychology was now waning, he nonetheless included measurement of patients' mental functions as part of their workup. He sought to engage bright young psychologically oriented physicians such as Willy Hellpach (who like Kraepelin had studied with Wundt[109]) to foster his larger plan of a comprehensive psychiatry ranging from the patients' dreams to their cerebral cortexes. Yet the emphasis was to be neither on psychology nor neuroanatomy but on the patient's course of illness across the years.

Looking at outcomes in psychiatric illness, and differentiating distinct diseases on the basis of those outcomes formed the essence of the Kraepelinian revolution. As the principal vehicle for disseminating his ideas, Kraepelin chose not scholarly articles but successive editions of the textbook he had begun in 1883. Starting with the third edition in 1893, new editions of this manual began to follow each other in close succession. So startling were the views Kraepelin began announcing that the entire psychiatric world would follow each new edition with rapt interest.[110]

Consider the state of psychiatric diagnosis before Kraepelin went to work. A half century of research in neuroanatomy and neuropathology had produced almost nothing in the way of concrete utility to clinical psychiatry beyond a picture of neurosyphilis. The biological psychiatrists had spawned a sprawl of clinical disease labels, each based on the particular circumstances associated with an illness ("masturbatory insanity," "wedding-night psychosis") or on the particular combination of symptoms ("chronic delusional disorder"), with almost no correlation to brain pathology. Multi-infarct dementia, neurosyphilis, thyroid deficiency, and the like were the only exceptions.

Yet before Kraepelin went to work, several fundamental issues had already been clarified. The notion of classifying diseases on the basis of course, or outcome, had already been raised by Karl Kahlbaum, one of the most neglected figures in the history of psychiatry. As a young physician at the Prussian state asylum at Allenberg, Kahlbaum had been irritated by Heinrich Neumann's assertion in 1859 that psychotic illness could not be

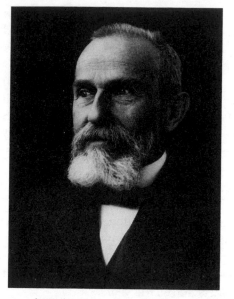

Eugen Bleuler, professor of psychiatry in Zurich 1898–1927, as seen around 1920. Bleuler coined the term "schizophrenia" in 1908 and was friendly for a while to Freud and the psychoanalytic movement (courtesy Psychiatrische Universitätsklinik Zurich).

subdivided into distinct diseases because there was only one "unitary psychosis" (Einheitspsychose).[111] In 1863, Kahlbaum responded that indeed there were many distinct illnesses, one of which was psychosis in the young, which Kahlbaum called "hebephrenia."[112] Three years later, he left the public sector for the private, becoming assistant physician at a private nervous clinic in Görlitz. Taking over the clinic himself in 1867, Kahlbaum added a youth division, a "Medical Paedagogium," which gave him plenty of opportunity to see psychotic patients in their teens and early 20s. As Kahlbaum became the chief at Görlitz, he brought over from Allenberg a 24-year-old colleague, Ewald Hecker. The two worked together, and in 1871 Hecker wrote an article applying Kahlbaum's notion of hebephrenia to several clinical cases, describing in detail a malady specific to the young, resulting in mental disorientation and psychosis, and having a downhill course.[113] This was the first clinical description of schizophrenia with the claim that it represented a distinctive disease. Thus Kraepelin had Kahlbaum and Hecker to build on.

He also had the work of two physicians at the Salpêtrière—Jean-Pierre Falret and Jules Baillarger—who had established in the early

1850s that mania and depression often occur not merely as isolated symptoms but in tandem with one another, alternating over a person's life course as "circular insanity."[114] (In 1899, Kraepelin would rebaptize this as "manic-depressive illness.") These French physicians had thus handed Kraepelin another building block, underpinning the notion that psychiatric illness consisted of an edifice of such building blocks, independent disease entities different in their symptoms and their outcomes.

Kraepelin and his residents would typically fill out a card for each patient and put them in the "diagnosis box." After they had had a chance to study the patient, they would take the cards out again and enter on a list the patient's name and revised diagnosis. When the patient was discharged, the end result would be noted on the list. "In this manner we were able to get an overview and see which diagnoses had been incorrect and the reasons that had led us to this false conception."[115] On vacation, Kraepelin would take the lists and cards away with him and try to sort things out.

Only in the 1893 edition of his textbook did he discover that his file cards had started to make sense. In the preface, Kraepelin emphasized that all he knew he had learned from experience, that data gathered from patients lay behind every assertion, and that his ultimate objective was to try and cut nature at the joints: to identify natural disease entities.[116] Kraepelin's classification at this point was quite conventional, mostly concepts taken over from his predecessors. His typology did, however, contain one of the products of his card file: "psychic processes of degeneration," meaning illnesses that end in dementia. One subcategory of these was "premature dementia," or *dementia praecox.*

Kraepelin did not acknowledge, if he in fact knew, that Morel had first used the phrase dementia praecox in writings in 1852 and 1860.[117] But even before Morel—and later quite independently of him—other psychiatric writers had been talking about adolescent insanity. In 1873, Edinburgh psychiatrist Thomas Clouston described the "insanity of pubescence," which he also termed somewhat reluctantly the "hereditary insanity of adolescence."[118] In 1891, Clouston took another stab at the subject, calling it now "adolescent insanity and its secondary dementia."[119] Other physicians chimed in too. In August 1890 at a psychiatry meeting in Rouen, Parisian psychiatrist Albert Charpentier gave a paper on "les démences précoces," among which were included "les démences de la puberté."[120] By 1893, the notion of "démence précoce" was more or less in the psychiatric air.

Kraepelin's 1893 textbook was a historic document. He described in great detail what Hecker—whom Kraepelin believed to be the major previous authority—had only adumbrated in 1871. Kraepelin thought that the cause of dementia praecox was biological, using the term "psychopathic predisposition" (the 1890s equivalent of the 1990s euphemism "neurodevelopmental in origin").[121] The achievement of this 1893 work was formidable. In giving a careful account of dementia praecox, or schizophrenia, as a distinct disease, Kraepelin had handed psychiatry its most powerful term of the twentieth century.

Surprises continued to unfold in later editions of this famous textbook. In 1896, in the reshuffling of file cards that produced the fifth edition, Kraepelin scrapped the part about degeneration. Dementia praecox was now a "metabolic disorder," set, to everyone's astonishment, next to thyroid psychosis and neurosyphilis. Yet what gripped his readers' attention most was his declaration in the preface that he was tired of grouping disorders according to their symptoms; he wanted to get to the inner nature of the illnesses, "as manifest in their course and outcome." "I have abandoned any effort to classify [psychosis] on the basis of the clinical presentation."[122] This was a decisive statement of Kraepelin's shift from studying the presumed causes of psychiatric illness, such as genetics, brain biology, and so forth, to concentrate on classifying illness in a way that would let one predict outcome. Prognosis, not cause, is the single most important word in understanding Kraepelin.

In this fifth edition in 1896, Kraepelin declared he was starting to put biological psychiatry behind him, deciding to concentrate instead on a psychiatry based on bedside observation of patients over time. He was not denying the validity of biological psychiatry, but simply declaring himself agnostic: "As long as we are unable clinically to group illnesses on the basis of cause, and to separate dissimilar causes, our views about etiology will necessarily remain unclear and contradictory."[123] In other words, cause is something that we, in our present state of knowledge, cannot know.

In the sixth edition of 1899, Kraepelin's ideas reached their definitive form, resulting in a classification of illness that provided the basis of the later *Diagnostic and Statistical Manual of Mental Disorders* of the American Psychiatric Association, the authoritative guide for world psychiatry in our own time (see pp. 565–580). Yet the point of all this classification, Kraepelin stressed, was not just ivory-tower pigeonholing but producing a psychiatry meaningful for patients and their families. Identifying natural disease entities should permit the physician to answer the question: Will my husband recover from his illness? As Kraepelin said in 1899, "The doctor's first task at the bedside is being able to form a judgment about the probable further course of the case. People always ask him this. The value

106

of a diagnosis for the practical activity of the psychiatrist consists of letting him give a reliable look at the future."[124]

Kraepelin decided to divide all psychiatric illness into 13 big groups, most of which were familiar (neurosis, febrile psychosis, mental retardation, and the like). Only two of the groups electrified his readers, and this is because Kraepelin had now split the vast world of those psychotic illnesses without an obvious organic cause into two neat camps: illnesses involving an affective component, and those without an affective component. (Affect means mood, whether the patient is depressed, manic, or anxious.) As he justified this dramatic compression of almost all affective illnesses into a single disease he said, "In the course of the years I have become more and more convinced that all [of the periodic and circular psychoses plus mania] are really just manifestations of a single disease process."[125] This process he labeled "manic-depressive psychosis" *(das manisch-depressive Irresein)*.

This division of insanity into two big groups made diagnosis quite simple. If the patients were melancholic or euphoric, cried all the time, were always tired without a cause, or displayed any of the other signs of depression or mania, they were classed as "manic-depressive illness." If they were psychotic in the absence of an affective component, they had dementia praecox. If they were manic-depressive, they would probably get better; if they had what everybody was soon abbreviating as "d.p.," they probably wouldn't.

Thus by 1899, Kraepelin had elevated the two greater nonorganic ("functional") psychoses—manic-depressive illness and schizophrenia—to the top of the pyramid, where they remain in only slightly modified form to this day as the object of endeavor of serious psychiatry. "Old maid's insanity," "monomania," "moon madness," and the rest of it had been reduced to these two diseases, whose diagnosis could be made on the basis of the patient's history and current symptoms, and whose course could be predicted. The concept of prognosis was the vaulting stone of the entire arch: Patients with manic-depressive illness had a circular disorder that naturally would improve; patients with dementia praecox would deteriorate into what Kraepelin considered to be "dementia," or at least three-quarters of them would; a quarter of Kraepelin's dementia praecox patients recovered. Rather than reassuring patients and their families, Kraepelin's classification terrified them—unfairly so in retrospect. In fact, patients with schizophrenia do not become demented, they retain their intelligence, although their thought processes may become disorganized.

In recognition that these patients were not demented and that the onset was not necessarily early, in 1908 Zurich psychiatry professor Eugen

Bleuler—who considered himself to be a faithful student of Kraepelin's—proposed the term "schizophrenia" for what Kraepelin had been calling dementia praecox.[126] Yet at the meeting of the German Psychiatric Society at which Bleuler made this suggestion, and later in his 1911 book on "schizophrenia," Bleuler did shift the discussion somewhat from physical symptoms such as catatonia (rigid postures) to imputed psychological processes such as the French psychiatrist Pierre Janet's "splitting" of consciousness.[127] The term schizophrenia was probably an unfortunate choice, for subsequent generations of physicians and nonphysicians alike would associate it with some kind of splitting or divided consciousness. In schizophrenia, nothing is split. The disease is characterized by delusions, hallucinations, and disordered thought.

Yet these are lesser details. The main point is that the majesty of Kraepelin's overall structure transfixed the psychiatric world. For one thing, the interpretation of mental symptoms had been dethroned. The content of the psychosis no longer mattered. The precise symptoms the patient evidenced were unremarkable unless they gave evidence of the cause (neurosyphilis, thyroid disorder, etc.), or the course and outcome. Gasped Adolf Meyer in 1904, "The terms of a tradition of over 2,000 years are overthrown."[128]

In addition to providing a new way of classifying illness, Kraepelin's structure insisted that there were a number of discrete psychiatric illnesses, or diseases, each separate from the next. Depression, schizophrenia, and so forth were different just as mumps and pneumonia were different. Finally, being "Kraepelinian" meant that one operated within a "medical model" rather than a "biopsychosocial" model, as the battle lines later became drawn. A medically oriented psychiatrist believed in approaching psychiatric illness just as a cardiologist would approach heart disease, while remaining mindful that the psyche is subject to cultural shaping in ways that the heart is not. A psychiatrist attuned to Freudian or Meyerian biopsychosocial views might see illness more as the result of one's personal misadventures than of constitutional forces.

Kraepelin's doctrines were not received with complete approbation. Some psychiatrists refused to accept giving up syndromes (symptoms that seem to hang together reliably whatever the long-term outcome) and balked at subordinating all illnesses to these two huge categories. Alfred Hoche, the Freiburg psychiatrist who was proud of his own doctrine of supposedly immutable syndromes, sneered at Kraepelin's "annual opinions," a reference to how the textbook kept changing.[129] Others resented Kraepelin's self-assured didacticism, the worldly Viennese psychiatrist Constantin von Economo calling him, "a North

German village schoolmaster writ large."[130] The biological psychiatrists were unhappy at the dismissal of their doctrines: Wernicke scorned Kraepelin's work as "facile" (*feuilletonisch*).[131]

Internationally, Kraepelin's schema encountered greatest resistance among the French, who clung determinedly to Magnan's elaborate distinctions long after they had been abandoned elsewhere. There was a wonderful encounter in Paris as Nissl took the young American psychiatrist Clarence Farrar on an excursion to see Magnan's clinic. "Magnan," said Farrar much later, "had dropped everything to give us a field-day in his clinic. . . . The high point of the day was a brilliant, detailed demonstration of a very special case by Magnan himself."

Magnan demonstrated a patient as an "indubious example" of the chronic delusional disorder with downhill course (*délire chronique à évolution systématique*) that he himself had described. "Nissl listened with closest attention, now and then nodding appreciatively as the Frenchman made some fine psychological analysis of symptoms. The presentation complete, Magnan hopefully awaited Nissl's comment."

It was brief and direct: "A quite typical case of dementia praecox."

Farrar and Nissl learned the next day that after they had left, "Magnan had gone to his office, bowed his head over his desk, and wept."[132]

Kraepelin and his coworkers put an end to biological psychiatry as the dominant school, although individual representatives of this first biological school lingered on adjusting their microscopes into the 1920s. And it was not just because Kraepelin, agnostic about cause, had declared anatomy to be unimportant. It was because Kraepelin's microscopist colleagues themselves, such as Nissl, also helped to extinguish the notion that all psychiatric disorders had to have a basis in the brain. What Nissl and Alzheimer could find under their microscopes they declared "neurology." What they couldn't find was psychiatry. As Nissl said in 1908, "It was a bad mistake not to realize that the findings of brain anatomy bore no relationship to psychiatric findings, unless the relationships between brain anatomy and brain function were first clarified, and they certainly have not been up to the present."[133] In the second biological psychiatry, people would realize that Nissl had given away too much.

An American Postscript

The story has an American postscript. Standing as a watershed in the United States was Adolf Meyer, a sort of American Kraepelin. Meyer's initial embrace of Kraepelin brought the doctrines of dementia praecox

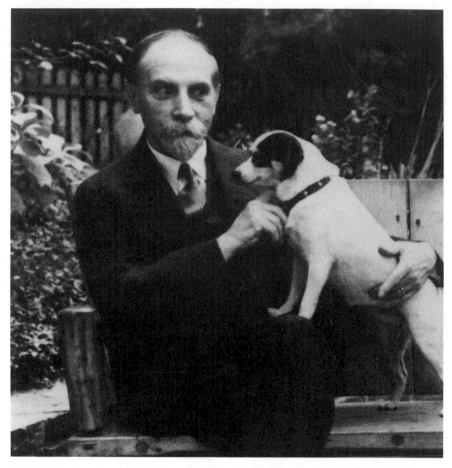

Adolf Meyer, professor of psychiatry at Johns Hopkins University 1910–1941. The most prominent American psychiatrist of his day, he indiscriminately advocated all forms of psychiatric thinking from the biological to the psychoanalytic (courtesy of the Alan Mason Chesney Medical Archives of the Johns Hopkins Medical Institutions).

and manic-depressive illness to the United States, breaking with the old biological psychiatry. And Meyer's later rejection of Kraepelin helped plunge the United States into its psychoanalytic adventure.

Meyer was not the only American psychiatrist to adopt Kraepelin's new system, as a whole squadron of young researchers regularly traveled back and forth from the Heidelberg clinic to their U.S. home bases. August Hoch, for example—who was originally Swiss but had a medical degree from the University of Maryland—had been hired in 1893 at the McLean Hospital in Belmont as a pathologist, a thoroughly biological type. After making several trips to Heidelberg, he started to lose interest (to the dismay of the McLean's superintendent) in laboratory studies and turned instead to "clinical" work, the kind of thing Kraepelin had been doing. In the mid-1890s, Hoch persuaded the hospital to adopt the Kraepelinian system, resulting in a reclassification of all the records.[134]

In 1896, Meyer himself imported the Kraepelinian system to the Worcester asylum, where he had been hired as pathologist.[135] And though it was largely forgotten in the later celebration of Meyer as an enthusiast of psychoanalysis, in the beginning Meyer was a confirmed Kraepelinian, writing in 1897 of Kraepelin's "excellent work concerning clinical psychiatry."[136] He remained for years under Kraepelin's influence. When he took the professorship of psychiatry at Hopkins in 1910, it was to help shape a German-style psychiatric clinic that had already been planned, and that would open its doors in 1913. The clinic was an elegant four-storied structure with windows guarded unobtrusively but not barred, a roof garden, and accommodations whose lavishness reminded more ribald staff members of "a general paralytic's dream."[137] There is no doubt that the model in Meyer's mind was Emil Kraepelin's brand-new psychiatric clinic in Munich (Kraepelin had gone from Heidelberg to Munich in 1904). The Phipps clinic, with its comprehensive facilities for both the psychological and the laboratory investigation of patients, had been very much cast in the Kraepelinian model.

But Meyer went further. He insisted on the integration of psychiatry into the rest of a general hospital, and treated psychiatry patients as "medical" in a way that went beyond even the Germans. Patients arrived at the Phipps clinic in an ambulance, for example, not in handcuffs, and usually were not under a certificate.[138]

It is puzzling, therefore, that Meyer later acquired the reputation of having always been anti-Kraepelinian.[139] One explanation is that his earlier writings had simply been forgotten, the bulk of his collected works appearing only after 1950, the year of his death. Certainly psychiatry's collective memory has blacked out that Meyer, the most honored American psychiatrist of the twentieth century, was once an ardent believer in degeneration. In 1895, for example, he called the ear a guide to nature's ample variety of types of "degeneration."[140] Meyer was even upset that Kraepelin had thrown out the notion of degeneration![141] Perhaps there was some amnesia.

An even greater obstacle to situating Meyer was Meyer himself. A second-rate thinker and a verbose writer, he was never, in his own mind, able to disentangle schools that were absolutely incompatible, and ended up embracing whatever new came along. Thus Meyer fervently saluted the maniacal Trenton psychiatrist Henry Cotton, who believed in pulling out his patients' teeth and removing their large bowels to cure psychiatric illness caused, as Cotton believed, by "autointoxication." Meyer urged that this work, the "remarkable achievement of the pioneer spirit," be continued after Cotton's death in 1933.[142]

Yet later in life, Meyer did reject Kraepelin. He also put biological psychiatry behind him, which is not at all the same thing. Meyer ventured forth his own psychosocial models of mental illness, and turned his back on Kraepelinian classification in favor of his own bizarre terminology of "reaction types," employing such neologisms as "ergasiology," "pathergasias," and "kakergasias."[143] (The notion of reaction types itself came directly from such German anti-Kraepelinians as Ludwig Binswanger.) As for the causation of psychiatric illness, Meyer ended up adopting the position that everything is very complex.[144] Although true at one level, this kind of throwing up of the hands in despair to concentrate on collecting even more "facts" (Meyer's wont) is poisonous to the advance of a scientific discipline.

For better or worse, Meyer's soaring reputation brought the advance of the first biological psychiatry in the United States to an end. By the 1940s, he would be calling schizophrenia "psychogenic" and urging psychotherapy as the treatment of choice.[145] On both sides of the Atlantic, looking for the causes of mental illness in the biology of the brain had become a thing of the past.

CHAPTER

4

Nerves

What was biological psychiatry for doctors was nerves for patients. Early in the nineteenth century, families brought patients to the asylum not for madness but for imputed nervous illness. Early in the twentieth century, it was nervous illness that provided the platform for private, office-based psychiatry in the treatment of the neuroses. Nerves are, then, central to the history of psychiatry, a great irony considering that diseases of the nerves, properly understood, lie in the province of neurology rather than psychiatry.

Here the social history of psychiatry enters in. Patients found the notion of suffering from a physical disorder of the nerves far more reassuring than learning that their problem was insanity. And until the victory of psychoanalysis in the 1940s, physicians were willing to go along with the fiction that both major and minor psychiatric illnesses were "nervous" in nature. Why psychiatrists were willing to concede to patients this fig leaf is an important issue, permitting us to understand some of the basic forces driving the history of psychiatry. For psychiatrists, the fig leaf of nerves offered a chance to escape the asylum for lucrative private practice with middle-class patients. For patients, this camouflage presented an opportunity to escape the opprobrium of madness and the implications of hereditary illness and degeneration. Unlike psychiatric illness, nervous illness was thought for the most part to be noninheritable and thus nonstigmatizing. In nervous illness, the symbiosis between doctor and patient was perfect: Psychiatrists (meaning the kinds of physicians who would be called psychiatrists after World War II) underwent a big leap up in their social stature and income as they became urban nerve-specialists, electrotherapists, neuropsychiatrists, and the like. And patients experienced the vast relief of knowing that their problems were really "organic" rather than constituting evidence of hereditarian family degeneration or being "all in their heads."

Nerves Better than Madness

"True!—nervous—very, very dreadfully nervous I had been and am," said the protagonist of Edgar Allen Poe's short story "The Tell-Tale Heart" in 1842, "but why *will* you say that I am mad?"

Why might he be thought mad? For one thing, he could hear from a distance the beating of the heart of the old man he was about to kill: "It grew quicker and quicker, and louder and louder every instant. The old man's terror *must* have been extreme! It grew louder, I say, louder every moment!—do you mark me well? I have told you that I am nervous: so I am."[1]

The pleading of this obviously distracted individual to be considered "nervous" and not insane echoed the pleading of a century, the nineteenth century as the nervous century. It is initially in the horror of the asylum and of the alienist that we can understand the insistence of the population on nervous disease.

From the beginning, the notion of being confined in an asylum evoked fear and loathing among the public. How could it have been otherwise with stories such as that of poor William Norris at Bethlem chained up for 10 years.[2] "The public asylum in Vienna," said Bruno Goergen in 1820, owner of a select private asylum, "just as perhaps all public institutions of this kind, is detested so widely in public opinion that it is scarcely necessary for me to enlarge upon the reasons for this detestation."[3] Public laments resounded down the decades: the asylum as a place of unlawful confinement, of abuse, and of scenes of horror. The alienists' vehement protestations that virtually no sane person was ever confined, or that psychiatrists were honorable physicians and not beasts, were unable to prevail against impressions created by such novels as Charles Reade's *Hard Cash*, published around 1863.

In *Hard Cash*, the wrongly confined Alfred attempts to bribe the attendant with a hundred pounds to let him out:

> A coarse laugh greeted the proposal. "You might as well have made it a thousand when you was about it."
> "So I will," said Alfred, "and thank you on my knees besides." Alfred protested that he had the money.

"Well, you are green," replied the attendant. "Do you think them as sent you here will let you spend your money? No, your money is theirs now."[4]

As the air filled with talk of degeneration after the 1860s, this fear of the asylum became a desperate panic to avoid at all costs the confinement of a relative in an insane asylum. The parents of a deeply melancholic young man in Zurich were, in the 1890s, anything but sympathetic when it was suggested to them that their son needed institutional care: "It's inconsiderate of him not just to pull himself together . . . because his three sisters are just coming into marriageable age and their suitors will surely be frightened off. Nobody wants to marry into a family with mental illness." Another set of parents decided to act only after their son had lain motionless in bed for three years, never speaking a word during this time. Still other parents summoned the resolution only after noting, as they told the clinic, "Our son imagines that he is a horse."[5]

The doctrine of degeneration meant that it was not merely the asylum that threatened the family and its honor but the psychiatrist and his menacing diagnoses. After the 1860s, the profession's conventional terms for psychiatric illness began to ring with awfulness. The notion that major psychiatric disorders came from poisoned heredity instilled in the public a kind of permanent dread. Never tell patients they have hypochondria, counseled the owners of a private nervous clinic in Austria: They will look it up in the dictionary and discover that it means "insanity."[6] Sir Andrew Clark, a distinguished internist at the London Hospital, was said in giving an opinion to have dropped the word "melancholia." "The outcome of that visit was disastrous, entailing serious trouble all round, in which even Sir Andrew himself shared, for he was pestered for weeks with letters to know whether in using the term 'melancholia' he had the idea of insanity in his mind."[7]

In Germany, turn-of-the-century psychiatrists were appalled at public benightedness in shunning the "odium psychiatricum."[8] People were willing to credit fantastical stories in which madmen switched identity with mayors. As a psychiatric editor recounted one such story: The Herr Bürgermeister was supposed to transport a madman to the asylum. "Underway he is said to have gone to sleep after a few glasses of beer, whereupon the patient exchanged papers with him. At the asylum the patient is reported to have legitimated himself as the mayor, handing over his horrified companion to the care of the institution. Only after a few days of greatest desperation is the misunderstanding said to have been clarified." Such reports actually circulated in the German popular press, fortifying the impression that psychiatry meant danger.[9]

It comes therefore as no surprise that turn-of-the-century Germany already had its own antipsychiatry groups. "What do we want?" asked the budding movement for the Reform of Psychiatric Law and Psychiatric Treatment in 1909. "We want to damn secretiveness, deception, and hypocrisy as unworthy of humankind." Its journal was filled with tales on the order of, "How Beuthen City Councilman Lubecki was Tortured in the Madhouse."[10]

With the press overflowing with stories of madmen switching roles with mayors and city councilpersons tortured in asylums, neither in Germany nor elsewhere did psychiatry have a terribly bright future. Unlike the rest of medicine, said Freiburg psychiatrist Alfred Hoche in his memoirs, the patient sees the doctor not as a friend but an enemy. Young doctors going into psychiatry had to understand, said Hoche, "that their relationship to the patient becomes a quite different one. Normally, patients see the physician as helper, because they hope he will remove their symptoms and effect a cure. But here they reject the idea that they are ill and need a physician's help. Indeed the doctor in their opinion is often the enemy." Then Hoche added an interesting observation: "This situation is not so apparent in the psychiatric clinics that treat nervous patients."[11]

It was not difficult to figure out that if psychiatry was to have a future outside the asylum, it must be under the rubric of nerves, and not under the proper descriptive term psychiatry. The latter had come to signify inexorable hereditary madness, while nervous illness implied merely an organic affliction of the nerves not necessarily hereditary in nature and not dangerous to the marriage prospects of one's daughters. This insight dawned on practitioners almost from the founding of the discipline itself, and the vast majority of psychiatric care in past times was delivered under the label nervous illness rather than psychiatry.

Although the category of nervous illness as a variety of psychoneurosis dated back to Cheyne in the 1730s, only in the first decades of the nineteenth century did nerves start to become a euphemism for psychosis. From the 1830s on, psychiatric illness—or "insanity"—became increasingly translated in the public mind as nervous illness. And psychiatrists in their communications to the public tended to use nerves, nervous, or some variation on this theme when they meant organic, brain, biological, constitutional, or some variation on that theme. This was a massive duplicity, a century-long deception of the public to the effect that illness meant a disorder of the nerves when in fact the brain was meant. While the patients believed their "nervous" problems stemmed from overwork (among the middle classes) and humoral imbalances (among the lower), doctors believed nervous problems to be constitutional in nature and possessing a heavy genetic component. Although both doctors and patients used the same terms, the malentendu could not have been more complete.

Why did this kind of deception—the kind of deception that occurs today when doctors tell patients they are suffering from "stress"[12]—seem necessary? There is always great pressure on physicians to tell patients what they want to hear, a pressure that affects psychiatrists in particular where an upbeat mood is supposed to be the outcome of therapy. What Bernard Shaw said in 1911 about the doctor-patient relationship in general was not necessarily intended for psychiatry, though it might well have been:

> The doctor who has to live by pleasing his patients in competition with everybody who has walked the hospitals, scraped through the examinations, and bought a brass plate, soon finds himself prescribing water to teetotallers and brandy or champagne jelly to drunkards; beefsteaks and stout in one house, and "uric acid free" vegetarian diet over the way; shut windows, big fires, and heavy overcoats to old Colonels, and open air and as much nakedness as is compatible with decency to young faddists, never once daring to say either "I don't know," or "I don't agree."[13]

The inference is that nineteenth-century psychiatrists felt themselves under much duress to convey to patients notions of the cause and nature of their illnesses that the patients wanted to hear.

"I was termed a nervous patient," said John Perceval, an English gentleman admitted in 1831 to the Brisslington private asylum. Perceval had been hearing voices and seeing visions. His mother "suffered from extreme nervousness" too, "during which she could scarcely endure, and even forbade a newspaper being unfolded in her room, so greatly did she feel the need of quiet."[14] Glad to accommodate such wealthy families as the Percevals, in 1835 Evans Riadore, a Harley-Street doctor in London, called nervous affections specially common "amongst the higher classes of society." These disorders "so embitter their lives, as to render their portion of worldly enjoyment nearly on a level with that of the poor and laborious."[15]

French writers chose to speak in these years not of melancholia—a psychotic illness apt for the asylum—but of "nervous erethism," a term encompassing irritability, emotional instability, and depression. Such erethism, situated particularly among urbanites accustomed to "luxury," was said to be on the rise.[16]

In Germany, with its large concentration of private clinics, this vogue for nervous illness began showing up early in institutional name changes. Dr. Adolf Albrecht Erlenmeyer's private asylum, founded in 1847 as a "Private-Institution for the Insane and Idiots," had 10 years later become a "Private Institution for Brain and Nervous Disease." In 1858, Dr. Erlenmeyer explained that his clinic was for "fully-developed forms of mental disturbance (curable and incurable) as well as for early forms, sufferers of which are starting to be designated with the name nervous patients [Nervenkranke]."[17] Sometime between 1858 and 1876, the private asylum in Eitorf in the Rhine province changed the wording of its admission policy from "insane only" to "nervous patients."[18] Were these changes the result of science on the march? As Ewald Hecker, who by 1881 had terminated his association with Karl Kahlbaum and was running his own private clinic for "nervous patients" in Johannisberg-on-Rhine, put it, "Among insiders it is an open secret that this designation has been chosen only euphemistically, in order to make it easier for the relatives of an insane patient [Geisteskranke], to whom the name insane asylum appears horrifying, to bring the individual for admission."[19] By 1900, virtually every major private psychiatric clinic in Central Europe had abandoned such terms as "mentally disturbed" (psychisch-gestört) and "insane" (Irre) in favor of self-descriptions involving disorders of "nerves" and "mood" (Gemüt). In the private sector, the fiction was complete.

Such was the public's revulsion from "psychiatry," that even in the public sector in Central Europe old-style descriptions were dropped for new. In 1906, psychiatry professor Robert Sommer in Giessen was able to persuade the health ministry to accept a name change for his university psychiatry department from "Clinic for Insanity" to "Clinic for Psychiatric and Nervous Disorders." He wished the change, he said, "out of consideration for the psychiatric and voluntary nervous patients, who did not wish to be considered 'mentally ill' [Geisteskrank]."[20] When Ferdinand Kehrer was able to establish a "neuropsychiatric clinic" in Münster in 1924, "it was for the sake of the public that we simply called it a 'Nervous Clinic' [Nervenklinik]."[21]

In England, there was no suggestion of naming comparable clinics "psychiatric." When a short-stay psychiatric hospital and outpatient department were added to the Edinburgh asylum at Morningside in the 1920s, it was decided to name the place "Jordanburn Nerve Hospital and Psychological Institute." Psychiatric wasn't even in the running; one authority said that even the term "nervous" has acquired an unfortunate "popular meaning or at least suggestion. But that is not fatal, and I should prefer 'nervous' to 'psychopathic,' which is horrible." The chief physician nonetheless put "nerves" in ironical quotation marks, for he knew very well what he was treating.[22]

All this renaming occurred for no underlying scientific reason. Doctors understood Griesinger's "nervous disease" to mean biological brain disease rather than disease of the peripheral nerves. The renaming was done for the sake of the public. The asylums in Germany continued to do the classic heavy lifting of psychiatry: psychosis. "Yet the public wants to call them 'nervous'-clinics, in order to avoid that harshly ringing term 'insane'-asylum or that foreign term psychiatric," as one asylum psychiatrist said after World War I.[23]

The flight from psychiatry also spilled over to internal medicine and general hospitals: Anyplace but the asylum! the families were crying. What is the logic for separating neurology from psychiatry? asked asylum psychiatrist Paul Näcke, who wanted them separate. "Nervous patients in particular find it undesirable to be on a psychiatric ward, even in separate units or in special houses, because it is well-known that many nervous people find the immediate presence of the mentally ill oppressive and start to be filled with dread, thus delaying their own recoveries." Näcke pointed out that having psychiatric units in general hospitals would let someone with an "acute psychosis recover unnoticed, without being branded in the public eye with the mark of shame of the asylum."[24] It had thus become impossible to practice psychiatry in a straightforward manner. Physicians wishing to treat major psychiatric illness among the middle classes, and minor psychiatric illness among any group of the population whatsoever, would have to find settings that fictionalized the nature of the illness.

The Flight of Madness into the Spa

Before the advent of the modern hospital around the time of World War I, the middle classes sought their health care at watering holes and spas. There were many reasons for this. Since ancient times, water itself had been assigned a therapeutic virtue, and the particle content of the mineral springs did help to get the bowels moving and overcome constipation. Some springs rich in iodine or iron would have relieved the medical conditions caused by shortages of those substances. The placid routine of the spa doubtless allowed many to unwind from the pressures of business and sociability. All of these factors help to explain why the custom of visiting spas for psychiatric conditions had remained intact since the eighteenth century (see pp. 23–24).

Yet in the nineteenth century, the frequency of spa-visiting vastly accelerated. Moreover, hydrotherapy became expressly associated with psychiatric illness rather than being a panacea for every condition imaginable. Here again, numerous social changes of the 1800s help account for this new popularity: the rising wealth of the middle classes (for spa-visiting previously had been a privilege of the nobility); middle-class interests in social improvement that translated ineluctably into self-improvement and into a heightened fascination with one's own body; better means of transport, particularly the extension after 1860 of the secondary rail network to small towns and villages having mineral springs. Demand soared. Water-therapy clinics sprang up, run by physicians who were able to give a commercial focus to the entire experience of spa-going. All of these circumstances operated in every country in the Atlantic community, making the spa by 1900 the elective middle-class site for the treatment of chronic illness. As the particular chronic illnesses addressed by spa therapy became increasingly psychiatric, the spa became the first place of refuge from the asylum.

The vogue for spa therapy was perhaps briefest in England. Although English invalids had always sought out such watering places as Bath, only in the 1840s did English spas become a medical rage in the form of "hydros," private clinics to which the middle classes could repair for comprehensive treatment. Joseph Weiss, an Austrian veteran of spa therapy, established the first English water-cure clinic around 1841 in Stanstead-bury in Hertfordshire, followed then by two Englishmen—James Wilson and James Gully—who opened for business in Malvern the following year.[25] By 1850, at least two dozen of these establishments existed in Britain. There is no doubt that among the thousands who flocked to them were a number of patients with some kind of major psychiatric problem, a trend no doubt accelerated by the passage in 1843 of an Asylum Bill that made it difficult for private asylums to admit patients on a voluntary basis: These patients would now seek other kinds of care where they had the assurance of being able to check out again voluntarily.[26] Charles Darwin's visits to Malvern for his chronic hypochondria are well-known. For a while, Edward Bulwer-Lytton, first Baron Lytton and well-known parliamentarian and author, also obtained relief at Malvern for symptoms that he considered nervous in nature:

Bulwer-Lytton, as he tells us in 1846, had been quite ground down by work, yet rest was of no avail. In his attempts at repose, "all my ailments gathered round me—and made themselves far more palpable and felt. I had no resource but to fly from myself—to fly into the other world of books, or thought, or reverie. . . . As long as I was always at work it seemed that I had no leisure to be ill. Quiet was my hell."

Then Baron Lytton began developing frank psychiatric symptoms as well. "The exhaustion of toil and study had been completed by great anxiety and grief." After the death of a family member, "I seemed

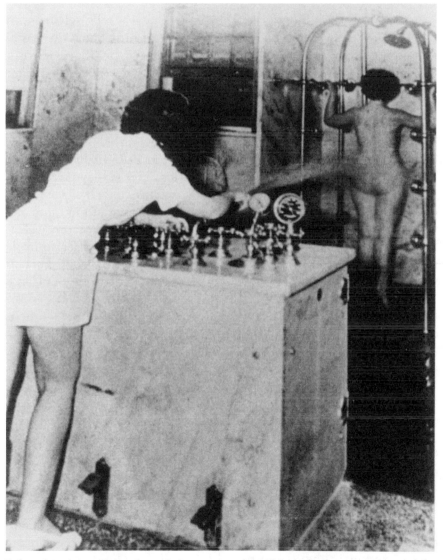

Before the advent of the physical therapies in the 1930s, hydrotherapy was one of the few means of calming agitated patients. Here the Mississippi State Hospital, Whitfield, c. 1920 (courtesy of Mississippi State Hospital).

scarcely to live myself." By January 1844, he was "thoroughly shattered." The least exercise exhausted him. "The nerves gave way at the most ordinary excitement," a result he believed of "a chronic irritation of that vast surface we call the mucous membrane." The obviously despondent Baron Lytton, like so many of his countrymen, was restored by the healing procedures of the hydro at Malvern.[27]

Yet the English fashion for local hydrotherapy was relatively brief. In the 1880s, wealthy English nervous patients, spurning domestic spas as impuissant or unchic, began searching out those on the Continent (since the 1820s the English had been wintering on the Continent for chest diseases). The vogue for nerves was new, and unwelcome to the foreign consultants who depended on chest complaints for their livelihood.[28] But with the efforts of the French in the 1880s to downplay tuberculosis (TB) (then known to be contagious) on the Riviera and to highlight nerves, English medical opinion lost its parochialism.

Leaders in this change were two generations of a Harley Street medical family named Weber, quintessential examples of physicians who, though apparently general internists (or the equivalent at the time), devoted much of their practice to psychiatry. The father, Hermann Weber, had been born in Germany and studied in the late 1840s under his uncle the Bonn psychiatrist Friedrich Nasse. After encountering Thomas Carlyle in the early 1850s in Bonn, Weber decided to visit England. There he married an Englishwoman and decided to stay on, able to practice medicine after becoming a licentiate of the Royal College of Physicians of London in 1855. Owing to his great personal charm, he acquired a carriage-trade practice, became physician to five prime ministers, and styled himself as a climatologist, a specialist in spas. In his widely read guide to spa therapy, published in 1880, Sir Hermann advised his medical readers to recommend the Italian Riviera for nervous disorders.[29] By 1898, when Weber senior and his medical son Frederick put out another edition of their guide, they had become much more favorable to the high country overlooking the Riviera beaches: "For neurotic patients and those suffering from neuralgic conditions, neighbouring more elevated regions are mostly preferable, such as Grasse and Cimiez."[30]

The records of Frederick Parkes Weber's extensive Harley Street practice have survived, and it is evident from them that many of the patients he was sending to these Continental spas had some kind of psychiatric problem. A not untypical example was Miss X, 25, of Durham, who had come down to London in October 1908 to consult Parkes Weber (as he was called, pronounced VAY-ber) about occasional pain around the site of an appendectomy she had had eight years ago. Parkes Weber detected a more immediate problem, however: This "rather slight, rather pale" young woman would vomit continuously after meals for about an hour. She was also "subject to headaches (and bursting sensation in head) this year." Parkes Weber diagnosed "nausea of incertain cause and mental depression," advising her to visit Friedrich Dengler's and Anton Frey's nervous sanatorium in Baden-Baden, or the Val-Mont, another nervous "san" in Territet, Switzerland, "with a winter season afterwards at St. Moritz."[31] It was thus under the influence of such consultants as the Webers that English patients with psychiatric conditions beneath the level of florid psychosis were diverted to watering places on the Continent.

England's own spa business underwent a fatal decline during World War I, never again to recover, at least as regards the carriage trade. In 1922, the special spa trains to Scotland that had run during the War were discontinued, now that "it is cheaper to visit a French or Swiss spa than to make this journey to Scotland," as a medical journal noted.[32] "Let there be no mistake about it," said one London society doctor, Continental spas were superior. "At the best of these establishments [on the Continent] treatment is carried to the nth degree."[33]

In France, spa therapy and water-cure clinics maintained their popularity far longer, partly because the country is blessed with a sunnier climate and a greater number of mineral springs, partly because the faith of the French in the curative power of waters that bubble from the deep was so fervent as to have survived to this day. "Thermal fever" began in the 1820s, the annual number of health-seekers accelerating from 31,000 in 1822 to 100,000 in the late 1830s, to 200,000 in the late 1860s. By the end of the century, French spas were receiving 300,000 to 400,000 visitors a year, and such watering-places as Aix-en-Savoie and Vichy achieved worldwide reputations.[34] These "rustic republics of water-drinkers"—the phrase comes to us from an account of a young woman suffering hysteric fits that later, at a spa, turn into multiple-personality disorder[35]—breathed the spirit of anxious hypochondria and neurosis.

French spas swam in nervous illness. Octave Mirbeau, in his 1901 novel "The Twenty-One Days of a Neurasthenic," allows spa "Dr. Triceps" to cry out, "Névrose! névrose! névrose! . . . Tout est névrose!"[36] At Royat in the Puy-de-Dôme department, the waters were said to help mainly "neuropathic manifestations" such as migraine, myalgia, and "certain psychopathic problems." Above all, according to Fernand Levillain, a hydro- and electro-specialist in Nice who consulted in Royat, the spa "offers the most help in neurasthenia." "Today [1894] this disorder has become extremely frequent and it is not rare to encounter isolated symptoms of neurasthenia in the majority of our rheumatic and gouty patients."[37] Thus Levillain, on the face of it a physical therapist with numerous orthopedic patients, was performing in Royat the duties of a psychiatrist.

If the fetish of English psychiatry was nonrestraint, that of the French was the notion that spas could be finely graded on the basis of indication, or presenting complaint. In the finest Cartesian manner, French spas in their hundreds were classified on the basis of what malady they were apt for. The therapeutic indications embraced all of medicine, from engorgement of the uterus, for which the spas at Salins in the Jura, Salies-de-Béarn, and Lamotte were said to be good, to engorgement of the liver, for which Bourbonne and Balaruc were recommended. Among this landscape of pseudo-uses, the indications that ranged above all others were psychiatric. If the patient was cachectic as a result of depression, the waters of Royat, Saint-Nectaire, Sainte-Marguerite, and Châteauneuf would suit. If nervous patients had stomach pain (enteralgia), they should try Néris, Bagnères-de-Bigorre, and Plombières. If "nervosisme" was the problem, Luxeuil and Luchon were indicated. If your nervous patients, doctor, were simultaneously hysterical, send them to Saint-Sauveur, Evian, and Ussat. On and on went these lists, through neuralgia, "softening of the brain," and paralysis: Paralysis from tabes was assigned to Lamalou (where to this day a statue of Charcot sits in the town square); paralysis from hysteria, Olette.[38] With these ultrarefined "indications," the spa-physicians of France put on a spectacular performance of making distinctions without a difference, for most of the healing waters, consumed today in bottles on the dinner table, were placebos. Often dictated by the physician who had the medical concession in the spa at that moment, the supposed indications were nothing more than a triumph of public relations.[39]

Spas in France and French-speaking Switzerland benefited greatly from the shift away from tuberculosis and toward nervous illness that began in the 1880s. The French Riviera suddenly discovered that its climate was indeed much more suitable for nerves than for TB.[40] Montreux experienced a huge increase in custom, from 22,000 visitors in 1896 to 62,000 in 1908, as it shifted indications from tuberculosis to nervous patients, "be they confirmed neurasthenics or patients suffering simply from exhaustion and overexertion."[41] The whole high Alps of France and French-speaking Switzerland opened up to nervous diseases as the tubercular were shunted into such highly circumscribed resorts as Leysin. By 1900, francophone Europe had become much more accommodating to the nervous than it had been a century earlier.

As in England, the medical center of a typical French watering hole became the private hydros, or water-cure clinics, that sprang up everywhere. Here the psychiatric essence of spa therapy saw its most perfect expression. Although hydrotherapy clinics were found throughout provincial French spas, the greatest concentration—some 40 in number by the turn of the century—was in Paris. It was in these hydros, where tap water and not mineral water was used, that the Parisian middle classes with diagnoses such as neurasthenia and hysteria congregated, exactly the same segment of the population that 70 years later would be seeking psychoanalysis. Typical was the *clinique hydrothérapeutique* of Alfred Béni-Barde, a hydrotherapist of four decades' experience who by the turn of the century had shifted from central Paris to the chic suburb of Auteuil. He described two patients who consulted around 1908: "[They were] twin sisters, one of whom offered the principal traits of hysteria, the other those of neurasthenia. Born in an aristocratic family tainted by numerous stigmata of nervosity and arthritis, they received an eccentric upbringing that exercised a disastrous influence on both of them." The one was sweet, sad, and contemplative, inclined to seek seclusion. She seemed to experience mental gaps and inexplicable lapses. The other was lively, alert, and loved the dirty stories told by her brothers. She was, however, subject to hysterical fits.

Béni-Barde adopted the appropriate hydrotherapeutic procedure for each. "For the neurasthenic we had recourse to a sedative shower, slowly moving over to more bracing temperatures. To treat the hysteric it was necessary to employ the Scottish douche [alternately hot and cold], the cold water obliging her from time to time to dive into a swimming pool filled with chilly water." Since these treatments, said Béni-Barde, both have been healthy, "though retaining a certain impressionability."[42]

Béni-Barde's theory of psychohydraulics was very straightforward: "The hybrid neuropathy that has seized [hysterics] does not require calming. These female patients must be tamed. That is why cold water succeeds."[43] Thus did the hydrotherapists articulate their theories of psychodynamics.

In the years before World War II, the French spas shared to some extent in the fate of the English. Both shed their upper-crust clientele to the great German *Weltbäder*, or internationally celebrated watering places.[44] In Central Europe, the tradition of hydrotherapy for psychiatric reasons ran broad and deep. Although the German spas reached back to the Middle Ages, it was the nineteenth century that saw them grow dramatically as the urban middle classes took up spa-visiting. And what the new spa guests brought was not fever, not acute infectious illness as the aristocracy had before, but neurosis. In the Bohemian watering place of

Karlsbad (Karlovy Vary), for example, the percentage of nobles among the visitors declined from 32 percent in 1793, to 11 percent in 1814, to 1 percent in 1911. The representation of businesspeople, by contrast, rose from 12 percent in 1814 to 59 percent in 1911.[45] The period of most rapid growth in the spas occurred after 1870 with the rising incomes that industrialization brought in tow and the expansion of the railnet. Between 1871 and 1911, visitors to Kissingen more than quadrupled, from 8,000 a year to 34,000; those to Wiesbaden, one of the main "nerve" baths, rose from 60,000 in 1871 to 127,000 in 1900; the number of "cure-guests" at Baden-Baden, another major nerve bath, was up from 50,000 in 1871 to 79,000 in 1911.[46]

The link between spa life and psychiatry established itself early. So puissant were the waters in Baden bei Zurich said to be that in 1818 one physician discouraged their use in patients who had "very weakened nervous systems, if drinking the waters increases the number of nervous episodes and causes prolonged nervous headaches."[47] Such defeatist notes, however, were soon drowned out by cries of jubilation. In a tour of the spa horizon in 1837, one doctor preached the virtue of Gleissen for "nervous weakness," another that of Teplitz for disorders of the "nervous system," specially for hysterical paralyses in young women. Meinberg's waters were said to be splendid for "hysterical incidents," again in young women, and Karlsbad's marvelous for hysteria in general.[48] What was any of this if not office-practice psychiatry?

Major psychiatric illnesses came to the spas as well though they were unwelcome. Until the appearance of the "open" private nervous clinics in the 1860s (meaning patients could be admitted without a certificate), alienists regularly sent psychotic patients to spas. Among the 7,063 patients seen personally by the local spa-doctor at Oeynhausen between 1858 and 1879, 2,111, or 30 percent, had psychiatric and neurological problems of some kind (neurosyphilis being the largest single category). Among those 2,111 there were 118 psychotics. Their number was not great relative to the total of nerve patients, but one imagines the significance for little Oeynhausen over those two decades of 118 individuals having hallucinations and delusions or who were severely thought disordered. The spa-doctor, however, reported good results even with them, particularly in cases caused by "previous masturbation."[49]

The actual spa therapy of the psychoses and neuroses would have been conducted not in the public bathhouses but in the hydros (*Wasserheilanstalten*), private residential clinics devoted ostensibly to water treatment but in reality offering a number of other procedures as well—

electrotherapy, massage, and the like. These clinics multiplied the various therapies to differentiate themselves from competitors in the fierce struggle for wealthy patients. Among the first Central European hydros was that established by Johann Christian Reil, one of the founders of modern psychiatry, at Halle in 1809. (Among Reil's early patients was the storyteller Wilhelm Grimm.[50]) Yet the craze for water-therapy clinics in Central Europe began only after 1833 as Vincenz Priessnitz, the nonmedical son of a peasant, opened a few lodgings in Gräfenberg, Austrian Silesia, for patients seeking water therapy. Thus began a movement tantamount to a secular religion on behalf of curing oneself through the application of damp packings, partial baths (arm, leg), and full baths in the cold waters of Gräfenberg.[51] The original operators of the hydros in England had been acolytes of Priessnitz, as were an entire generation of lay hydrotherapists and naturopaths who set up shop all over Central Europe.

Originally, the main candidates for these cold baths seem to have been patients with fevers, and the cold water did procure some subjective relief. But as time went on the febrile patients gave way to nervous ones, and the cold waters—more than a weakened nervous constitution could stand it was said—were warmed up. After Priessnitz died in 1851, the fashionable water-therapy centers shifted from the cold springs of the east, run by laity, to the warm springs of Baden-Baden, Wiesbaden, and other spas in the west, run by physicians.[52]

From the outset, the fashionable hydros of Vienna, Lake Constance, the Black Forest, and the Rhine Valley had a heavy psychiatric component. Psychiatry lurked in the background of even the most organic-appearing of them. Wilhelm Winternitz, was professor of hydrotherapy at the Vienna University and founded in 1865 a hydro in Kaltenleutgeben outside of Vienna. He prided himself on having put water treatments on what he considered a scientific basis. Yet Winternitz had previously worked as an asylum physician.[53] The Winternitz hydro included nerves in its advertised indications. It did not advertise for psychotics, although it got them too.

Thus early in November, 1894, Barbara T, age 41, checked into the Winternitz hydro with a feeling of "jerking in the limbs." There she received mild electrotherapy, becoming in the process "increasingly more agitated." She "holds long monologues, attempting to speak High German. At night she prays for hours. Turns her back when spoken to. In a loud voice she incessantly discusses events of her daily life, addressing an inkwell or a stone. She suddenly tries to take off her clothes.

Demonstrates erotic desires while being investigated," noted the physicians of the Vienna Asylum after Barbara T had been removed from the Winternitz hydro with a diagnosis of "mania."[54]

The world of the hydros was filled with Barbara T's, to the dismay of asylum psychiatrists who saw such hydro referrals as malpractice. Said one exasperated psychiatrist at a meeting in 1874, "The water-cure clinics and mineral spas do not represent appropriate treatment for patients with early signs of major mood disorder." Yet he noted that, "in the course of the previous year, at various places in Germany and Switzerland several water-clinics directed by trained psychiatrists have arisen that in fact target preferentially early mood disorders. But in order to conceal this purpose, and above all to avoid being branded as a kind of insane asylum, these institutions have assumed the 'mask of water-cure clinics.'"[55]

Yet the family might see the water-cure clinic as preferential to the asylum. And the director of a well-known private asylum in Bendorf-on-Rhine urged his colleagues to make referrals to such clinics: "[In a water-cure clinic] there are in fact numerous mental patients, and we know from experience that many are discharged as being well." The writer thought separation from the family the main factor in these successes.[56]

The water-clinic Marienberg in Boppard-on-Rhine was typical in every way of the middle-class hydro, and statistics from Marienberg show it was, without question, a primarily psychiatric facility. Of 1,185 patients seen there between 1883 and 1888, only one-fifth were somehow off the psychiatric spectrum (chest disease, anemia, overweight). Fifty-two percent of all patients at Marienberg had "neurosis" (neurasthenia, hysteria, hypochondria); 5 percent suffered from organic diseases of the central nervous system such as neurosyphilis; 13 percent were alcoholics; and 9 percent had some form of what was considered "psychosis," mainly obsessive-compulsive disorders and depression.[57] Thus Marienberg's patients were overwhelmingly psychiatric, and there is no doubt that by subsequent standards Marienberg's director Karl Hoestermann would have been considered a psychiatrist although he styled himself a hydrotherapist. Places like the Marienberg hydro must be drawn into any comprehensive history of psychiatry, for it was there that the middle classes received their psychiatric care.

By the turn of the century, the water-cure clinics had begun to lose their cachet, because the public, as one observer put it, "thinks of them as an ostensible entryway to the insane asylum."[58] It was time for middle-class psychiatric care to move on to other kinds of institutions where one would not be so readily hallmarked "insane."

Tired Nerves and the Rest Cure

At this point, the Americans rush on stage, defining a new disease, neurasthenia, and discovering rest as the means for its cure. "Tired nerves" and the rest cure were both American inventions. But they resounded upon the international scene, legitimating a new kind of open asylum for the care of psychiatric illness and drawing the attention of physicians to psychological means of effecting a cure.

Psychiatrists' vocabulary for describing the minor psychiatric ailments had really been rather limited. Nerves, hysteria, and hypochondria were all holdovers from the eighteenth century and more or less interchangeable: hysteria for women who had psychosomatic complaints or who seemed emotionally incontinent; hypochondria approximately the same for men; and nerves for everybody who experienced depression, compulsive behavior, or anxiety. These were all considered to be functional nervous diseases, meaning that they were hypothetically organic but demonstrated no tangible tissue changes.

Then in the second half of the nineteenth century, progress in clinical neurology started to make it easier to find something organic while the patient was alive, not just at autopsy. After the 1860s, multiple sclerosis could be distinguished from hysteria, or general paralysis from hypochondria. If the patients toppled over after you asked them to stand up straight with their eyes closed (Romberg's sign), they probably had neurosyphilis, not nerves.

These new discoveries made a number of physicians very uncertain. As the old Viennese clinician Salomon Federn (father of psychoanalyst Paul Federn) later put it, "There were all these new means of investigation, such as the reflexes, the different pupil reactions and the complicated examination of skin and muscles which were supposed to point to pathognomonic symptoms [symptoms specific to a given disease]. Many of these new diseases were still little known in the literature, and at the beginning there was probably no neuropathologist, to say nothing of a clinician, who was familiar enough with these processes to be able to make a certain diagnosis."[59] A weasel word was needed.

This climate of medical uncertainty about what was really organic and what was just hypothetically organic was a mirror image of patients' uncertainty about what was madness and what was nerves. Both doctors and patients required a bridge between these two uncertainties, an organic-*sounding* disease term to explain psychiatric-*looking* illness behavior. In 1869, New York electrotherapist George Beard supplied this bridge with his announcement of the discovery of neurasthenia, a supposedly distinctive disease entity. Neurasthenia, like its grandchildren chronic fatigue syndrome and multiple chemical sensitivities a hundred years later, served as a bridge between supposedly organic causes and symptoms involving mood and cognition. Beard declared that a large number of nervous symptoms were really owing to a physical exhaustion of the nerves, or neurasthenia. Unlike neurosyphilis, one could not see this physical exhaustion under the microscope, hence it was functional. But it must be real because the patients themselves seemed so genuinely afflicted. Thus neurasthenia became the prototype of the functional nervous diseases.

The range of symptoms the new diagnosis encompassed was vast. Said Beard: "[It] may give rise to dyspepsia, headaches, paralysis, insomnia, anesthesia, neuralgia, rheumatic gout, spermatorrhea [wet dreams] in the male and menstrual irregularities in the female." What was the cause, Dr. Beard? ". . . The central nervous system becomes dephosphorized, or perhaps, loses somewhat of its solid constitutents."[60] Beard's neurasthenia did not rest on the solidest of scientific foundations.

Yet the new diagnosis became wildly popular, particularly after Beard wrote a lengthy book on it in 1880. (He likened himself to the explorers of Central Africa, pushing into "an unexplored territory into which few men enter. . . .")[61] The book was immediately translated into German the following year and later appeared in numerous other languages. Until World War I, Beard's neurasthenia would be the standard diagnosis for all functional nervous diseases, lying as it did between major depression and psychosis on the one hand, and "hysteria," a term still preferred for women, on the other. Neurasthenia became the needed medical weasel word. As Federn said, "Neurasthenia dominated the realm of the chronic functional organ diseases just as the doctrine of bacteriology dominated that of infectious diseases."[62]

But let us say that we have a neurasthenic patient. What are we going to do for him or her? Here a second American nerve doctor weighed in, Silas Weir Mitchell, who created in 1875 a therapy called the rest cure that had almost as historic a trajectory as the disease of neurasthenia, which it was designed to combat.

Although Weir Mitchell's rest cure was probably the most famous rest cure in the history of psychiatry, it was by no means the first treatment prescribing rest. The therapeutic use of rest and isolation for nervous disease had a long previous history. In 1787, William Perfect had placed in his own home a psychotic male patient: "I . . . forbade all sorts of intercourse with his relations and acquaintances . . ." Perfect confined the patient "to a still, quiet and almost totally darkened room. I never suffered him to be spoken with . . . nor permitted by anyone to visit him." Not only did Perfect establish complete authority over this patient, isolating him from outside influences, Perfect also insinuated various dietary and physical therapies into the regimen, such as meals that were "light, cooling and easy of digestion" or warm footbaths. After four months of such treatment, the patient was restored to "a state of sanity."[63] This was Mitchell's rest cure in embryo. In the treatment of melancholia, there was a long Continental tradition of bed rest in a darkened room and seclusion from noise.[64] The notion of isolating asylum patients from friends and family was also very familiar.[65] Historically, these are techniques that each generation of psychiatrists invents for itself.

Mitchell merely described a variant on this age-old theme, but in 1875 it was an idea whose time had come, for the rest cure was ideally conducted in private clinics, and such clinics were just beginning to spring up. Born in 1829, Mitchell graduated in medicine from the University of Pennsylvania, then studied for a year with Claude Bernard in Paris. During the U.S. Civil War, he served as a surgeon with the Union army, at this point acquiring a lively interest in the nervous system as he encountered such phenomena as phantom pain in soldiers whose limbs had been amputated. But Mitchell had an arrogant pretentiousness that ill qualified him for military medicine and suited perfectly the needs of nervous female patients in the carriage trade. When he returned to Philadelphia, it was as a society nerve doctor that he made his name:

In January 1874, a Mrs. G from Maine became a patient at a private clinic that Mitchell helped run, the Infirmary for Nervous Diseases. She was suffering from deep exhaustion and was unable to walk up stairs, read, or write. "Any such use of the eyes caused headache and nausea." After unsuccessful rounds of spa treatment, she had accepted a life of isolation. But there was one positive note: "She was able partially to digest and retain her meals if she lay down in a noiseless and darkened room."

"I sat beside this woman day after day," said Mitchell, "hearing her pitiful story." He found it interesting that she could eat.

"Yes," she said. "I have been told that on that account I ought to lie in bed." But she disliked all this bed rest and pleaded with Mitchell not to put her to bed again.

Nonetheless he did so, whereupon, challenging his authority, she began throwing up all her meals. Now it struck Mitchell, not that there was a complex authority issue in the doctor-patient relationship at play here, but that she needed exercise. Rest plus exercise were required, he told himself. "How could I unite the two?" Then it occurred to him: Rubbing! She needed "exercise without exertion." So he trained a young woman to become a masseuse and rub Mrs. G. A couple of days later,

Mitchell hit upon the idea of using electricity as well. "Meanwhile, as she had always done best when secluded, I insisted on entire rest and shut out friends, relatives, books and letters." In 10 days, Mrs. G "blossomed like a rose." As Mrs. G was now able to keep her food down, Mitchell began "overfeeding" her with a diet heavy with milk fats. In two months, she gained 40 pounds and went happily home to Maine.[66]

Thus the Weir Mitchell rest cure was born, involving the components of seclusion enforced through bed rest, a milk diet, electrical treatments, and massage. Mitchell believed that his famous cure represented an organic treatment of an organic condition, and throughout his life he was tin-eared to the notion that a psychological component might be involved. He did concede that, for its successful conduct, the rest cure required a "childlike obedience"[67] and therefore worked better with females than males. Yet for Mitchell, organicity was the core: We've got to get the blood flowing again to those "spinal ganglia in the state of exhaustion," he explained to his colleagues in April 1875, the first outing of the rest cure in the medical community. In 1877, Mitchell published *Fat and Blood*, explaining the mechanics of the cure. The book became a sensation, and Mitchell's Infirmary for Nervous Diseases turned into a "Mecca for patients from all over the world."[68]

The rest cure required a good deal of money and was mainly restricted to an international elite of nervous patients, criss-crossing the oceans in search of relief. Physicians would ship patients far afield to a spa clinic for a rest cure of typically six weeks to three months. One of Mitchell's first patients was a referral from Hermann Weber. "She was entirely cured," said a surprised Weber.[69] Because the rest cure was so ideal for a private sanatorium, a symbiotic relationship soon developed among the spa clinics, the urban nerve doctors, and the nervous middle-class females of the Atlantic community. All flourished together: the private clinic boom of the late nineteenth century, the diagnosis of neurasthenia (the rest cure's target par excellence), and the profession of office-practice psychiatry (not called that).

In 1881, society gynecologist William Playfair, his office on Curzon Street in London's Mayfair district, gave the rest cure its proper introduction in England: "I have simply followed Dr. Mitchell's directions, but with results so astonishing and satisfactory to myself, in cases which were quite heart-breaking from their obstinate resistance to all ordinary management, that I am confident [Mitchell's plan] deserves a more extended trial."[70] Playfair apparently used private lodgings in London for the conduct of the cure, hiring the Amazon nurses needed to enforce obedience. His colleagues relied on nursing homes and "hysterical homes," or private clinics, which were better equipped to compel isolation, coordinate electrotherapy and massage, prepare the special diet, and then, toward the end of the cure, to reintroduce the patient to society at the common dinner table.[71]

Charcot brought the rest cure to France in 1885, though he did not acknowledge Mitchell's priority and insisted that he himself had discovered what he called the "isolation" cure.[72] He would refer patients to a network of water-therapy clinics and the like, then follow them from his seventh-arrondissement consulting room. The highly receptive German doctors required no official introduction, and by 1884 many private clinics had incorporated the "milk diet" (*Mastkur*), as some called it, or "Mitchell-Playfair Cure," into their palette of therapies for hysteria and neurasthenia.[73]

By 1900, the rest cure had become the treatment of choice for neurasthenia everywhere, for those who could afford it. The nicest of the new open asylums, nerve clinics, and general sanatoriums now sprouting in many countries would customarily feature the Weir Mitchell treatment. Although neurasthenia as a diagnosis never caught on in the United States as in Europe, it did have a certain vogue in connection with the rest cure. At "The Retreat" in Des Moines, Iowa, a private hospital for "nervous and mental" patients, "neurasthenic and mild mental cases" could obtain a treatment consisting of "rest, baths, massage, electricity . . . and suitable trained nurses." The "Crystal Springs Sanitarium for Nervous and Mental Diseases" in Portland, Oregon, claimed to relieve "nervous states, notably the insomnia of neurasthenia," with electrotherapy and similar treatments in "cottage homes."[74]

In Central Europe, the choice was limitless. The Marienberg water-clinic in Boppard made much of its "Playfair Cure" in the treatment of neurasthenia. At Richard Jaenisch's sanatorium in Wölfelsgrund, from among many therapies neurasthenics could choose the code-named "milk diet."[75] The rest cure was thus adopted worldwide.

But it soon became apparent to many doctors that the essence of the Weir Mitchell cure was the physician's authority, and not the specific physical components of the cure itself. What made patients better, in the view of contemporaries, was the act of submission to the doctor. This was a psychological not a physiological component. Harley Street nerve doctor Alfred Taylor Schofield described one of his "neuromimetic" patients whose nerve power had so seeped from her that she was unable to walk. He ordered that she be driven to some secluded gardens and propelled along by two nurses. "That night the patient tried to jump over the banisters and break her leg so that she could not walk; and, failing to do so, refused all food and actually had to be fed for a fortnight by tube through the nose before she would give in. She tore the dress of one nurse to ribands, but at last was overheard one Sunday morning whispering to herself: 'Annie, you've met your match'; and then out she went and soon walked three miles on end."[76] The entire rigmarole was intended to produce in the patient a confession of surrender to medical authority. That it was highly effective reminds us how different the social climate of the day was from our own.

In practice, the rest cure worked as the Anglo-American actress and novelist Elizabeth Robins explained in a fictionalized account of a six-week isolation cure that "Dr. Garth Vincent" (in reality a West End consultant named Vaughan Harley) put her on.

"No letters, no telegrams, no messages, no daily papers, no communication of any sort for six weeks," he instructed. Exceptionally, she was attempting the rest cure in her own house, supervised by a nurse.

The nurse arrives and is uneasy about whether she should let "Katharine" read. "It is very seldom [Dr. Vincent] consents to take a real Rest Cure patient that is not nursed at the Home."

Why is that?

"Because—well you see, at the Home everything goes by rule, it's all like clockwork. He thinks that people, especially women, haven't enough sense of discipline to carry out orders for themselves."

Then Dr. Vincent arrives for a visit. "He had come swiftly in, seemed not even to look at her, went straight to the nearest window, already down an inch from the top, and pulled it open a foot and a half. 'You're too hot in here,' he said, and stood an instant taking a stethoscope out of his pocket and fitting it together, frowning down upon it. Katharine was conscious of a little shudder passing over her."

There were struggles over food, for Katharine had been eating little. That evening Katharine had not eaten her butter. The nurse warned that Dr. Vincent might have to return.

"Come here? again? to-night?" asked Katharine.

"Yes," said the nurse. She'd have to phone him.

"Did you ever have to do that?"

"Oh yes," said the nurse.

"What happened?"

"He is always in one of his black rages, when he's sent for."

Katharine began spreading the butter on her toast.

After six weeks of struggles over massage, milk diet, and so forth—all of which Katharine loses—her neurasthenia gets better. She learns that she can get up and look at her letters tomorrow. How excited she is at the thought of going out, her old symptoms now cast behind her. At the end of the story she cries out joyfully "I'm a new creature."[77]

As a physician, one would have to be psychologically unminded indeed to care for such a patient and still believe neurasthenia an organic disease of the nervous system curable with a milk diet. Katharine clearly owed her improvement to her psychological surrender to the medical martinet Dr. Vincent. As the physicians of the United States, France, Britain, and Germany administered thousands and thousands of such cures, a collective lightbulb started to go on: They were dealing with a disorder having a major psychological component.

Just before going down from Paris to his new practice in Nice, Charcot's student Fernand Levillain, who deemed himself a physiatrist and "clinical neurologist," wrote a précis of the Weir Mitchell cure for French physicians. The specific components such as electrotherapy were really secondary, said Levillain. The central component of the rest cure was isolation from the outside world, for the conferral of "psychological force . . . against certain psychological forms of neurasthenia."[78]

In the United States, as well, practitioners began to recognize the psychological component. Neurologist Francis Dercum, professor of nervous diseases at Jefferson Medical College in Philadelphia, was on the whole a big believer in organicity. Yet he thought the rest cure mainly a phenomenon of suggestion. Full-feeding and the other features served mainly to "untie" the patient's "pathological associations," Dercum declared at a Boston psychiatric meeting in 1908.[79] Soon thereafter, another doubting neurologist, Harvard's George Waterman, speculated that Weir Mitchell's own strong personality was probably the curative factor in his famous cure. "The general result . . . owes its success rather to the suggestive influence than to any physical change that takes place."[80]

In Britain, Edwin Bramwell, a member of Edinburgh's famous medical dynasty of that name and lecturer on neurology at the university, debunked this supposedly neurological cure designed by America's most famous neurologist: "Even at the present time," Bramwell said in 1923, "there are many who fail to recognise that when isolation is employed in the treatment of the neuroses, it is merely an adjuvant. . . . In the majority of cases in which a rest cure is advised, the purpose of isolation is to give the physician free play, so that the impression which he makes by the persuasive measures he adopts may not be weakened by countersuggestion."[81] It is important to emphasize that all these thunderers against the organicity of the rest cure were neurologists, not psychiatrists. They were not long in drawing the conclusion: If the rest cure was psychological in nature, then neurasthenia could be treated with psychotherapy.

The significance of the rest cure, neurasthenia, and the rise of private clinics supposedly for medical and neurological disease, is that these apparently organicist concepts helped open the way for psychotherapy and broke ground for the insight that certain forms of psychiatric illness may yield to the healing power of the human voice. This is why the rest and isolation cures claim such historic significance: They treated the mind in the context of a one-on-one relationship between doctor and patient. The biological model, as it had evolved by the end of the nineteenth century, was much lacking in any understanding of the mind as the intervening link between brain and behavior. Light on the importance of this link started to glimmer in the private clinics as doctors saw such placebos as a milk diet completely transform patients' lives.

Neurology Discovers Psychotherapy

Psychiatry outfitted with biological assumptions bore a strong resemblance in those days to neurology. Not that in office practice it mattered so much. In the absence of qualifying exams for either discipline, physicians were pretty much what they called themselves. In practical terms, a "psychiatrist" or alienist was someone who had spent a good deal of time in asylums, a "neurologist"—the original term meant a specialist in the anatomy of the nerves[82]—someone who had trained in general pathology and internal medicine. Psychiatrists were clearly identifiable as an asylum-based speciality: Of 124 physicians attending the annual meeting of the American Medico-Psychological Association in 1910, for example, only 4 were not identified with an asylum or private nervous clinic.[83] Yet from early on, neurologists too constituted an identifiable speciality, based in private offices rather than institutions. American neurologists formed their own organization in 1875, German neurologists in 1907.[84]

What interested these early neurologists was not so much "nerves" but the neurological implications of such diseases as thyroid deficiency, beriberi, stroke, kidney failure, and the like. Yet they were obliged by their patients to attend upon nerves, nervous disorders being far commoner and more remunerative than the neurological complications of uremia. It was the patients' fearsome rejection of anything "psychiatric" that forced neurologists willy-nilly to become involved with the world of psychoneurosis. If the mad-doctors were unsuitable for the middle classes, the nerve-doctors would have to serve.

Thus from the very beginning the cure of psychoneurotic illness had a heavily neurological slant. Freud, Janet, and Charcot, the great names in the understanding of hysteria, were all neurologists. The private nervous and organic clinics that after the 1880s took the baton from the water-treatment clinics were virtually all premised on the assumption of treating organic nervous disease and were staffed by physicians whom the public believed to be neurologists. What anxious turn-of-the-century nervous patient would not be comforted to hear, entering the "Sanatorium Friedrichshöhe" in Wiesbaden, that Richard Friedländer, owner and chief physician, treated "hypothyroid disease, St. Vitus Dance, peripheral and central paralysis, tabes, neuritis, loss of muscle bulk, and morphinism." Of course Dr. Friedländer also accepted cases of "nervosity, neurasthenia, hysteria, hypochondria, and melancholic depression." We offer, said Friedländer, all of the water therapies, thermal therapy, pine-needle baths and many kinds of other baths, electrotherapy of various kinds, massage and physiotherapy. It all sounded so marvelously organic, especially when he added, "The mentally ill are absolutely excluded from admission."[85]

One of Dr. Friedländer's therapies, however, did not sound so organic. "Psychological influencing plays a cardinal role in the treatment," he said. It was indeed physicians like Friedländer, essentially neurologists, who dipped into psychotherapy rather than mainline psychiatrists. The reason was that neurology offered patients the necessary fig leaf: We believe your problems are organic but we may be able to help you with this new kind of influencing. This cover permitted neurologists to take over the minor psychiatric illnesses under the guise of treating somatic complaints of the central nervous system.

Psychotherapy arrived in medicine by two routes, neither of them particularly psychiatric. Initially, the early hypnotherapists convinced physicians that patients' symptoms could be abolished through suggestion, both hypnotic and nonhypnotic. Then along came the psychological-milieu therapy of the private "neurological" clinics.

It is actually the last chapter of the hypnosis story that concerns us here.[86] Medical hypnosis had begun at the end of the eighteenth century with Franz Anton Mesmer and his French followers. Hypnotism then experienced various ups and downs over the course of the nineteenth century and was finally headed for oblivion, just as the French medical community revived it in the 1880s (it would vanish largely from the medical screen in the decade before World War I). The revival in France involved two rival groups of physicians: Jean-Martin Charcot, leader of the Salpêtrière school, and Hippolyte Bernheim of the Nancy school, Nancy being the capital of the eastern French province of Lorraine whither the Faculty of Medicine of Strasbourg had fled after the Germans annexed Alsace in 1871. Charcot believed hypnotizability to be evidence of hysteria, seeing no therapeutic use for it save confirming the diagnosis that the patient was indeed hysterical. On the other hand, internist Bernheim believed that hypnosis could be used for medical therapy, there being nothing specifically hysterical about it (Bernheim thought the phenomenon of suggestion to be characteristic of all psychoneuroses: If patients could be suggested into them, they could also be suggested out of them). Bernheim, who had instructed himself in medical hypnotism under the tutelage of an old country doctor named Ambroise-Auguste Liébeault, applied hypnotism with varying degrees of success in a number of organic and psychological conditions. But he soon realized that nonhypnotic suggestion—meaning a good talking-to—was just as effective, particularly among middle-class patients who resisted the pretentious imposition of medical authority that full-blast hypnosis required. After 1883, Bernheim began preaching nonhypnotic suggestion as well, marking the true beginning of modern medical psychotherapy.[87]

The next chapter of the story moves to Amsterdam. A young Dutch medical student named Frederik Willem van Eeden had gone to Paris in November 1885 to collect material for a dissertation on tuberculosis. He happened to audit some of Charcot's lectures and became highly enthusiastic about hypnotic suggestion. After graduating from Amsterdam in 1886, van Eeden returned to Paris, and went also to Nancy. "I had now seen," he later wrote, "that the body could be cured by the mind, and this I felt to be the only true and lasting cure."[88] Back in Amsterdam again, van Eeden met up with another enthusiast of hypnotism, Albert Willem van Renterghem, who had just been to France to visit Liébeault.[89] Van Renterghem had set himself up with a hypnotherapy practice in a small Dutch town and had been run off his feet by avid patients. Later that year, van Eeden and van Renterghem decided to found in Amsterdam an outpatient hypnotherapy clinic, and in August 1887 their "Clinic for Psychotherapeutic Suggestion" opened its doors, van Renterghem handling the business side, van Eeden doing the hypnosis.[90] The clinic thrived although van Eeden, who treated the poor free of charge in any event, refused to collect fees from the rich either. He left it after seven years to retire from medicine and become an author. This Amsterdam clinic, which evidently employed only hypnosis, represents the first modern use of the term "psychotherapy."[91]

After van Eeden, psychotherapy in the form both of hypnosis and non-hypnotic suggestion began a tour through the world of psychoneurosis.[92] Psychotherapy at this point was not at all incompatible with biological psychiatry for it spoke to the issue of treatment rather than causation. A more dyed-in-the-wool organicist than August Forel, Zurich psychiatry professor between 1879 and 1898, would be hard to imagine. Forel spent much of his time doing neuroanatomy, and his correspondence with colleagues reflects far greater interest in frog brains than in clinical psychiatry. Yet Forel was a master hypnotist.[93] So great was his reputation that one colleague referred to him a woman whom another hypnotist had put into an evil hypnotic trance, with the request that Forel lift the trance.[94] Later in life, Forel even went beyond hypnotism to talk about the therapeutic uses in the doctor-patient relationship of "love" and "intimate knowledge" of patients' lives. Yet at the same time, he referred to the "pathology of brain life."[95] Thus for Forel, there was no contradiction between a neuroscientific view of psychiatry and psychotherapy.

Outside the universities as well, psychotherapy spread among doctors identified with the organic side of psychiatry and with neurology. But it was not the psychotherapy of later "systems," such as family therapy, group therapy, depth therapy, and the like. At its birth, psychotherapy was understood in its Bernheimian sense as the therapeutic use of the doctor-patient relationship, applied in an intimate and informal context.

In Central Europe, with its great concentration of private clinics, psychotherapy first caught on in the open hospitals for nerves and the general sanatoria, almost all of them run by neurologists and internists. Heinrich Obersteiner in Vienna, a psychiatrist so neurologically oriented that he donated to the university a laboratory for brain research, seems to have been among the first to apply hypnotism. He did so at his elegant private nervous clinic in the Viennese suburb of Ober-Döbling, going public on the subject in 1885 with an address to Vienna's "Scientific Club."[96] Six years later, he explained his conception of "psychotherapy" as basically "calming and diverting" the patients, adding that the staff also did some hypnotism and suggestion on nervous patients but that psychotic patients were accessible to neither.[97] Richard von Krafft-Ebing evidently used "psychical therapy" at the private nervous clinic he had founded in 1886 in a suburb of Graz.[98]

Many smaller clinics followed in the footsteps of these two influential Viennese organicists. Rudolph von Hösslin, who had studied with Charcot and then served as an assistant in the university psychiatric department in Munich, used hypnotism as early as 1887 at the "Neuwittelsbach" clinic he had opened in a Munich suburb.[99] Karl Gerster featured hypnotism at the sanatorium he founded in 1893 in Braunfels-on-Lahn (later he turned to psychoanalysis).[100] The notion of "psychic treatment" was becoming so chic that staff physicians of a private asylum in Berlin could use it as a label for entertaining patients with concerts and amusements.[101] By the mid-1890s, psychotherapy in one or another of its senses had arrived in the private clinics in Central Europe.

In France, with its lack of private clinics and emphasis on state medicine directed from Paris, psychotherapy burst first into such centers as the Salpêtrière. Yet a word of caution: The tradition of moral therapy in French psychiatry ran so deep that the French did not need to import "psychotherapy" from a couple of very junior Dutch hypnotists. Morel, the degenerationist, had invoked in 1857 "the phrase moral therapy that we employ in our asylums to define the action that the physician seeks to exercise on a portion of the degenerates. . . ."[102] Two decades later, physiologist Claude Bernard conducted an investigation of hypnotism, by implication an informal form of psychotherapy. Starting in 1881, Amédée Dumontpallier taught hypnotism at the Pitié Hospital.[103] Nonhypnotic suggestion would enter Paris medicine in 1888 with a "Clinique de Psychothérapie" that Edgar Bérillon, a pupil of Dumontpallier's and follower of the Nancy school, opened in the rue Saint-André-des-Arts on the Left Bank.[104] Dumontpallier and his students, it must be emphasized, were neurologists and internists, not psychiatrists.

The great French neurologist Charcot had little interest in one-on-one relations with his patients, but after he died in 1893 psychotherapy moved into the medical wards of the Salpêtrière. Pierre Janet, a psychology graduate, had come to the Salpêtrière under Charcot in 1890 to do psychological studies. Janet became a medical student (MD, 1892) and went on to a career as a psychologically minded neurologist. He left the Salpêtrière in 1895 to teach at the Collège de France although he retained a clinical connection in the service of neurologist Fulgence Raymond, Charcot's successor. In the Charcot days, Janet was certainly interested in psychotherapeutic approaches to the neuroses, though doubtless out of deference to the master he used the phrase "psychological treatment" rather than psychotherapy. He also relied heavily on hypnotism.[105] So Janet is really the first big name in France in the history of psychotherapy.

The second big name, Jules-Joseph Dejerine, came to the Salpêtrière in 1895, the year that Janet left. Dejerine, 46 at the time, had been born in Geneva but was trained in medicine in Paris and served in various hospitals as an internist and as a neurologist in the true sense, not the German sense, doing research on polio, diseases of the spinal cord, and the like. Yet he was drawn to psychoneurosis in the way of most other neurologists of his day, simply because the patients sought out such doctors, and because much psychoneurosis has what neurologists like to call a pseudoneurological presentation: It looks and feels like organic disease.

What probably drew Dejerine to psychotherapy was the personal interest he took in his patients. One American physician—Smith Ely Jelliffe of New York—recalls Dejerine as "a great big, simple-hearted fellow weighing 250 pounds, 6 feet 2 inches in height," known for his "gusto and a laugh and not afraid of a Rabelaisian reference."[106] Jelliffe found Dejerine's probing of the emotional life of his patients akin to Sigmund Freud and Josef Breuer's "cathartic therapy" (see p. 157).[107] Dejerine did little more than articulate as psychotherapy his own natural clinical style: The sympathetic expression of interest in patients plus the willingness to take time with them and let them talk were the essence of his technique.

After arriving at the Salpêtrière, Dejerine turned Charcot's famous "hysterics' ward" in the Pinel wing into an "isolation service" for a modified version of the rest cure. This involved keeping the curtains drawn about each patient's bed, as well as providing enforced rest, hyperfeeding, and psychotherapy. Dejerine's isolation service marked the first time that the normally very expensive Weir Mitchell rest cure became available outside the setting of the private clinic. It met with great success.[108] Yet the secret to Dejerine's success was not the rest cure as such but his patient and attentive listening to what sick people had to say. He describes his morning rounds on the hysteria ward: "The psychotherapeutic method that I employ has nothing in particular about it. It is as simple as can be, for it is based on reasoning and persuasion, supported by firm but benevolent discipline. On morning rounds I ask each patient how she spent the night. I explain patiently to her that the symptoms of which she complains do not have the significance that she attributes to them. And I do not go on to the next patient until I see by her answers that conviction is sprouting in her mind."[109]

Jelliffe had watched Dejerine at work: "He would sit on the edge of the bed with the poor little seamstress or the little cellar rat . . . and go over their life's history, their family troubles, difficulties in collecting their bills, how the children's teething kept them up all night, and so on and so on. He poured out a sympathetic emotional type of reaction to them. He was the indulgent humorous father, and the hospital the warm embracing mother with its staff of nurses trained by him."[110] (Jelliffe had become a psychoanalyst by the time he wrote these lines.) It was Dejerine's deliberate use of one of the standard components of the doctor-patient relationship—the benevolent expression of interest—that made his form of psychotherapy well known abroad, especially in England.

When Raymond was chosen instead of Dejerine as Charcot's successor, Dejerine had something of a nervous breakdown.[111] In his misery, he turned for help to a boyhood friend from Geneva who in the meantime had become professor of neurology in Berne: Paul Dubois. Whereas Dejerine had drifted toward Paris, Dubois earned his MD at Berne in 1874, going on in internal medicine. Having acquired a large reputation as an internist, Dubois became involved with electrotherapy, the perfect placebo for an internal-medical practice. So prestigious did he become as an electrotherapist that in 1902 Berne created a chair of neuropathology for him.[112] Although Dubois lived in German-speaking Switzerland, his professional horizons were turned toward France, and he and Dejerine remained close friends, influencing each other over the years (which is my justification for discussing Dubois in the section on France). Dejerine was said to have taken his psychotherapeutic ideas from Dubois. In 1904, two years after gaining his professorship, Dubois published (in French), what was to become the most influential book on psychotherapy written before Freud. Dubois offered a highly rationalistic philosophy of "persuasion," using the doctor-patient relationship to persuade the patient to change his or her ways in a kind of Socratic dialogue in which medical advice constantly tugged patients toward betterment. Dubois had no use either for hypnotism or for the notion of an unconscious mind. "For neurasthenia," he said, "there is another psychotherapy altogether [than Bernheim's suggestion], a psychological training that does not try to conjure away fatigue but to make it disappear by slowly suppressing its principal cause: emotivity."[113] The "rational psychotherapy" of Dubois was a bit too preachy even for Dejerine's liking.[114] But the names of Dubois and Dejerine are linked together as offering the principal form of psychotherapy available before Freud.

This horde of neurologists and internists rushing into the private practice of psychotherapy touched off a terrific turf struggle in France. In 1911, Dejerine, just having received the Charcot chair of neurology, tried to reach out to the younger generation of family doctors, assuring them that through such tactics as putting the patient at ease and expressing sympathy, they would be able to get the "neuropaths" back on their feet.[115] Gilbert Ballet, the professor of psychiatry, would have none of these neurological pretentions: The psychoneuroses belong to psychiatry, he claimed. "Thus, gentlemen," said Ballet, "the field of psychiatry embraces the study of all the disorders of the mind [psychisme intellectuel]" and everything related to these disorders. Psychiatry, claimed

Ballet in prophetic words, must not be limited to the study of psychotic illness. Whatever brain mechanism neurotic illness possessed was unimportant. As long as the symptoms were "psychic," the patient belonged to psychiatry.[116] To this cool challenge, Dejerine responded rather lamely that psychiatry should limit itself to mental illness, while neurology would take the "neuropaths."[117] The exchange is exquisite in its foreshadowing of the future: Ballet's views would ultimately win, conquering for psychiatry the garden-variety neuroses of modern life. Dejerine's views would ultimately lose, as neurology became a rarified specialty dealing, it is only a slight exaggeration to say, with unusual and incurable diseases of the central nervous system.

Yet in the years before World War I, it was the neurologists who triumphed by acquiring office-practice psychotherapy. Private-practice psychotherapy, the basis of late-twentieth-century psychiatric practice, began with the neurologists, not the psychiatrists.

Harley Street in London and Queen Street in Edinburgh became Britain's psychotherapeutic epicenters. Although the British shunned specialization well into the twentieth century, Dejerine and Dubois were widely read and cited among British physicians who styled themselves simply as consultants with no mention of specialty. Just as soon as Edinburgh internist Byrom Bramwell had read of Dejerine's therapy in 1903, he astonished the medical students by putting the new psychotherapy into practice to cure a patient with a hysterical paralysis. After isolation and milk feeding, she was soon hopping about the corridor.[118] By contrast, psychiatry in Britain remained in the asylums virtually until World War II.[119] "The only psychiatrists I can recall in private practice," said psychoanalyst Ernest Jones, "were those who had retired from the position of superintendent at Bethlehem."[120] (Among them, Jones mentioned George Savage, known for having attended Virginia Woolf in bouts of depression.[121]) The distinctive British contribution to office-practice psychotherapy had always been the suggestive effect of a brass plate on a Harley Street door, and would remain so for many years.

Efforts of American neurologists to snare the lucrative carriage trade went back at least to 1879 when William Hammond, a New York neurologist and former surgeon-general, suggested treating "mental aberrations" at home.[122] The big American cities contained many "neurologists" who in fact were the equivalent of today's psychiatrists. It was at the instigation of neurologist-internists such as Lewellys Barker of Johns Hopkins—and not psychiatrists such as Adolf Meyer—that Dejerine and Dubois were enthusiastically received. Barker had visited Dejerine in Paris in 1904, then read up on Dubois and Janet. "During my first year in the

[Hopkins] clinic," said Barker, "we had more than eighty cases in which psychotherapy was the main influence in treatment." Barker set out to bring the message to family physicians that nervous patients could be helped.[123]

In the decade before World War I, the new doctrine of psychotherapy spread rapidly among internists and family physicians in the United States.[124] In 1913, Charles Dana, professor of neurology at Cornell Medical College in New York City, looked to the future: Neurology has passed, he said, from the microscope and the autopsy suite to "the study of psychoneuroses." The neurologist now had to contend with "subjective states and the importance to all neuroses of environment, education . . . the character, temperament and social conditions of his patients." Why? Because "nervous diseases are so largely social." Therefore, the neurologist should follow his patients from youth, "advise them as to marrying, even marry them at times and tell them about the management of the children." An overwhelming role indeed for specialists who only recently were cutting sections of spinal cords. "He must be a kind of superman," Dana concluded, "one with higher ideals, more potent inhibitions and wiser in life and wider in outlook than those whom he is trying to guide."[125] What lends this grandiosity its humor is that, after World War II, it was precisely the psychiatrists who began demanding this role.

The initial diffusion of psychotherapy had nothing to do with the discipline of psychiatry. The doctrine of "madness" had driven the patients from psychiatry, the panache of "nerves" luring them to the neurologist and the internist. By World War I, in every country in Western society psychiatry had become marginal to the mainstream of medicine and to the ebb and flow of dysphoria in daily life. Intellectually, it was being gobbled up by medical specialties whose very premise was organicity. To survive as a discipline, psychiatry had to break free of insanity and of organicist assumptions about the nature of "nervous disease."

5

The Psychoanalytic Hiatus

M any histories of psychiatry see psychoanalysis as the end point of the story, the goal to which all previous events had been marching. Yet with the hindsight of half a century since Freud's death in 1939, we are able to achieve a different perspective, in which psychoanalysis appears not as the final chapter in the history but as an interruption, a hiatus. For a brief period at mid-twentieth century, middle-class society became enraptured of the notion that psychological problems arose as a result of unconscious conflicts over long-past events, especially those of a sexual nature. For several decades, psychiatrists were glad to adopt this theory of illness causation as their own, especially because it permitted them to shift the locus of psychiatry from the asylum to private practice. But Freud's ideas proved short-lived. In the longer perspective of history, it was only for a few moments that the patient recumbent upon the couch, the analyst seated silently behind him, occupied the center stage of psychiatry. By the 1970s, the progress of science within psychiatry would dim the lights on this scenario, marginalizing psychoanalysis within the discipline of psychiatry as a whole. In retrospect, Freud's psychoanalysis appears as a pause in the evolution of biological approaches to brain and mind rather than as the culminating event in the history of psychiatry.

Yet it was a pause of enormous consequence for psychiatry. Freud's psychoanalysis offered psychiatrists a way out of the asylum. The practice of depth psychology, based on Freud's views, permitted psychiatrists for the first time in history to establish themselves as an office-based specialty and to wrest psychotherapy from the neurologists. Moreover, psychiatrists aspired to a monopoly over this new therapy. In the mind of the public, psychotherapy and psychoanalysis became virtually synonymous. If patients wanted one of the fashionable new depth therapies they would have to go to a psychiatrist for it, for the American Psychoanalytic Association initially insisted that only MDs could be trained as analysts, and later that only psychiatrists could be so. In retrospect, this insistence was bizarre, for psychoanalysis required no more medical training than astrology, and the attempt to impose a medical monopoly over Freud's technique was a self-interested ploy to exclude psychologists, psychiatric social workers, and other competitors from the newly discovered fountain of riches.

Ultimately, psychoanalytically oriented psychiatrists were unable to preserve their monopoly. After the 1960s, all manner of nonmedical types demanded admission to the training institutes, for there was no intrinsic reason why professors of English could not do analysis as well as psychiatrists. Even worse, what had previously passed for the scientific basis of psychoanalysis began to collapse. It could not be simultaneously true that one's psychological problems were caused by an abnormal relationship to the maternal breast and by a deficiency of serotonin. As evidence began to accumulate on the biological genesis of psychiatric illness, psychiatry began to regain the scientific footing it had lost at the beginning of the analytic craze: The brain was indeed the substrate of the mind. By the 1990s a majority of psychiatrists considered psychoanalysis scientifically bankrupt.

Thus Freud's model of the unconscious and the elaborate therapeutic techniques he devised for laying bare its supposed contents failed to stand the test of time. Accordingly, analysis largely vanished from psychiatry, discredited as a medical approach to the problems of mind and brain, although nonmedical psychoanalysis continued to flourish. The whole affair turned out to be the artifactual product of a distinctive era. Psychoanalysis failed to survive because it was overtaken by science, and because the needs that it initially met became dulled in our own time.

Freud and His Circle

Freud's psychoanalysis said that repressed childhood sexual memories and fantasies caused neurosis when reactivated in adult life. Such neurosis could be cured by an elaborate technique emphasizing dream analysis, free association, and the working through of a "transference-neurosis" (in which the analyst represents one of the patient's parents as a love-object,

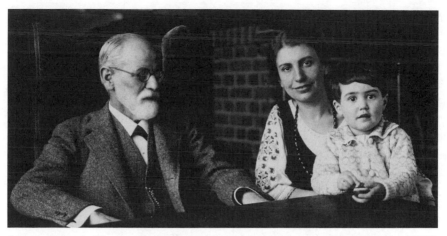

Sigmund Freud, (the founder of psychoanalysis) was born in 1856 and died in 1939. Here he is seen later in life with his daughter Anna Freud. The child is unidentified (courtesy of the Library of Congress, Prints and Photographs Division).

the patient then living out earlier childhood attitudes). Thus psycho analysis was intrinsically very psychiatric, in that it addressed disorders that doctor and patient agreed were disorders of the mind.

Yet ironically, the doctrine of psychoanalysis had its origin among nonpsychiatrists: neurologists, family doctors, and specialists in physical medicine whose patients craved some kind of caring, intimate, and ongoing contact with their physicians. The problem was that the placebo therapies these doctors used, such as hydrotherapy, electrotherapy, or dietetic therapy, often failed to transmit the message that care was being conveyed as well as treatment. In psychoanalysis by its very nature, doctor and patient communicate in the enterprise of soul-searching, creating the suggestion that one is being cared for emotionally. Thus psychoanalysis became popular initially because it filled a sentimental gap in the consultation. It offered a doctor-patient relationship in which patients basked in what they believed to be an aura of concern.

Numerous physicians other than Freud understood these psychological cravings, but Freud was the first to elaborate a therapy that would appeal to middle-class sensibilities, in particular to the desire for leisurely introspection. Yet his theories possessed a powerful additional resonance because, owing to his own ethnic origin and social position, he had privileged access to a group of patients who were especially needy in psychological terms: middle-class Jewish women in families undergoing rapid acculturation to West European values. The story of Freud's life is a familiar one.

Sigmund Freud was born in 1856 in the small town of Freiberg in Moravia, the son of merchant Jacob Freud and his third wife Malia. Four years later, the Freud family moved to Vienna, the city where Freud grew up and the centerpiece of the story of psychoanalysis. Though the Freuds arrived under somewhat reduced financial circumstances, they remained thoroughly middle class—never being without servants in the household for example—and the history of psychoanalysis would always reflect the experiences of people like the Freud family: educated, well-off, psychologically sensitive, and secularized.

Although by 1860 every city in Western Europe had a contingent of Jews, the Jews of Vienna were distinctive in constituting virtually the city's entire middle class. Whatever circle one examines—journalists, bankers, businesspeople, academics—all had a significant Jewish component by the end of the nineteenth century. This tremendous preponderance of Jews in the middle classes reflected the great social progress the Jews of Europe had made since the end of the eighteenth century, when they lived largely sequestered in the small towns of Poland, Russia, and the Ukraine. As a result of the Jewish emancipation of the nineteenth century, the small-town Jews of the east flocked to the cities of the west, using the high-school diploma as a launching pad for careers in the liberal professions. In 1890, for example, 33 percent of students at the Vienna University were of Jewish origin.[1] Fully one half of the professors of Vienna's medical faculty were Jewish.[2] As many as two-third's of the city's physicians were Jews.[3] Thus, rather than being marginalized or scorned for his ethnic background as some have claimed, the young Sigmund Freud found in Vienna an intensely Jewish setting where he had every prospect of advancement through dint of hard work.

In 1881, Freud graduated in medicine, having taken eight years to complete the degree because of repeated distractions caused by his scientific curiosity. One of these distractions had been research on the nervous systems of lower forms of sea life, and Freud went on to do a residency in neurology, in the course of which he spent five months on Meynert's service in the Vienna General Hospital. In 1885, just after receiving his title as docent, Freud traveled to Paris and was permitted to observe at Charcot's clinic through the winter of that year—a period when Charcot himself was just at the height of his obsession with "hysteria." Freud then returned to Vienna to set himself up in the private practice of neurology.[4]

As Freud opened his office, he was just one among many conventional neurologists, and he used the standard treatments of the day on the dysphoric, largely female population that was then the mainstay of private-practice neurology. Freud hypnotized his early patients, trying to cure the highly neurotic Elise Gomperz, wife of professor Theodor Gomperz, through suggestion. (Her husband complained that the hypnosis had made her worse.)[5] He also applied electrotherapy to his patients; in 1894, for example, he treated the supposedly "neuralgic" arm of Erwin Stransky's father with faradization (Stransky's father had cancer).[6] Because business was so poor, at one point Freud contemplated hiring on at a water-cure clinic.[7] For many years, Freud maintained a run-of-the-mill neurology practice.

But one aspect of, or misadventure in, his professional life was not conventional. Just after returning from Paris in 1886, he was asked by his former chief Meynert to give a lecture on hysteria to the Society of Physicians. In front of an audience who considered themselves the elite physicians of the Western world, Freud waxed fully about the wonders of Charcot's approach. "This went down poorly with the Vienna greats," psychiatry professor Julius Wagner-Jauregg recalled many years later. "[Heinrich] Bamberger and Meynert gave Freud a big rap on the knuckles in the discussion, and Freud fell almost into disgrace within the faculty." Then, continued Wagner, a distinguished Viennese family doctor with an extensive consulting practice in the Jewish community named Josef Breuer took pity on Freud "as a neurologist without patients." "Breuer now came up with work for Freud in referring hysterical Jewish girls to him for treatment."[8] In 1895, Freud and Breuer published a book together, *Studies on Hysteria*, containing Breuer's history of a young woman he named "Anna O," as well as Freud's account of several other cases.[9] (Breuer's approach to the case became christened "cathartic therapy.")

Freud was struck by what he believed to be a sexual element in the stories of these young women. There was, for example, Elisabeth von R, who later remembered, after finding her sister dead, that she had previously longed for her sister's husband. She thought guiltily to herself, "Now he is free again and I can be his wife." Freud believed that the patient developed a hysterical paralysis as a result of dealing with this conflict.[10] These experiences could be generalized, Freud thought. He theorized that much hysteria and anxiety could be explained on the grounds of patients' early experiences with sexual trauma and with adult experiences of sexual abstinence, masturbation, and such practices as coitus interruptus. After 1897, Freud came to believe that it was not actual sexual trauma but fantasies of incest in childhood that opened the wellsprings of neurosis in his adult female patients.[11]

Thus in his practice, Freud began talking to his bewildered patients ever more about sex. As he wrote to his friend Wilhelm Fliess in 1893, a

Berlin family doctor whom Freud had chosen as a special confidant, "The sexual business attracts people who are all stunned and then go away won over after having exclaimed, 'No one has ever asked me about that before!'"[12] But in eliciting all these sexual memories—in a population of young middle-class women with presumably normal hormonal drives who were cloistered in conservative Jewish families—Freud pressed his patients very hard, to the point of suggesting them into recalling events that may not have occurred or of vastly exalting the importance of trivia. By applying pressure to one patient's forehead, he was able to get her to bring an aria from *Carmen* into association with a longing for sexual caresses. The patient fled the interview.[13]

. This urgent dredging for sexual material became characteristic of the early days of psychoanalysis. Budapest analyst Sandor Ferenczi would plunge immediately into sexual matters in the clinical interview. He was once called to the bedside of a young woman who had become delirious after breaking a leg on a bobsled run. When the patient proved resistant to the sexual line of interrogation, Ferenczi began quizzing the patient's mother, who reported that the patient had once fainted while out on a drive. Ferenczi interpreted this as evidence of the patient's desire for sex with the coachman.[14]

The early analysts became well known for searching out sexual material. Viennese psychiatrist Emil Raimann, who knew Freud and his patients well, complained that Freud was able to persuade these complaisant and easily suggestible young women to say anything he wished them to. "The patients who consult Freud know in advance the information he wants to extract from them. These are patients who have let themselves be convinced of the causal significance of their sexual memories. Individuals in whom sexual motives play no role are aware that they would consult Freud in vain." (Raimann noted that in working-class families in Vienna there was plenty of sexual contact, even incest, but no hysteria. Yet among the closely guarded young women of the city's better families, where there was no possibility of sexual trauma, hysteria flourished.)[15] In the late 1890s, Raimann had worked summers at a private nervous clinic at Purkersdorf near Vienna, and was quite familiar with the middle-class families from whom Freud recruited his patients: "Once he [Freud] had called their attention to sex, this would automatically replace any other variety of pathogenic memory." Among these patients, said Raimann, "little remained in the way of daily concerns save sexual matters, resulting in an ennui and boredom that the patients tried to drown out by reading the latest and most arousing novels. . . . In these circles Freud quickly became well-known and valued as a sex researcher."[16]

Yet the culture of the European middle classes at the *fin de siècle* was receptive to sex. Although the young Freudians did not claim to monopolize the subject, they were nonetheless the only ones to offer a road map of how one got from sexual desire and repression of it to neurosis. On the basis of this map, psychoanalysis, a term Freud first used in 1896, would turn into a movement.[17] It launched itself on the world as a group of doctrines comprising three main areas: study of the patient's resistance to thoughts that attempted to press into the conscious mind from the unconscious; concentration on the causal significance of sexual matters; and an emphasis on the centrality of early childhood experiences.[18] The core doctrine, from which Freud never wavered, was that neurotic symptoms represented a trade-off between sexual and aggressive drives and the requirements of reality.

In 1902, Freud set up a discussion group that met on Wednesday evenings in his home. This was his first attempt to go beyond communicating with his (by now ex-) friend Fliess and to recruit a group of followers. The schisms and rivalries that plagued this Wednesday group in its brief existence before World War I illuminated the basic problems that dogged psychoanalysis throughout: Freud was so intent on propagating his own views that, by turning psychoanalysis into a movement rather than a method of studying subrational psychology, he denied analysis the possibility of ever acquiring a scientific footing.

The master's insights were to become articles of faith, incapable of disproof. And the efforts of others to criticize Freud's wisdom would always be considered evidence of "resistance," of personal pathology, never as scientific hypotheses to be dealt with in the way that science treats all hypotheses. Alfred Adler fell away, as did Wilhelm Stekel, Freud's physician-patient who had suggested establishing the Wednesday group in the first place. Such far-distant fans of analysis as the Zurich academics Carl Jung and Eugen Bleuler would soon turn heretic, as did later many others. The efforts of all these critical individuals to nudge Freud away from the bedrock of childhood sexuality on which he built his theories would fail. But a core of faithful remained. And it was these loyal captains who, in the belief that they possessed an inner truth, took psychoanalysis to the wide world.

The Berlin analyst Franz Alexander, who in the early 1930s established a beachhead for psychosomatic medicine in Chicago, explained how it felt to be "a member of such a courageous pioneering group." "In the main, *you* were right and the *world* was wrong. Even at the first rough approach to your subject, there was sufficient evidence for your teachings. You knew positively that . . . repressed sexual impulses were the main sources of neurosis of the Victorian and post-Victorian Westerner, and, above all, that sexuality was there from the beginning of life, and its objects in the infant were incestuous."[19]

Did Freud and his followers really know these truths? Or were they simply self-suggesting one another into accepting highly dubious propositions as being somehow "confirmed"? Freud tended to see himself more as an adventurer than a scientist, once telling Fliess flatly, "I am actually not at all a man of science, not an observer, not an experimenter, not a thinker. I am by temperament nothing but a conquistador—an adventurer, if you want it translated—with all the curiosity, daring, and tenacity characteristic of a man of this sort."[20] His inner circle was rife with toadyism, for the other analysts were economically dependent on Freud for referrals. (He kept a pile of their calling cards in his drawer, and would dole them out to patients according to his whim.)[21] "Freud never realized how much of a suggestive impact he had on his followers," writes historian Paul Roazen, "and therefore could be led to think that his findings were being genuinely confirmed by independent observers."[22] The issue of validity would therefore haunt psychoanalysis until its eclipse within psychiatry.

A second troubling issue was the extent to which psychoanalysis represented a specific therapy as opposed to a worldview. It offered indeed a comprehensive picture of human connectedness within society, able to account for the shapes of water faucets (penislike) as easily as explaining the fear of intimacy (suppressed homosexual longings). But Freud himself was uneasy about whether psychoanalysis could actually make people better. He published few case histories and seems to have felt most comfortable with analysis at the societal level, of which the best known example is his book *Civilization and Its Discontents*, written in 1930.[23] After a colleague told him about a therapeutic success, Freud is reported to have looked up almost astonished and said, "Oh yes, you can also cure people with analysis."[24] On another occasion, Freud confided to Ludwig Binswanger, the superintendent of a luxurious private nervous clinic in Kreuzlingen, Switzerland, "I often console myself with the idea, that even though we achieve so little therapeutically, at least we understand why more cannot be achieved. In this sense our therapy seems to me to be the only rational one."[25] As psychoanalysis set out to take over psychiatry, therefore, it was with a doctrine that was therapeutically uncertain, intellectually highly speculative to say the least, and best adapted to the psychological needs of a deracinated group in transition: young middle-class Jewish women who aspired to be like their non-Jewish counterparts. It would be hard to imagine a therapy less appropriate for the needs of people with serious psychiatric illnesses.

Given the intrinsic inappropriateness of psychoanalysis for psychiatry, there must have been some other force driving it forward in Europe than the power of the idea itself. That force was middle-class enthusiasm. Freud's ideas proved tremendously popular among the educated classes as a codification of the kind of search for self-knowledge that had run through bourgeois culture throughout the entire second half of the century. Psychoanalysis was to therapy as expressionism was to art: Both represented exquisite versions of the search for insight. Psychoanalytic ideas were sufficiently *à la page* in prewar Berlin that the readers of Grete Meisel-Hess's novel *The Intellectuals*, published in 1911, would have resonated to "Erika's" psychiatric adventures:

> "I am sick," she decided. "I must go to the doctor." As she had long been curious about "this psycho-analytic" procedure, she sought out a "famous psychiatrist."
>
> After hearing her tale, he told her, "You have repressed your painful sexual experiences instead of overpowering them. . . . *Nicht wahr?*"
>
> Erika nodded. He continued, "It's important to open your eyes and to recall into your consciousness that repressed experience in its true form." He used the verb "abreact" and explained to her basic notions about dreams and her erogenous zones. He gave her a gynecologic exam, apparently on the theory that a tilted uterus might be causing her hysteria.
>
> "Since everything's in order down there," he said, "I will need to treat you only psycho-analytically." He told her that her "hysterical affective psychosis" was curable and that he would hypnotize her.
>
> The consultation came to an end after he awakened her from hypnotic sleep by touching her eyelids. Erika was well again.[26]

We recognize this as a travesty of psychoanalysis in the form that Freud's doctrine was later codified—Freud stopped hypnotizing patients late in the 1890s—and psychoanalysis did not incorporate hypnosis. Yet this is how psychoanalysis was understood before the analysts founded their own training institutes to standardize the technique. Berlin's psychoanalytic society, the first in Central Europe, was founded in 1908 (after 1920 actual training was conducted in a psychoanalytic outpatient clinic).[27] By 1925, psychoanalysis had become so fashionable among the Berlin middle classes that people would chat about their "Minko's," short for "Minderwertigkeitskomplex," or inferiority complex.[28]

In Vienna, too, the "psychoanalytic infestation" (as novelist Elias Canetti put it) had taken firm hold. "At that time you couldn't say anything in conversation without having it nullified with some kind of facile reference to unconscious motivation. The unspeakable boredom that these people gave off, the sterility that resulted from this, was of apparent concern to few."[29] When Canetti himself had some kind of absence fit, the kindly old family "Dr. Laub" was summoned. He reassured Canetti's mother: Just let him be. "That's good for the Oedipus."[30]

Regular psychiatrists were bemused at the grassfire spread of psychoanalysis within the middle classes. One physician at the Budapest psychiatric clinic tried to account for it along the following lines: "The flood of patients seeking salvation through psychoanalysis is explainable partly from the publicity, partly from the receptiveness of our time to introversion and introspection." It was a procedure of obvious appeal to "hypersexual neurotics," he said.[31] Thus we have a core of physicians dubious, even contemptuous of "hypersexual neurotics" and their problems, and an educated middle class keening at the doctor's office for further self-insight. The stage was set for the virtual destruction of traditional, asylum-based psychiatry.

The Battle Begins

How psychoanalysis grew into a movement is a story in its own right. What interests us here is its efforts to take over psychiatry. Between the late 1890s, when Freud's new notions of therapy started to interest outsiders, and the 1960s, the high-water mark of the psychoanalytic movement, Freudian doctrine made deep inroads into psychiatry. These analytic incursions provoked a tremendous struggle within psychiatry, a discipline previously oriented to biology and not to psychology. If in the end analysis won, it was not necessarily because of the power of Freud's ideas but because analysis opened the road to private practice.

What most physicians understood initially by psychoanalysis was not its classic form, meaning 50-minute hours five days a week, a silent psychiatrist seated behind a patient on a couch who was reciting dream memories or doing word associations. That form tended to be disseminated by the psychoanalytic training institutes that flourished in the big cities after the 1930s. The early form of analysis, disseminated by Freud's own writings, emphasized interrogation of the patient about his or her erotic life in the context of a close doctor-patient relationship. Freud himself was actually quite "unorthodox," often going to his patients' homes, socializing with them, and indulging in behavior that would later have been considered unconventional.[32] Yet the early Freud did not offer some anodyne version of psychotherapy. Rather it was a thorough grilling on such matters as coitus interruptus, masturbation, and early memories of sex and desire.

As psychiatry resisted the psychoanalytic incursion, two main themes came to the fore: skepticism about Freud's views on the sexual causes of mental illness, and the professoriate's reluctance to see psychiatry diverted from psychosis to neurosis.

The battle was joined first in Central Europe. Among those who opposed Freud, the dominant note was simple disbelief in Freud's sexual reductionism. It is inconceivable, said Gustav Aschaffenburg, a former assistant of Kraepelin and, in 1906, psychiatry professor in Cologne, that masturbation causes "the repression of affect." Nor did Aschaffenburg find it likely that sexual abstinence was the main cause of anxiety. Freud must be getting his results by putting words in the patients' mouths, Aschaffenburg said, and concluded that the whole edifice of psychoanalytic theory was a triumph of suggestion.[33] Adolf Friedländer, chief physician at a private clinic near Frankfurt, was judged in the psychoanalytic movement to be a notorious enemy of Freud. Yet Friedländer had sinned mainly by skewering various figures within psychoanalysis for their negative statements about women.[34] His position was actually quite moderate: "Psychoanalysis [meaning psychotherapy] is in and of itself indispensable for neurologists and psychiatrists. But *sexual* psychoanalysis strikes many of us as doubtful or unnecessary."[35] These comments are typical of a whole range of reaction in Germany, a disbelief that stemmed not necessarily from prudishness, for many critics of psychoanalysis had nothing against other forms of psychotherapy in which intimate details might also emerge, but from sheer unwillingness to accept that neurotic pathology boiled down to sex.

The professors represented a slightly different source of hostility. The analysts claimed quite correctly that most of the chair-holders in psychiatry were lined up against them, with the well-known exception of Eugen Bleuler in Zurich and the less-well-known exception of Karl Bonhoeffer in Berlin. (In 1914, for example, Bonhoeffer asked candidates for medical-officer-of-health posts to write an exam question on "The significance of psychoanalysis for psychiatry."[36]) To be sure, the professors, like most other observers, disliked the movement's sexual reductionism. Thus Germany's leading neuropsychiatrist, Adolf Strümpell, called the Viennese obsessed by sex.[37] "I find this Freudian cult nauseating," said Zurich psychiatry professor August Forel in 1907, and later told of patients whom psychoanalysis had worsened by fixating them upon sexual matters.[38]

Yet sex was not the sticking point for most of the professoriate. And if Otto Binswanger, Oswald Bumke, Alfred Hoche, Emil Kraepelin, Konrad Rieger, and others saw fit to attack psychoanalysis, there must have been some other circumstance. These men without exception had backgrounds in asylum psychiatry. For them mental illness meant psychosis, a disorder requiring institutional care. Seeing the younger psychiatrists abandon the psychoses and chase after a doctrine that promised relief mainly for neurotic illness was probably more than the senior professors could stand. It represented a renunciation of their life's work and of their sense of the very mission of psychiatry. For they quite correctly perceived Freud and the analysts to be redirecting the discipline toward the understanding and therapy of the psychoneuroses—the psychiatric disorders of daily life seen outside the asylum.

There was almost a professorial bewilderment at seeing psychiatry's entire center of gravity shift.[39] Würzburg professor Konrad Rieger captured this regret perfectly in 1896: "I cannot imagine that an experienced alienist would be able to read [Freud] without sensing true disgust. And the reason for this disgust would be that the author assigns great importance to paranoid chatter of a sexual nature . . . even when it has not been wholly invented. This kind of effort can only lead to a ghastly 'village-crone psychiatry [Altweiber-Psychiatrie].' "[40] The problem with village-crone psychiatry was that it addressed people who were unhappy but not mad.

Rieger and company did well to be alarmed, for in the years before World War I, younger psychiatrists were indeed flocking to psychoanalysis as a form of psychotherapy. There are two themes here: first, the willingness to use some form of analysis as a way of prying open the doctor-patient relationship, of introducing psychological sensitivity to psychiatry without necessarily becoming a "psychoanalyst" oneself; second, the embracing of Freud's doctrine willy-nilly because it appealed to patients and had started to become celebrated in the patients' world. As internist and psychiatrist Viktor von Weizsäcker said of his youthful encounters with psychoanalysis, "Medicine as it was practiced in university clinics then [around 1914] awakened in me and in many other young physicians the greatest doubt. Rounds were becoming increasingly impersonal; the wards, the dominance of laboratory tests and [electrocardiogram] curves revolted me. There was never a one-on-one conversation between doctor and patient. . . . What a contrast with what the psychotherapists were doing, who had spent their entire lives just having intimate dialogues in their practices!"[41] For Weizsäcker, it was important not to become a formal psychoanalyst but to use this new perspective as a way of talking with patients. He belonged to a whole cohort of young physicians who saw in analysis not a holy shrine but a way of communicating.[42]

Another group of psychiatrists, perhaps less psychologically minded but more profit oriented, embraced psychoanalysis because they wanted to attract patients. These were the owners of the private nervous clinics. And their fondness for what they advertised as "psychoanalysis" was the supply-side response to the rising demand for "Freudianism" among the middle classes in the years around World War I. For these were the classes that became patients in such clinics. The highly competitive private clinics would generally offer whatever therapies seemed trendy, diet therapy in the 1890s or "sun and air" cures in the belle époque.[43] After around 1910, it was psychoanalysis that was in fashion.

Freud's and Breuer's version of psychotherapy as enunciated in 1895 was called cathartic therapy. It was picked up immediately in the world of the private clinics. As early as 1900, Wolfgang Warda, owner of a private nervous clinic in Blankenburg, a spa in Thuringia, was telling colleagues of his success with the "cathartic method of Breuer and Freud."[44] After Freud abandoned the notion of catharsis as curative and went over to insight-oriented therapy, his supporters in the private sector began to multiply. After visiting Freud in Vienna in 1907, young Ludwig Binswanger at the Bellevue Clinic in Kreuzlingen became an adept. After the death of Binswanger's father Robert in 1910, Ludwig took over the clinic and began advertising to doctors and patients his enthusiasm for the new therapy. "In those days," said Binswanger, "I was still convinced that every psychoneurosis, and many psychoses and psychopathic personalities, could be healed or at least improved with psychoanalysis."[45] Despite demands by mainline psychiatrists to boycott such clinics, Bellevue flourished with the new approach.[46] There were several other prewar examples like Binswanger, such as Otto Juliusburger, a founding member of the Berlin psychoanalytic society. On staff at a large private asylum in the Berlin suburb of Lankwitz, Juliusburger was very sensitive to the accusation that psychoanalysis and Jewishness somehow ran together.[47]

World War I made a big difference in public acceptance of psychoanalysis, perhaps because Freud's views of the death instinct and aggression seemed to illuminate the war's awesome irrationality. (In 1920 Freud argued that two fundamental instincts existed—the life and death instincts, or Eros and Thanatos, rather than just the sexual instinct as he previously believed.) After the war, it became the rage to include psychoanalysis in one's therapeutic palette. Many clinics that previously would have nothing to do with psychotherapy were now proclaiming their attachment to psychoanalysis. By 1927, for example, Wilhelm Rohrbach was insisting that he offered "psychoanalysis" in his establishment in the Kassel suburb of Wilhelmshöhe among a long list of therapies that otherwise included "all varieties of baths, modern light and air treatments, electrotherapy in the newest forms, terrain therapy, gymnastics and massage . . . and hypnotic and nonhypnotic suggestive treatments."[48] (Rohrbach had taken the clinic over just after the war from a former owner who had disgraced himself by assaulting the patients.) With the Nazi seizure of power psychoanalysis vanished from private clinics of Germany.

A final domain of psychiatry into which psychoanalysis pushed was the public asylum itself. Here it was mainly keen young physicians, avid to try anything new, who picked up Freud's doctrine. A typical early instance: In 1903, a junior physician, Hans Eglauer, at the Lower Austrian asylum of Kierling-Gugging outside of Vienna, noted in a patient's chart that he had attempted to investigate her "inner life" (*Seelenleben*), but had little success because she appeared to him too unintelligent and uneducated.[49] Eglauer was almost certainly influenced in this enterprise by Freud's teachings, which by 1903 had become celebrated in Vienna. Novelist and psychiatrist Alfred Döblin, who before the Nazi takeover worked in the asylum of Berlin-Buch, gave in his 1929 novel *Berlin Alexanderplatz* what may have been an autobiographical account (from a prewar experience) of two young psychiatrists trying to use psychoanalysis on a psychotic patient, the mythical "Franz Biberkopf."[50] The novel reads:

> "[The young doctors] are inclined to consider Franz Biberkopf's trouble as psychogenic, that is, his rigidity comes from the soul, it is a pathological condition of inhibitions and constraints which would be cleared up by an analysis (perhaps it emanates from early psychic states)." Yet they cannot get Biberkopf to talk. The analysis fails.
>
> The young doctors then talk the case over with the weary old chief physician of the asylum. He laughs at their efforts: "When a confirmed jail-bird like him sees two young gentlemen who talk a lot of rubbish about him . . . and want to do some prayer-healing with him, well, take it from me, you're simply soft mash for a chap like that."
>
> The young doctors protest, "But he's inhibited, sir, in our view it is a repression, conditioned by a psychic crisis, a loss of contact with reality, due to disappointment, failure, perhaps infantile and instinctive demands on reality. . . ."

158

"Psychic crisis be damned," says the old physician. "You're really a master-healer, three cheers for the new therapy, and you can send a telegram of congratulation to Freud in Vienna."[51]

Elsewhere, enthusiastic young efforts to bring psychoanalysis to the asylum also met with similar rebuffs. Around 1907, Arthur Muthmann attempted to import analysis to Basel's Friedmatt asylum, but was rejected by the chief physician, who apparently thought so little of Muthmann's judgment that he refused to sponsor Muthmann's postdoctoral habilitation research.[52] Another junior Swiss doctor, Karl Gehry, on staff at the Rheinau asylum near Schaffhausen, was so enthusiastic about Forel's work on the psychic life of ants that he decided to read Freud's *The Psychopathology of Everyday Life,* published as a book in 1904. Encouraged by his colleague Franz Riklin, a well-known advocate of analysis, Gehry began attending Jung's and Bleuler's psychoanalytically oriented seminar at the Burghölzli, the university psychiatric clinic in Zurich. The contagion seems to have spread to the entire Rheinau staff except for the medical director who, Gehry said, "had on blinkers when it came to sex." Gehry abandoned Freud, however, when all of his efforts to analyze these very ill patients failed.[53]

Thus in Central Europe the efforts of psychoanalysis to press into psychiatry ran along three lines: attempts to make the doctor-patient relationship psychologically more sensitive, to improve one's competitive position in the private sector, and to achieve some glimmer of therapeutic hope in the public sector. All three would help lay the basis for office practice, as physicians who had trained in these various settings understood how much wider the sweep of psychiatry became once the discipline absorbed a psychological approach to neurotic illness.

By the first annual meeting in 1926 in Baden-Baden of the General Medical Congress on Psychotherapy, an organization whose inspiration was heavily psychoanalytic, psychotherapy in Central Europe had come to mean applying in private practice some kind of technique derived from psychoanalysis. Of the nearly 500 physicians attending that congress, 70 percent were in private practice. And while a few pediatricians and dermatologists did take part, the majority of doctors present were psychiatrists.[54] Thus by the mid-1920s in Central Europe, the spirit of psychoanalysis had made great inroads into psychiatry.

The main points of the general story are evident from this account of events in Central Europe, which it is unnecessary to extend to all other countries. After World War I, young psychiatrists everywhere who were interested in office practice based on psychotherapy started thinking psychoanalytically, though not necessarily seeking to become full-fledged analysts themselves. By the end of the 1920s, what they were reading about psychotherapy and the like was heavily analytic in nature.[55] This was a trend in which every country shared and illustrates the extent to which psychiatry was coming to mean some kind of therapy based on the doctor-patient relationship as opposed to dumping patients into baths in an institution.

By the 1920s, psychiatry was blossoming outside the asylum. The intellectual trend giving energy to this blooming was psychoanalysis. Until this point, the center of gravity of the story had been Europe, for it was mainly in Central Europe that the beat to the international stride was drummed. Yet in the 1930s, the history of psychiatry underwent a momentous change. The rise of Nazism in Germany and Austria snuffed out literally from one moment to the next the rich scientific discipline of psychiatry that had flourished on that soil for a century and a half. Many of its distinguished Jewish practitioners were murdered in the Holocaust or dispersed their energies in the chaos of emigration. By 1945, psychiatry as a discipline was dead in Germany and Austria.

After the 1930s, the world epicenter of psychiatry shifted to the United States. It was in America that psychoanalysis flourished beyond the wildest dreams of its Viennese founders. In the United States, psychoanalysis took over the profession of psychiatry for a period of about three decades. Only in the 1970s would American psychiatry begin to recover from its analytic infatuation. And because postwar America replaced Central Europe as psychiatry's driving force, what happened in the United States had a capital importance for the evolution of the discipline in general.

American Origins

Psychoanalysis had great significance for the history of psychiatry in the United States. Under the influence of Freud's teachings, American psychiatry accomplished the switch from psychosis to neurosis as the object of study, and from the asylum to Main Street as the venue for practice. The price of this advance was that psychoanalysis infiltrated American psychiatry far more deeply than elsewhere, causing scientific stagnation and increasing disengagement from the rest of medicine.

Psychoanalysis was important in anchoring American psychiatrists in the office. Yet the trend from asylum to private practice began before that period and for independent reasons. As early as the 1880s, psychiatry started to establish a freehold in the form of outpatient clinics, some based in asylums and some not. In November 1885, Philadelphia's John Chapin, superintendent of the Pennsylvania Hospital for the Insane, opened a clinic in the outpatient department of the Pennsylvania General Hospital, the parent organization of the asylum. The clinic saw about a hundred patients a year, half of them psychiatric, half neurological.[56] This was the first significant American facility for treating noninstitutionalized psychiatric patients. Twelve years later, in 1897, Walter Channing established a "mental clinic" at the Boston Dispensary to enable giving clinical instruction to medical students and young doctors. Channing was the owner of a private nervous clinic in the suburb of Brookline and taught psychiatry at various institutions in the area. "There is a big field for the psychiatrist outside of the hospital," he said.[57]

Indeed. Around the turn of the century, psychiatry began to care for patients in the community on a number of fronts. In 1906, for example, in New York State a charitable association initiated a program of aftercare for discharged patients under the guidance of Louise L. Schuyler. Before World War I, several psychiatric hospitals opened their own outpatient clinics, the Henry Phipps Psychiatric Clinic in Baltimore under Adolf Meyer being the first university hospital to do so.[58]

Psychiatry further reached out with the founding in 1909 of the National Committee for Mental Hygiene. A book by ex-psychiatric patient Clifford Beers, *A Mind That Found Itself* (published in 1908), prompted a number of prominent figures such as Meyer and William James to promote the concept of "mental hygiene." In subsequent years, the mental-hygiene movement involved psychiatrists in numerous plans to improve the "mental health" of Americans through various well-meaning efforts.[59]

Thus even before psychoanalysis, private-practice psychiatry, dedicated to the lesser but extremely common psychiatric illnesses, was acquiring a Main Street beachhead. By 1927, George Kline, commissioner of the Massachusetts department of mental health and then president of the American Psychiatric Association, was able to write, "The past decade has witnessed a remarkable extension of the sphere of psychiatry beyond the walls of the mental hospital."[60] Of psychiatrists attending the annual meeting of the American Psychiatric Association in 1910, only 3.2 percent were in private practice. By 1921, the figure had risen to 7.3 percent.[61] Yet it was psychoanalysis that permitted this beachhead to be expanded into a victorious onmarch that would ultimately sweep almost the entire discipline. Psychoanalysis was the caisson on which American psychiatry rode triumphantly into private practice.

From the very beginning, Freud's writings were received enthusiastically in America. Well before the organization of local psychoanalytic societies, individual physicians who themselves often spoke and read German as a result of postgraduate training in Berlin or Vienna were picking up Freud's works and trying to apply them. Around Boston, for example, Freud first started to be read around 1894—a year before the publication of *Studies on Hysteria.* Harvard psychologist William James went on to kindle interest among a small number of physicians who formed a discussion group meeting in the home of Morton Prince, a professor of neurology at Tufts University. (Prince, who founded the *Journal of Abnormal and Social Psychology* in 1906, became well known among American physicians and psychologists for importing a psychological, semi-Freudian perspective into the study of neurosis.) James Jackson Putnam, professor of neurology at Harvard, contributed a paper to the first issue of this journal on his experiences with what he called "psychoanalysis" at the Massachusetts General Hospital. This represented the official launch of Freud's doctrines in America though that had not really been Putnam's intention; he was interested in experimenting broadly with psychotherapy as opposed to psychoanalysis in particular.[62]

In New York large numbers of neurologists and family doctors acquainted themselves with Freud's techniques. In 1909, Abraham Brill, an Austrian-born neurologist who had emigrated to the United States at the age of 15, translated Freud's *Studies on Hysteria* into a rather clumsy English. Brill had traveled back to Austria and Switzerland, knew Freud (he considered his chats with the Professor to be a training analysis), and claimed credit as the actual founder of psychoanalysis in the United States.[63] Analysis flourished particularly among New York's society neurologists who, as in Europe, had been the principal previous practitioners of psychotherapy. By 1922, there were said to be more than 500 "unofficial" analysts in the city.[64]

In September 1909, accompanied by Jung and Ferenczi, Freud came to the United States to lecture at the invitation of Stanley Hall of Clark University. The tour gave a great boost to psychoanalysis among American physicians and the public. Freud however hated the United States, despising many of his American enthusiasts. (He considered Prince "an arrogant ass who would be conspicuous even in our menagerie.") Yet the press interviews that he gave aroused great curiosity. In the immediate wake of the visit, there was a spurt of medical praise of analysis, and psychoanalysis became launched as a movement in the United States.[65]

The building of the psychoanalytic movement was accomplished in two steps. First came the founding of local psychoanalytic societies, the professional organizations of the analysts themselves. Second came the psychoanalytic training institutes, usually but not always under the control of the local societies. These served to educate future generations of analysts in the intricacies of psychoanalytic theory and technique, so that a commonly understood body of doctrine could be handed down from one generation to the next. As in Europe, the societies and training institutes were separate from each other. Unlike Europe, however, in the United States only physicians were eligible to apply for training. Although there was no good reason why nonphysicians could not do analysis just as effectively—there being nothing intrinsically medical about plumbing the unconscious mind—American medical psychoanalysts had a horror of lay competition. And from their viewpoint, rightly so. Given that psychoanalysis had been psychiatry's ticket out of the asylum, the last thing the American analysts wanted was to break their monopoly by sharing it with psychologists and social workers avid to have a go at analysis themselves.[66]

The first local psychoanalytic society in the United States was founded by Brill in New York in February 1911. At the outset, the theme of escaping the asylum was significant. Of the 15 founding members, 10 were associated with the Manhattan State Hospital.[67] Another member, Bronislaw Onuf, was chief physician at Knickerbocker Hall in Amityville, Long Island, a private nervous clinic that would soon start offering psychoanalysis, if in fact Onuf was not already applying it in 1911.[68] "These matters were eagerly discussed at our staff meetings, and at the Ward's Island Psychiatric Society," said David Henderson, an Edinburgh physician who between 1908 and 1911 was doing a psychiatry residency on Ward's Island. At one meeting of the society, Adolf Meyer gave a paper entitled "A Discussion of Some Fundamental Issues in Freud's Psycho-Analysis."[69] So there is no doubt that asylum psychiatry was heavily implicated at the very birth of American psychoanalysis.

In May 1911, Ernest Jones came down to Baltimore from Toronto, where he was then in exile from England, and arranged for the founding meeting of the American Psychoanalytic Association. Here Jones and associates were building on another organization, the American Psychopathological Association, which Putnam, Meyer, August Hoch, Jones, and others had founded in Washington the previous year. In 1911, the new psychoanalytic society would meet at the same time and in the same Baltimore hotel as the psychopathological society.[70] The American Psychoanalytic Association was not to be a local society but was open to anyone in the country who declared an interest in Freud's ideas.[71] Until 1932, this nationwide organization amounted to little, controlled as it was by

New Yorkers who additionally had their own robust local society. It was peopled by the somewhat quirky and reflective physicians who in those days tended to express an interest in Freudian ideas.

Other local societies were soon established elsewhere. Washington, DC, acquired its initial psychoanalytic society in 1914 (which flickered in and out of life until being solidly refounded in 1930). Boston's first psychoanalytic society was founded in 1930, Chicago's in 1931, numbering among its members such European heavyweights as Franz Alexander and Therese Benedek.[72] In 1932, the American Psychoanalytic Association reorganized itself as a federation of local societies, and from that point on, national standards became applied to local organization and training. The training institutes founded in the 1930s applied these standards with a vengeance. Soon an orthodox template for conducting psychoanalysis began to press individual idiosyncrasies about hypnotism, cathartic therapy, and the many other practices once identified as "psychoanalysis" into a uniform pattern that would be recognizable from coast to coast.

From the viewpoint of the history of psychiatry, the most interesting aspect of the history of psychoanalysis is its efforts to take over psychiatry. How does a small discipline set out to engulf a big one? Overlapping membership is one tactic. Ideally, all the analysts would end up as psychiatrists, and vice versa to a lesser extent. Starting in the 1920s, big psychoanalytic names showed up increasingly at psychiatric meetings. At the 1928 psychiatric meeting in Minneapolis, for example, present among the 32 psychiatrists in private practice were such figures as Leo Bartemeier, who years later would help found the Detroit psychoanalytic group, or Clarence Oberndorf, a founding member of the New York Psychoanalytic Society.[73]

More and more analysts were becoming psychiatrists. They had no choice. In 1938, the American Psychoanalytic Association required candidates for a training analysis to have completed at least one year of a psychiatric residency. During the 1940s, several local institutes raised this requirement to two years, and the association began encouraging psychiatry residents to commence simultaneously a training program at a nearby psychoanalytic institute (if one were in fact nearby). By 1944, 70 percent of American psychoanalysts had qualified in psychiatry (sometimes in neurology as well: a common examination board for psychiatry and neurology was established in 1934). By 1953, 82 percent of the members of the American Psychoanalytic Association were simultaneously members of the American Psychiatric Association. The psychoanalytic association had by now stipulated that would-be analysts must complete at least three years of a psychiatric residency before commencing psychoanalytic training.[74] The analysts had thus joined psychiatry.

The psychiatrists and psychoanalysts moved closer together in organizational terms as well. From 1924 on, the American Psychiatric Association and the American Psychoanalytic Association would hold their meetings at the same time in the same city. Nine years later, in 1933, the American Psychiatric Association started a special section of psychoanalysis for interested members.[75] Although there initially had been a huge fight on the APA's executive board about embracing analysis, the psychiatric organization could see which way the wind was blowing. It was blowing toward private practice, and that meant encouraging psychotherapy.

In the late 1930s, the analysts themselves were pushing hard for their movement's breakout into general psychiatry. Lawrence Kubie, president of the New York Psychoanalytic Society, urged that the psychoanalytic education of psychiatrists be carried on in units attached to mental hospitals and medical schools. "In this way training in psychoanalysis could gradually become part of the training of the house-physician in every mental hospital," he argued.[76] As Franz Alexander of the Chicago institute declared in a 1939 letter to Ernest Jones, "[Psychoanalysis] is rapidly becoming part of general medical practice and training."[77]

By the entry of the United States into World War II, psychoanalysis had captured the basics of training in psychiatry at the undergraduate and graduate level. In 1942, a major study of psychiatric education concluded that, while one could not turn all medical students into analysts, "one can have no quarrel with the introduction of at least the basic psychoanalytical concepts in the course of psychopathology [for the medical students], and indeed it is difficult to see how psychopathology can be taught without these concepts."[78] The psychiatrists who went marching off to cure combat fatigue during the war were armed with psychoanalytic doctrine.

With analysis skyrocketing in psychiatry, the public was not long in latching onto this appealing new therapy, at least those who could afford it. Just as the middle classes of Berlin had chattered about their "Minko's," middle-class Americans were breathless about their unconscious "defenses" that required dismantling. In Sally Pierce's 1929 memoir of her encounter with nervous disease, she describes having tried first one exclusive private nervous clinic then another. The rest cure, the being-yelled-at cure, the Dubois-style cure of rational persuasion: All had failed her. Then she stumbled into the hands of "Frank Gaylord," the psychoanalyst.

"No permanent cure of a neurosis could take place," Dr. Gaylord told her, "until each unconscious cause of each neurotic symptom had been discovered and brought up into the patient's consciousness; not only brought up into consciousness, but discussed, examined, appraised, and finally understood and recognized by the patient for what it was: infantile, regressive stuff that blocked a progressive, adult living of life." Dr. Gaylord told her she would need daily appointments of an hour each time, stretching over many months. Finally after her "unconscious defenses" against the intrusion of reason had been broken down, she would be well again. Indeed after months of analysis, she did become well again. Here was apparent evidence that psychoanalysis worked. The American public that feasted on this and similar accounts increasingly put behind them the world of the private clinic with its amazonian nurses enforcing rest cures and embraced the Park Avenue practitioners of psychoanalysis.[79]

In 1935, *Fortune* magazine in a piece entitled "The 'Nervous Breakdown'" explained soberly that, "The suppression of the sexual instinct in childhood pushed certain experiences and desires deep into the unconscious, where they reappear in the adult as neuroses."[80] For the first time in history, the depressed businessman or the anxious housewife would seek out the services of a psychiatrist, and if the psychiatrist lived in New York, Boston, or Washington, chances were that he would be oriented to psychoanalysis.

The Arrival of the Europeans

History moves in odd ways. What ultimately converted a chic therapeutic boomlet into a mass ideology shaping almost every aspect of American thought and culture was the Holocaust. In the 1930s, fascism drove many analysts who were Jewish from Central Europe to the United States, where they lent the strippling little American movement the glamour and heft of the wide world. On the face of it, this massive transfer of culture from the German-speaking world to the English had positive results for psychoanalysis, reinforcing the homespun American heterodoxy with the prestige of internationally acclaimed figures.[81] In the long run, however, the migration of the European analysts proved fatal for psychoanalysis in the New World, for the refugees brought with them a stifling orthodoxy, a reflexive adherence to the views of Freud and his daughter Anna that American analysis was never able to outgrow and that ultimately caused, within medicine at least, its death from disbelief.

The number of refugee analysts from Europe was not large. Set against the 4,000 physicians from Germany and Austria who found shelter in the United States between 1933 and 1944, there were not more than 250 psychiatrists. And of these 250, not more than 50 were psychoanalysts.[82] Yet many were very well known. Consider who emigrated from the Berlin Psychoanalytic Society. Franz Alexander, whose name became synonymous with psychosomatic medicine, accepted a visiting professorship in psychiatry at the University of Chicago in 1930 (Alexander insisted that it be in "psychoanalysis"). Two years later, he founded a psychoanalytic training institute in Chicago. After the Nazi seizure of power, Alexander was no longer able to return. Sandor Rado of Berlin had initially been lured to New York in 1931 to organize a Berlin-style institute. Events would bar his return too. Otto Fenichel, who had written the first textbook of psychoanalysis, left Berlin in 1933, ending up in 1938 in Los Angeles where he worked as a training instructor.[83] When in May 1940, the Emergency Committee on Relief of the American Psychoanalytic Association inventoried refugee analysts with whom it recently had been in contact, there were eight names from Berlin on the list.[84]

Things were not easy for the new arrivals. Even though they read English, they often spoke the language poorly. When Fenichel, for example, visited at the Menninger clinic in Topeka, he was asked to give a lecture. Aware that he often mispronounced words, he asked another emigré, Martin Grotjahn, for help. Grotjahn later recalled that Fenichel wanted to talk about something called "penis envoy." "That did not sound right," said Grotjahn, "and I tentatively suggested . . . 'penis ivy.' A suggestion by another immigrant 'envy' was rejected as too unlikely by Otto and me." Fenichel's talk was "respected by all and understood by none. 'Penis envoy' finally brought down the house."[85]

Despite their linguistic deficiencies, the luminosity of the emigré analysts made them much in demand: Hermann Nunberg had left Vienna in 1932, initially for Philadelphia, then secured for himself a society practice on Park Avenue in New York; Freud's physician Felix Deutsch and his analyst wife Helene left Vienna in 1935 for a lovely home in Cambridge, Massachusetts. A swarm of analysts escaped Vienna in the great panic following the Nazi invasion of March 1938. Freud's lieutenant Paul Federn arrived in New York where he was, according to his friend psychiatrist Heinrich Meng, "at once counted among the leading psychiatrists of the country."[86] Heinz Hartmann ended up as a training analyst in New York. Lay analyst Ernst Kris became a professor at the New School for Social Research in New York (he had a PhD in art history, and had begun medical school, which he did not finish, in 1933). Beate ("Tola") Rank landed at the Judge Baker Guidance Center in Boston.[87]

One can only imagine the circumstances in which these men and women left Vienna, on a day's or hour's notice. Viennese dramatist Franz Werfel portrayed the scene, in which august and by-now middle-aged individuals, the Nazi tanks rumbling on the streets outside, would suddenly receive a phone call:

The doctor: "You mean it's got to be tonight, over the border, no other choice? . . . Otherwise . . . What do you mean the worst can happen? . . . That's terrific you'll take me in your car."

The elderly physician begins to throw a few things together, then stops. He goes into his library and with hands shaking, starts taking down books. "What'll I take along?" He runs to his desk, "At least my medical diploma."

Here Werfel permits himself a bit of fantasy. The streetlights come on, lighting up the bust of the doctor's old teacher. The physician hears in the room the teacher's voice: "Antisemitism is just a cyclical psychosis, from which manic-depressive nations suffer from time to time."

The doctor [addresses the bust]: "It's easy for you to make diagnoses, Herr Professor, because first of all you're not Jewish and second you're dead."[88]

That most of these very real emigré psychiatrists and psychoanalysts not only flourished but became the trend-setting force in the New World is a tribute to their energy and their bravery.

The emigré analysts had a major impact on American psychiatry and psychoanalysis. Paul Schilder, a member of the Vienna Psychoanalytic Society whose interests embraced the entire range of biological and dynamic psychiatry, left Vienna temporarily in 1928 for a post at Hopkins, from which he went in 1930 to a professorship at New York University and directorship of the clinical psychiatry division of Bellevue Psychiatric Hospital. Astonishingly, Schilder was rejected for membership by the New York Psychoanalytic Society on the grounds that his procedures were too unorthodox (he didn't see his patients five times a week for fifty-minute hours and insisted, moreover, upon giving them advice). Nonetheless, he spoke up for psychoanalysis as a way of untangling problems of the mind-body relationship, and at Bellevue nurtured a whole flock of younger psychiatrists who went on to become famous in their own right, such as John Frosch, founding editor in 1953 of the Journal of the American Psychoanalytic Association.[89] It might be argued that Schilder was not a true refugee, having left in the late 1920s by his own choice. Yet his departure was owing to the refusal of the anti-Semitic professor of psychiatry, Julius Wagner-Jauregg, to advance him,[90] and there is no question that Schilder, like Nunberg, Alexander, and the others who emigrated, while not being, strictly speaking, refugees, felt the bite of anti-Semitism.

The newcomers were accepted as stars. Else Pappenheim of Vienna was 28 when she arrived in 1939 at the Phipps Clinic in Baltimore. Back home, she had been a mere psychiatry resident and moreover was still in the middle of her own training analysis. But at Hopkins, she soon became an object of wonder. "As a physician from Vienna, I was accepted professionally immediately, even to the point of being hero-worshipped," she said.[91] Such was the prestige of Vienna-style psychoanalysis at the Phipps that, at rounds, Meyer would always ask New Yorker Joseph Wortis, who had spent four months in Vienna being analyzed by Freud, "And what would Freud have thought about that?" Wortis confided to Pappenheim that he always bluffed some kind of answer.[92]

The refugee analysts played a particularly important role in alliance with the younger generation of Americans in forcing the training institutes that had budded in the 1930s to ensure the orthodox teaching of a given body of doctrine, in contrast to the eclectic, haphazard, and often eccentric training that had previously prevailed. What became orthodoxy in the United States was the "ego psychology" that Freud had first proposed in 1923 on the structure of the psyche (in which the ego and the id struggle over unbearable ideas). Freud's daughter Anna became the chief standard-bearer of ego psychology.

In the United States, ego psychology broke away from the sexual doctrines of id psychology to emphasize the adaptation of the adult patient to social demands. It was a doctrine that suited the American analysts as progressive in spirit and practical in the prospect of improving patients' lives, as opposed to Freud's own pessimistic views about the inevitability of repression in civilized life. Ego psychology was also a particular gift that the younger emigré analysts were able to bring in their luggage. Ego-psychologist Heinz Hartmann, one of the last candidates to receive a training analysis from Freud himself in Vienna, became known as "the American prime minister of analysis." Ernst Kris and Rudolph Loewenstein joined with Hartmann in becoming a triumvirate reigning over ego psychology in the 1950s and 1960s.[93] Thus the young Americans who were just founding training institutes, such as Ralph Kaufman and Ives Hendrick in Boston or Lawrence Kubie and Bertram Lewin in New York, made common cause with the refugee Central Europeans to capture psychoanalytic training.[94]

The European newcomers also overwhelmed the Yankees by virtue of their sheer prestige. The writings of none of the American analysts were known abroad. By contrast, many of the new arrivals from Central Europe were international celebrities. When in 1966, Arnold Rogow asked a sample of 31 psychoanalysts to name "the most outstanding living psychiatrists and psychoanalysts," six of the top seven names were European refugees[95]: Anna Freud was in first place, followed closely by Heinz Hartmann and Erik Erikson. American-born Phyllis Greenacre was number four, known for her work on the psychoanalytic study of the child. Fleshing out the list were Rudolph Loewenstein, who had studied medicine and psychoanalysis in Berlin in the early 1920s, ending up, after a 13-year interlude in Paris, in a Fifth Avenue practice in New York, where he wrote about ego psychology; the Viennese René Spitz, who came to New York via Paris and became known as an authority on nurturing children; and Robert Waelder, a nonmedical Viennese analyst who had settled in Philadelphia and became a popular interpreter of Freud. When in 1980, the members of the New York, Boston, and San Francisco psychoanalytic institutes were asked to identify the profession's leaders, six of the seven top figures were again refugee analysts, the list being similar to the preceding one.[96]

Thus the handful of refugee analysts from Europe had succeeded in imposing themselves as the leaders of American psychoanalysis. "These analysts formed a kind of bodyguard around an imaginary Freud," wrote Martin Grotjahn many years later—himself a Berlin psychiatrist and analyst who in flight had landed initially at the Menninger Clinic in Topeka. "They tried to keep psychoanalytic theory, technique, therapy, and training unchanged for years to come." Instead of "the relaxed and free debating atmosphere of the psychoanalytic coffeehouses in Berlin," Grotjahn found a "frighteningly standardized" American product,[97] one little capable of change or adaptation to scientific findings about the nature of cognition and psychotherapy. By helping to turn analysis into a temple devoted to the last remaining dinosaur ideology of the nineteenth century, the refugee analysts unwittingly guaranteed that the temple would soon come crashing down.

Triumph

But first intervened the years of triumph from the late 1940s to the late 1960s. As Seymour Sarason, who had observed these events from a catbird seat in the Yale psychology department, looked back in retrospect,

"American psychiatry before World War II was biological psychiatry and within a few years after the war it was largely a psychoanalytical psychiatry."[98] The rising influence of psychoanalysis was expressed partly in numbers. The American Psychoanalytic Association grew from 92 members in 1932 to around 1,300 in 1968, at which time there was roughly one psychoanalyst for every 13 psychiatrists.[99] By the 1960s, in what Lewis Coser calls "the golden age of psychoanalysis in America," there were 20 training institutes, 29 local societies,[100] and a climate of opinion in which psychoanalysis was the therapy of choice for dysphoric members of the middle classes. This boiling growth was fueled partly by the GI Bill of Rights, which paid for psychiatrists' psychoanalytic training as long as it took place in institutes. But the real motor of growth was the analysts' unremitting mandate to extend Freud's domain to all of psychiatry and to the American public.[101]

Starting from the early 1940s, psychoanalysis began taking over the prestigious psychiatry chairs and university departments. Each new conquest was celebrated as a triumph within the movement. Because New York—which in 1940 contained over a third of the analysts in the entire country[102]—was the movement's epicenter, the takeover began earliest and penetrated most extensively there. New York saw the foundation of a series of training institutes. In 1941, Karen Horney left the New York Psychoanalytic Society, taking a group of adherents with her to found the rival American Institute for Psychoanalysis. In 1942, this new institute was able to insert its training program in the New York Medical College.[103] In June 1942, a second group of schismatics from the New York Psychoanalytic Society led by Sandor Rado founded yet another rival organization, the Association for Psychoanalytic Medicine. Rado's people then pulled off a real coup in 1944 by persuading the department of psychiatry of Columbia University to agree to the establishment of a psychoanalytic training institute there, the first in the United States situated within a major institution.[104] After the American Psychoanalytic Association changed its charter in 1946, permitting the establishment of more than one training institute in a given city, the Psychoanalytic Clinic of Columbia University became a powerful bastion of university-taught psychoanalysis.

After the war, the takeover of university departments began outside New York. At Yale University, the Institute of Human Relations had long been, in Sarason's phrase, a "buzzing center of psychoanalytic thinking."[105] Then in 1948, a group of young psychoanalytically oriented psychiatrists ousted Eugen Kahn, a student of Kraepelin from Munich, who had come to the United States in 1930 and whose special

171

research interest was the genetics of schizophrenia. Frederick ("Fritz") Redlich, an analyst from Vienna, became chairman of the psychiatry department, situated in the building of the Institute of Human Relations. At this point, virtually every prestigious chair of psychiatry in the country fell into the hands of an analyst: Kenneth Appel became chair of psychiatry at the University of Pennsylvania in 1953; Royden Astley (a member of the Philadelphia society) got the professorship at Pittsburgh in 1956; in that same year Western Reserve in Cleveland asked Maurits and Anny Katan, also members of the Philadelphia society, to run a new psychoanalytic training institute within the school of medicine (Maurits became the professor of psychiatry).[106] The list could be extended at length.

The emigré analysts, with memories still live of their craft being spurned by the European professoriate, were astonished at these developments. Edith Weigert had been a resident physician at Ernst Simmel's psychoanalytic sanatorium in Berlin in the early 1930s and fled Germany in 1938. As she reported to her German colleagues in 1953 (now that she was chair of the Washington Psychoanalytic Institute), "Psychiatry chairs in outstanding universities are increasingly being filled with psychoanalysts or with psychiatrists who recognize analysis." She might have had in mind people such as John Whitehorn at neighboring Johns Hopkins University, who was sympathetic to analysis though not himself a psychoanalyst. He had replaced Meyer in 1941, and it was under Whitehorn that the department of psychiatry at Hopkins got its first full-fledged analyst, Theodore Lidz, who began his psychoanalytic training in 1947.

"Psychoanalysis in the United States," continued Weigert, "has not descended to the status of serving maid of psychiatry, as Freud feared it might . . . but instead has tended to become psychiatry's highly respected pathfinder."[107] Swiss psychiatrist Henri Ellenberger, who in 1953 had taken a post at the Menninger Clinic in Topeka (and who in 1970 would establish for himself a towering reputation as a historian of psychiatry), noted there were many areas in which American psychiatrists were not strong: They were poor in classifying illness (nosology), poor in "phenomenology" (the patient's actual experience of symptoms), poor in "constitutional" approaches, nil in psychiatric genetics. But in psychoanalysis they were tops. "Of all the countries of the world," wrote Henri Ellenberger in 1955, "America is the first to have adopted a dynamic psychiatry [psychoanalysis] as its leading psychiatric trend."[108]

As the analysts reached for the university chairs, they grasped for control of the discipline of psychiatry as a whole. In organizational terms, psychoanalysts and analysis-sympathizers took over much of the apparatus of the American Psychiatric Association. In the late 1940s and early

1950s the organization had a spate of presidents who themselves were either analysts, such as William Menninger, the younger of the two Menninger brothers, or strongly sympathetic to it, such as Whitehorn. Then in the 1960s, the APA presidents became uniformly analysts or members of organizations closely affiliated with analysis.[109]

One such organization was the Group for the Advancement of Psychiatry (GAP), founded in 1946 at a meeting of the American Psychiatric Association by a group of Young Turks whose leader was William Menninger. Its purpose was to bring social activism and encouragement for psychoanalysis to the parent Association. For example, in 1950 a GAP manifesto stated that social reality could influence anxiety (true enough) and that such reality "also exercises a selective influence on the choice of defense against anxiety (projection, reaction-formation, symptom formation, sublimation, and others)."[110] This kind of formulation was mother's milk to a Freudian, and GAP took a strong position in favor of psychoanalysis. Of 177 GAP members in 1948, 30 percent held posts in the American Psychiatric Association. This was three-quarters of all the committee posts in the APA.[111]

Yet the surest route to controlling the discipline of psychiatry was not to capture its professional organization but rather take charge of psychiatric training. Psychoanalysis was able to exercise such an enormous influence on American psychiatry not because the number of full-time analysts was so large but because analysts wrote the textbooks, staffed the university departments, and sat on the examination boards. In 1953, of 7,000 U.S. psychiatrists only about 500 were psychoanalysts.[112] Yet the influence of analysis ranged far beyond these numbers. From the 1940s to the 1970s, American psychiatrists, generally speaking, were not psychoanalysts as such but were psychoanalytically *oriented*.

The infiltration of psychiatry by analysis accelerated in 1952 with a joint report of the American Psychiatric Association and the national body of medical educators, the Association of American Medical Colleges. Everybody now agrees, the report said, that a competent psychiatrist has to understand "the principles of psychodynamics," including "Freudian concepts." There simply were not enough psychoanalytic training institutes to go around and so ways must be found to infiltrate psychoanalytic knowledge into the graduate curriculum. ". . . Such knowledge finds its way into the content of residency training programs through many different practices—supervised therapy, analytically oriented case discussions. . . . Better scientific communication about . . . the supervision and structuring of so-called 'psychoanalytically oriented therapy' is greatly to be desired."[113] As Karl Menninger noted in 1953,

"Gradually the dynamic concepts have gained complete supremacy."[114] (Dynamic was a code word for psychoanalytic.)

Meanwhile, the analysts had convinced the public that Freud's teachings contained the secret of happiness. Market forces therefore would also contribute to the new supremacy of analysis within psychiatry. Residents demanded psychoanalytic training simply because the public now expected psychoanalysis and a good income was to be made in satisfying that demand. As a 1951 survey of 42 psychiatry residents at the College of Medicine of the State University of New York and Columbia concluded, "Since training in a psychoanalytic institute is considered the stamp of being a 'first-class' citizen, it is inevitable that none wants to be considered a 'second-class' one."[115]

Yet it was not just "the New Yorker Syndrome," as this hunger for analysis would later be called.[116] Residents everywhere desired psychoanalytic training. GAP was writing for the whole country when it said in 1955, "At present the prestige value of being a psychoanalyst is high, and it appears to offer greater financial rewards." Of 165 psychiatry residents polled by GAP, "All . . . indicate their desire for personal psychoanalysis and psychoanalytic training." Of those residents, 20 percent were currently having a training analysis, and 26 percent were receiving psychoanalytic training in their residency.[117]

Established analysts were just as avid to teach Freud as residents were to learn. Of a sample of staff members polled in 1951 in various psychiatry departments, 56 percent had received formal psychoanalytic training including a personal analysis (and a further 11 percent had had a personal analysis without formal training, a practice the national psychoanalytic association thundered against for years).[118] When in 1955 the GAP surveyed 14 graduate programs in psychiatry, "all indicate that their training program is based on psychodynamic theory."[119]

What were the most influential books in teaching psychiatry around 1965? In more than half of all programs, the basic list consisted of 17 titles, almost all of which were works of psychoanalysis ranging in alphabetical order from August Aichhorn's *Wayward Youth* to Gregory Zilboorg's *History of Medical Psychology*.[120]

The payoff from this approach was that by 1966, a third of American psychiatrists had received some kind of psychoanalytic training, and 67 percent said that they employed "the dynamic approach" with their patients.[121] By the mid-1960s, psychiatry had come in the mind of the American public to mean psychoanalysis. The seizure of power was virtually complete.

The most baleful aspect of the takeover of psychiatry by psychoanalysis was the analysts' ambition to extend their theories to the diagnosis and treatment of psychotic illness. If one is going to take over psychiatry, one has to have something to say about psychosis which, until the 1920s, was the discipline's core interest. From the very beginning therefore, analysis had toyed with explanations and treatments of schizophrenia, mania, and psychotic depression. And although Freud publicly discouraged his followers from burning their fingers on psychotic patients, in private he was more permissive, and members of his inner circle had no compunctions about taking on the major psychiatric illnesses.

In 1908, Ferenczi became keen on treating Frau M., who suffered from paranoia. Yet first Ferenczi sought the Professor's opinion: Did Freud think she needed to be treated in an institution, or would an outpatient basis suffice? Freud replied, "I've seen Frau M. She has frank paranoia, and probably is beyond the border of treatability; still, you can have a go at it and learn from her at all events. Her brother-in-law, who is accompanying her and is a doctor, is an ass. He will probably advise something other than what I've proposed. I demanded that she enter the Budapest [private] asylum and there let herself be treated by you."[122] Freud's disciple Paul Federn proposed a formal psychoanalytic assault on psychosis, becoming known as the great analytic advocate of reaching beyond neurotic patients.[123] Yet these European efforts to apply psychoanalysis to psychosis usually petered out after a trial or two, and in Europe analysis remained *grosso modo* an approach to the neuroses.

It was in the United States that psychoanalysts made their strongest attempts to treat psychosis. The seminal figure here is Adolf Meyer, an early member of the American Psychoanalytic Association and a large presence in the local Washington-Baltimore society. Although Meyer claimed to practice "objective psychobiology" and not psychoanalysis, he often sent patients to analysts. It is characteristic of Meyer's own constitutional state of confusion that he clarified his stance toward psychoanalysis thus: "I feel but rarely the urge to go far ahead of the attitude of inquiry to a need of finality which will take care of its own lack of necessity."[124] (At the same time that Meyer was sending some patients to psychoanalysts, he was referring others to Henry Cotton at the Trenton State Hospital to have their teeth or colons removed for madness.) As early as 1909, Meyer toyed with psychoanalysis as a way of understanding schizophrenia, and such students of Meyer's as Edward Kempf (who left Meyer's department in 1914 to become a full-time psychotherapist at the government asylum, St. Elizabeths Hospital, in Washington) and C. Macfie Campbell (later director of the Boston Psychopathic Hospital) were ardent fans of applying analysis to patients with psychotic illness.[125]

Thanks to Meyer, the tradition of using psychoanalysis on patients with major mental illnesses rooted itself firmly in the Washington-Baltimore area. It was here that two private nervous clinics—Chestnut Lodge in Rockville, Maryland (founded in 1910 by Ernest Luther Bullard) and the Sheppard and Enoch Pratt Hospital in Towson, Maryland (opened in 1891 as the Sheppard Asylum), became the American flagship hospitals for applying psychoanalysis to gravely ill patients. In December 1922, Harry Stack Sullivan, perhaps the most famous figure in the psychoanalytic treatment of the psychoses, arrived at the Sheppard.

Sullivan had received his analysis training in 1916 and 1917 from Clara Thompson, one of the strong female figures in the history of American psychoanalysis and a confederate of Horney. He had become interested in psychosis while on staff at St. Elizabeths Hospital under the tutelage of director William Alanson White, one of the best-known American psychiatrists to acquire an early interest in analysis. Sullivan came to the Sheppard with the understanding that he would have a free hand. He created a special six-bed ward where he achieved quite good results with patients he had diagnosed as "schizophrenic." (These were the days when American psychiatrists used the diagnosis of schizophrenia far more frequently than their colleagues elsewhere.) In Sullivan's view, schizophrenia was an unsuccessful reaction to anxiety. He was known for the hours of sympathetic care he would give his patients, many of whom responded gratefully to the attention.[126] Although he was not a strictly orthodox analyst, he nonetheless became the spark plug in touching off interest in the psychoses within American psychoanalysis in general.

In 1930 Sullivan left the Sheppard, establishing himself in private practice in New York and Washington. Later in the 1930s, he would also found his own school of psychiatry and his own journal. Midst all this activity, large crews of psychoanalytically oriented psychiatrists and psychoanalysts began mustering at the Sheppard and at Chestnut Lodge (by 1938, for example, six analysts from Chestnut Lodge alone belonged to the Washington-Baltimore Psychoanalytic Society).[127]

The situation took a new turn in 1935 with the arrival at Chestnut Lodge of Frieda Fromm-Reichmann, a refugee German analyst with a long history of private-clinic work. (Frieda Reichmann was married briefly to analyst Eric Fromm.) She became influenced to some extent by Sullivan's ideas, given that he was the chief figure in the Washington-Baltimore region. Yet she went a step farther.[128] Fromm-Reichmann did not just believe in standard psychoanalytic notions about anxiety and such as the cause of schizophrenia. She knew that it was the work of the mother in particular. Generations of American mothers had to suffer unwarranted reproaches as "schizophrenogenic mothers"—to use Fromm-Reichmann's notorious phrase—after her writings on this subject began to appear in 1948. What was the problem in schizophrenia? "The schizophrenic is painfully distrustful and resentful of other people," said Fromm-Reichmann, "due to the severe early warp and rejection he encountered in important people of his infancy and childhood, as a rule, mainly in a schizophrenogenic mother."[129] There one had it. The mother must not leave the side of the child. The psychoanalytic incursion into psychiatry, much like Napoleon's invasion of Russia, had reached its furthest point.

Far from being marginalized, Sullivan's and Fromm-Reichmann's teachings on the causes and treatment of psychotic illness became widely adopted in psychiatry. Fromm-Reichmann's schizophrenogenic mother became the basis of "family systems theory" in the treatment of schizophrenia, and such therapists as Gregory Bateson at the Mental Health Research Institute in Menlo Park, California, postulated a complex "double bind" theory of the disease, in which the mother emerged as the sickest member of the family. "It became standard practice," wrote one scholar, "to believe that mothers were the cause of their children's psychosis."[130]

Beyond schizophrenia, analytic interpretations of other psychotic illnesses became standard dogma within American psychiatry. The cause of mania? An oral triad of "a wish to eat, a wish to be eaten . . . and a wish to go to sleep," said New York analyst Bertram Lewin in 1951.[131] Depression? "A despairing cry for love," said Sandor Rado. The ego tries to punish itself to forestall punishment by the parent.[132] Paranoia? It arises in the first six months of life, said London analyst Melanie Klein (who had come to England from Budapest via Berlin), as the child spits out the mother's milk, fearing the mother will revenge herself because of his hatred of her.[133] When in 1958 the American Psychoanalytic Association organized a program to import the teaching of these doctrines into mental hospitals, the campaign by psychoanalysis to take control of psychiatry had shattered the last resistances.[134] A psychiatry resident from abroad recalled the scene at Delaware State Hospital once the analysts had taken control of it: "The training in individual and group psychotherapy was given over to psychiatrists who came from the various university clinics in nearby Philadelphia. Their teaching model was psychoanalytic psychotherapy. It was urgently driven home that we should view institutional psychiatry merely as a brief transitional stage for us. We should begin our training analyses as soon as possible. Our ideal professional goal was doing psychoanalysis in private practice in combination with supervising training at one of the psychoanalytic institutes independent of a university department. From the viewpoint of the psychoanalytic theories of the 1940s, our daily therapeutic activities [at Delaware] were considered highly questionable. The somatic therapies, so we were told, were stopgaps. They concealed instead of uncovering. Ordering a sedative for even an agitated psychotic patient was not therapeutic for the patient but considered an anxiety reaction on the part of the doctor. Whoever expressed the slightest doubt about psychoanalytic interpretations, making reference to other theories, was considered to be neurotically disabled from overcoming his resistances."[135] Into these analytic hands, the discipline of psychiatry had been delivered.

What is ironic, given the attempt of analysts to dominate psychiatry, is their contempt for the precise diagnosis of psychiatric illness, the intellectual core of psychiatry over the previous hundred years. Psychoanalysts ridiculed attempts to divide mental illness into specific categories, as Kraepelin had done on the basis of course and outcome. According to Karl Menninger in 1956, "The old Kraepelinian terms have largely disappeared."[136] But not just the Kraepelinian terms: Gone was any sense of well-defined disease entities. Menninger: "Gone forever is the notion that the mentally ill person is an exception. It is now accepted that most people have some degree of mental illness at some time, and many of them have a degree of mental illness most of the time."[137] We are all, in other words, a little bit schizophrenic or a little bit manic-depressive (an assertion that

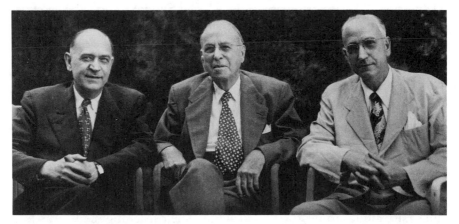

The Menninger family as seen in 1951. In the middle the father, Charles F. Menninger, who along with his son Karl (on the right) founded the Menninger Diagnostic Clinic in Topeka, Kansas, in 1919. On the left is C. F.'s other son William, who helped found the Group for the Advancement of Psychiatry in 1946 (courtesy of the Menninger Clinic).

would rule out a genetic basis for those illnesses). Menninger once told refugee psychiatrist Lothar Kalinowsky, who had a strong background in organic psychiatry, "I consider you to be an intelligent individual and cannot understand why you are interested in questions of classification."[138]

Behind the analysts' indifference to the fine Kraepelinian distinctions between affective and nonaffective psychosis was the conviction that only one form of psychiatric illness existed, and that this form exhibited mere quantitative differences on the basis of how severely one had failed to adapt to the environment. Since there was only a slippery slope rather than an absolute line between the ill and the well, the analysts considered it pointless to talk of curing "disease." We were all the walking wounded, normal neurotics. Rather, the purpose of psychiatry was to understand the meaning of the symptom and "undo its psychogenic cause"—in the words of one observer—"rather than manipulate the symptom directly through medication, suggestion, etc."[139]

The analysts' indifference to determining what "disease" the patient suffered infiltrated all of American psychiatry. "In Europe," reflected Ellenberger, "people go to the psychiatrist because of a *symptom*, in America because of a *problem*."[140] Symptoms came from disease, problems from society. The whole concept of disease implied brain lesions, disorders of neurotransmitters, genetic loading, and the like. If psychiatric illness were psychogenic, the product of anomalous childhood socialization exacerbated by the inability to adapt, psychiatric disease did not actually exist unless one had neurosyphilis. Continued Ellenberger, "I remember the consternation of a German psychiatrist hearing that certain American colleagues consider manic-depressive psychosis as a form of schizophrenia; for him this was about as fantastic as the assumption that a camel is a subspecies of the elephant. On the other hand, Americans can hardly understand the strenuous efforts of the Europeans to isolate and individualize mental diseases; they have the impression that the Europeans are satisfied with merely labeling the disease. Nosologic [classificatory] discussion of whether paranoia is a subform of schizophrenia, or a specific disease, appears as ridiculous to them as the Middle Ages' theological controversies on the sex of angels."[141]

This incuriosity about the nature of illness meant that when the analytically trained psychiatrists encountered patients with serious disorders, they were baffled. Lawrence Kubie and Sandor Rado would refer patients to the psychosurgery unit that Columbia University's Department of Neurology ran in common with the New Jersey State Hospital at Greystone Park (the "Columbia-Greystone Project") with a diagnosis of "pseudoneurotic schizophrenia." The meaning: We know something serious is wrong with these people but we can't tell what. These referrals were not innocuous for the patients because they may have subsequently undergone lobotomy, surgical excision of brain matter.[142]

The flip side of misdiagnosing major psychiatric disorder was in the inappropriate application of psychobabble to individuals who were well but different in background from the analyst. Here is a group of psychoanalytically oriented psychiatrists in 1955 in Cleveland at the bedside of a 75-year-old black laborer who had undergone a prostate operation, and whose behavior in the hospital had apparently prompted the surgeons to request a psychiatry consultation. Although the psychiatrists found the man "normal," which they put in quotation marks, they nonetheless found pathological his "pride in being 'the man who worked' in his family," as well as his belief in getting up as soon as possible "because lying around weakened a man, and in his concern about having enough 'pep' postoperatively." They took all these as "evidences of pseudomasculinity."[143] The message: Black laborers who want to retain their pride are being pseudomasculine (and would benefit from psychoanalysis if they could afford it).

In any event, analysts for the most part had little interest in treating black laborers. Analytic practices had a much larger proportion of professionals, executives, and the like than did practices that used a variety of therapies excluding analysis.[144] The psychiatry of those years distinguished between "good" patients and "bad." Good were those who, as Herman van Praag—later head of psychiatry at Albert Einstein College of Medicine—put it, were "fairly young, quite intelligent, and introspective." They tended to be educated and middle class. Bad were the seriously ill and chronically disabled, the schizophrenics and the addicts, the patients who were often uneducated and poor. "In other words, the patient had to fit the treatment, rather than the treatment being adjusted to the patient."[145] For thoughtful clinicians such as van Praag, the discipline of psychiatry had become an embarrassment, a mockery of medicine.

By the 1960s, psychoanalysis was at the apogee of its success within psychiatry. Although analysts numbered only about 10 percent of all psychiatrists,[146] the influence of psychoanalysis reached into most of the private practices in the country. The biological psychiatrists, in contrast, had been limited to unglamorous posts in state hospitals. Analysts were being consulted by government agencies and the Congress. Being "shrunk" became the ne plus ultra of upper-middle-class American life.

Under the influence of psychoanalysis, American psychiatry completed its long march from the asylum to Main Street. Analysis could only be done in private practice, midst the hubbub of middle-class life. In 1917, only about 8 percent of American psychiatrists were in private practice, a figure that had increased only to 31 percent by 1933.[147] In 1941, psychiatrists either entirely in private practice or in institutions with a private office on the side numbered only 38 percent of the total.[148]

The balance then shifted dramatically during the heyday of psychoanalysis. By 1970, at least 66 percent of all American psychiatrists were in private practice, in reality doubtless more because many of those with appointments in hospitals and universities also had private offices on the side.[149] Of those psychiatrists who in 1941 had been entirely in hospitals and asylums, by 1962 half had gone over to private practice. (Interestingly, with the decline of analysis in the 1970s and beyond, the percentage of psychiatrists in institutional settings would again rise: 11 percent of the total in 1988 were in private, free-standing psychiatric hospitals.)[150] The victory of the psychotherapeutic model seeded psychiatrists throughout the middle classes of the big cities. An analytically oriented therapist would be almost as close at hand as an optician or a lawyer in case of trouble.

This apparent indispensability in the crises of middle-class life brought to psychoanalytically oriented psychiatry its own arrogance. Its lieutenants dealt swiftly with doubters by giving them psychiatric diagnoses or simply by shouting them out of court, as Hopkins child psychiatrist Leon Eisenberg discovered in 1962 when he ventured a few critical remarks about the scientific nature of psychoanalysis at a medical educators' meeting. "There was a veritable stampede of Department Chairmen to the floor microphones. . . . Just about every eminent figure present rose to defend the primacy of psychoanalysis as 'the basic science' of psychiatry."[151] When in 1964 *Fact* magazine polled 2,400 psychiatrists about whether Senator Barry Goldwater, a Republican, could safety be elected President over Lyndon Johnson, 1,189 pronounced Goldwater "psychologically unfit to be President."[152] The hubris of the analysts was extraordinary. Shortly, it would all come crashing down.

Psychoanalysis and the American Jews

It is impossible to understand the extraordinary rise of psychoanalysis in terms of "internalist" perspectives alone, meaning developments within a discipline such as the evolution of ideas or the succession of personalities. So hallucinatory did the sexual perspectives of psychoanalysis seem that its ascent and triumph could not possibly be explained merely on the basis of sound ideas driving out invalid ones. Events in the external world helped make possible its ascendancy, granting it a momentum that its internal dynamic would never have achieved. These are "externalist" perspectives on the history of psychiatry. Various such factors made a difference, from a rising affluence among the middle classes that permitted such personalized care, to the desire for introspection that humanistically educated people often bear away from the university. Some observers have commented on the lack of authority of the American professoriate, which let academic objections to psychoanalysis be swept aside, whereas in Europe the professoriate were able to hold up the onmarch of analysis.[153] One historian sees the "hothouse" nature of American family life creating a kind of "oepidal" nest into which a belief in analysis could burrow.[154] I want to call attention to yet another external factor, not because it is necessarily the most important one in the rise and fall of analysis but because it runs like a silver thread from the beginning of the story to the end: It is the history of the Jews in Europe and North America.

From the viewpoint of the history of psychiatry, the vicissitudes of the Jews in the Old World and New were a matter of capital importance. The common theme linking the misadventures of psychoanalysis on both sides of the Atlantic was the desire of recently acculturated middle-class Jews for some symbol of collective affirmation. Although Freud sought mightily to downplay any kind of ethnic specificity in psychoanalysis, the subtext of Freud and his followers to the non-Jewish charter culture was: We Jews have given this precious gift to modern civilization.

Why would Jews need such a symbol any more than any other ethnic group? In the history of modern times, Jewish people have had to endure not just one but two great shocks. Every people that undertakes the long journey from small-scale life in the traditional village to middle-class life in the big city undergoes one major shock: the shock of assimilation and integration, the psychological upheaval that goes with newness of arrival. In their move from shtetl life in the small towns of eighteenth-century Poland and the Ukraine to such bustling cities as Berlin, Frankfurt, and Vienna, the Jews underwent this shock just as everybody else did. But then a second shock lay in store for the Jews, the Holocaust, and the forced transplantation of hundreds of thousands of individuals who themselves had only recently become middle-class, from a comfortable and bourgeois European existence to the nightmare of scrambling for a passage to America. This second shock was experienced by no other cultural group.[155] It profoundly shaped the desire of the American Jews for some kind of a special symbol of self-affirmation, a collective badge of pride in the chaos of the living city. That symbol, I argue, was psychoanalysis.

At the turn of the twentieth century, the Jews of Central Europe were experiencing the cultural confusion of a massive deracination. Between the 1860s and 1900, countless numbers of people were torn from the ghettoes and shtetls of Eastern Europe, without becoming as yet newly rooted among the middle classes of the West. Many of the Jews of Berlin and Vienna had left their religion behind and were rapidly trying to assimilate by changing their names and by converting to Protestantism (less so to Catholicism). Yet despite their best intentions, despite their knowledge of the plays of Schiller and of the refinements of the German language, they encountered a baffling wall of anti-Semitism.

There was something about psychoanalysis that made it, according to historian John Cuddihy, a "plausible ideology for [a] decolonizing people."[156] Jewish patients with psychoneurosis were therefore drawn to it. Perhaps psychoanalysis was seized upon because it extended the possibility of finding one's identity from within, as opposed to the external signposts that orthodox Judaism offered. And it may have appealed to Jewish women in particular. Perhaps these cloistered but well read and highly curious women—members of a "middle-class drenched in spirit" in the words of Viennese novelist Robert Musil—were simply more self-reflective, more psychologically minded that the women of the non-Jewish lower-middle classes below them who worked alongside their husbands in shops, or the women of the nobility above, busy with the social whirl of the salon.[157] Or perhaps Jewish men and women alike adored psychoanalysis because it was "our thing." In any event, psychoanalysis in the early days had a very specific social address.

It was above all among the middle-class Jews of Berlin, Budapest, and Vienna that psychoanalysis proved such a hit. Historian Steven Beller finds the Jews of Vienna, as outsiders, using psychoanalysis to "make a political attack on Viennese society by an alliance of scientific rationality with instinct" against the city's traditional sensual baroque culture.[158] In Budapest, there were descriptions of psychoanalysis in the Jewish quarter, the Leopoldstadt, as an almost "incomprehensible and impenetrable secret doctrine or ceremony. . . ."

Historian Paul Harmat concludes, "Psychoanalysis was most popular among enlightened Jewish circles as a result of their minority situation."[159] Of course, non-Jews had recourse to analysis as well. Yet among patients, there seems to have been a kind of Jewish tropism.

The analysts themselves also tended heavily to be Jewish, and many of them assumed that Jewishness helped one to appreciate Freud's wisdom fully. As Freud said in 1908 to the Berlin analyst Karl Abraham, on the occasion of a malentendu with Carl Jung (then one of the few non-Jews in the movement), "Please be tolerant, and don't forget that it is actually easier for you than for Jung to follow my ideas . . . because you stand closer to me as a result of racial affinity, while he, as a Christian and son of a pastor, finds the way to me only in the face of great inner resistance." On another occasion, Freud reassured Abraham, "May I say that what attracts me to you are our related, Jewish characteristics. We understand each other."[160] Freud's inner circle was almost entirely Jewish, and Ferenczi said to Freud of the one non-Jewish member, the Londoner Ernest Jones, "It has seldom been so clear to me as now what a psychological advantage it signifies to be born a Jew. . . . you must keep Jones constantly under your eye and cut off his line of retreat."[161]

Within the middle-class Jewish public, psychoanalysis became signposted as belonging to some larger Jewish worldview. Humorist Salomo Friedländer, writing in the 1920s under the pseudonym "Mynona," made analysis the portal through which Christians who wanted to convert to "true Judaism" must pass. In one tale Friedländer allows the wildly anti-Semitic Count Reschock to fall in love with the beautiful Rebecka Gold-Isak. Losing his bearings completely, the Count decides to convert to Judaism to win his prize. Rebecka insists that he must become truly Jewish before she will accept him. The Count's first step on the path of a Jewish identity is an analysis with Professor Freud. "This destroyer of fig-leaves," as Friedländer termed Freud, "robbed the noble Reschok soul of its protective coat with such anatomical certainty that the Count fell with a cry into the arms of his alarmed servant." (Reschock goes on to have a famous surgeon convert him from a blonde Prussian warrior into a "Jewish Torah-student.")[162] Jewish and non-Jewish readers alike found the Friedländer fable delicious, yet accepted implicitly its premise that psychoanalysis was identified with Judaism. If psychoanalysis is written as a history of ideas, these social themes are unimportant. But if we try to understand its rise and decline as a movement, the singular tropism that many Jews felt toward analysis, both as doctors and patients, is of considerable significance.

With the passage of time, in Europe at least, psychoanalysis lost its Jewish stamp. Although it had originated among the Jews of Vienna and Berlin, as it developed, it ceased to be their property. There was certainly no Jewish tropism among the chief physicians of the many private clinics that offered psychoanalysis. And in Switzerland and England, psychoanalysis was known to be a specifically non-Jewish affair. As Swiss psychiatrist Max Müller commented of the 1920s, "It was characteristic of the psychoanalytic movement in Switzerland that, unlike other countries, it did not consist predominantly or almost exclusively of Jewish physicians and lay-analysts."[163] And the two most prominent advocates of analysis in Switzerland before 1914—Eugen Bleuler and Carl Jung—were if anything anti-Semitic. (It is perhaps indicative of the mood of the Bleuler household that, upon discovering that Viennese psychiatrist Erwin Stransky was Jewish, Bleuler's wife expressed great astonishment and said, "Well then you must at least have an aryan soul in you.")[164] Commenting on the plethora of Jews in psychoanalysis generally, Ernest Jones noted, with relief, that apart from the refugees, "in England . . . only two analysts have been Jews."[165]

Before 1933, a number of Jewish physicians figured prominently among the opponents of analysis. In Central Europe, for example, Gustav Aschaffenburg, Adolf Friedländer, and Erwin Stransky—all Jewish—were among Freud's most outspoken enemies, as were Boston's Abraham Myerson and New York's Bernard Sachs in the New World. (Stransky took this to mean that no one could accuse the opponents of psychoanalysis of being anti-Semitic.[166]) It could be argued that by 1933 in Europe and even in America, psychoanalysis had shed its initially Jewish imprint.

After 1933, all this changed. As a movement, analysis in Europe was destroyed. Its main representatives who fled to the New World were Jews. For these battered and profoundly disoriented survivors, psychoanalysis became one of the Jewish accomplishments that could be presented to the host population as a ticket of entry. Among the refugee Jews, both physicians and nonphysicians—psychoanalysis became a badge of Jewish solidarity in the face of a population of Anglo-Saxons perceived to be racially hostile, psychologically insensitive, and culturally backward. Said Martin Grotjahn of his fellow emigré analysts, "Psychoanalysis symbolized for them the light of the Old Country to be carried to the New Country."[167] But it was a light that Jews had created, and in whose warmth they would bask for several decades.

The American Jews had not experienced the trauma of emigration. Yet they too had arrived as outsiders, and as psychoanalysis acquired new prestige in medicine after the Second World War many Jewish physicians and patients alike were drawn to it as a symbol of collective self-affirmation: This is what we have created. By it we shall become better and in doing so bring enlightenment to others. After 1945, American Jews took on psychoanalysis as a kind of *mission civilisatrice*, a healing gift to all the world, which is not at all an overwrought formulation considering the prose with which Jewish analysts themselves described their mission to humanity. How things have changed for us, Franz Alexander assured his colleagues in

185

1953, "as soon as all that you professed is accepted and the world is asking you sincerely and avidly to explain the new truth. They turn to you now: 'Please tell us all about it. How does the new knowledge help us, how can we use it constructively to cure a neurotic or psychotic patient . . . to alleviate social prejudice and international tension, and to prevent war.'"[168] Is it any wonder that Jews themselves would preferentially have recourse to this new knowledge?

Why had psychoanalysis spread so rapidly after World War II? asked psychologist Seymour Sarason. "Most analysts (and a significant portion of the psychiatrists who received training during the war years) were Jewish. For them, Hitler and fascism were not abstractions but threats to existence. And for them, Freud represented a Moses-like figure whose contributions had opened up new vistas about the nature of humans. . . ."[169] For Sarason and Alexander, Jews were a gifted but marginal population, still ill at ease and unintegrated.

Surveys establish the extent to which Jewish physicians predominated in the practice of psychoanalysis. In 1959, two researchers drew up a profile of psychiatrists who believed in psychoanalysis: Eighty percent of them were of Jewish origin and tended to be upwardly mobile, insight-oriented, and deracinated (in contrast to the biologically oriented psychiatrists in the sample, who tended to be mainly Protestant). On a number of characteristics, the psychoanalytically inclined Jewish psychiatrists stood out from the non-Jews: They were agnostic, as opposed to the organically oriented Protestant psychiatrists who retained some shreds of their religious faith. They were more leftist, and they were more aware of the importance of social class, as opposed to the Protestant group who were somewhat embarrassed by the subject.[170] When Arnold Rogow quizzed a sample of 35 psychoanalysts and 149 nonanalyst psychiatrists in 1965, he found 26 percent of the analysts willing to declare they were Jewish; a further 17 percent were willing to say they had Jewish mothers; a third were unwilling to say anything about religious affiliation. (By contrast, the figures for the nonanalyst psychiatrists were lower in all three categories.)[171] On the basis of these statistics, it is fair to infer that a majority of the practitioners of psychoanalysis were of Jewish origin though of course numerous non-Jews entered the field as well. How about patients? It seems to be the case that Jews overconsume most psychiatric services in proportion to their numbers in the population. This is certainly true of psychoanalysis. In Rogow's study, one third of the analysts said they had practices consisting heavily or overwhelmingly of Jews.[172] A variety of other studies revealed the same finding in other ways.[173] Most dramatic perhaps was a random, nationwide survey of the adult American population in 1976, which found that 59 percent of Jewish respondents had at some point in time received psychotherapy (in contrast to the non-Jewish help-seeking rate of 25 percent).[174] In other words, more than half of all American Jews had sought out psychotherapy at a time when psychotherapy was overwhelmingly psychoanalytically oriented. It is not stretching the facts to refer to psychoanalysis in the middle decades of the twentieth century as a kind of Jewish "our thing."

This is not the place for a comprehensive account of the decline of psychoanalysis (see pp. 305–313). Many factors were involved, such as the advent of effective new medications that obviated long sessions of therapy, a new model of psychiatric illness stressing neurogenesis rather than psychogenesis, and the rise of alternative systems of psychotherapy. Compared with these changes, developments within the Jewish community, previously an important bastion of psychoanalysis, do not bulk large. Yet since Jews are under discussion here, this might be the place to mention the role that the loss of a social base appears to have played in the plunging popularity of analysis. In my opinion the main source of this loss was the increasing social assimilation of the American Jews. They no longer required psychoanalysis as a badge of collective identity because they were no longer affirming themselves. Instead they were becoming like everyone else.

Consider the experience of "Deborah" in *I Never Promised You a Rose Garden*, Joanne Greenberg's semi-fictionalized account of her own psychotic illness, published in 1964:

> Greenberg was born in 1932 into families of recent immigrants on both sides. In 1944, around the age of 12, she started to fall ill with symptoms of what was undoubtedly a genuine psychosis. The Greenberg family consulted Richard Frank, a New York psychoanalyst specializing in children, and when Joanne was sixteen, Frank had her admitted to Chestnut Lodge. He had encouraged the family to hold out until then because the Lodge did not admit children under that age and Frank evidently wanted his young patient to be treated psychoanalytically.[175]

The world the Greenberg family inhabited in those years was an intensely anti-Semitic one. In the novel, Deborah is cursed by her playmates at a "cruelly anti-Semitic" camp as a "stinking Jew." In their New York suburban home, the well-to-do Greenberg family (in the novel at least) had anti-Semitic slogans painted on the wall and rats flung at the porch. Is it any wonder that the Greenbergs encapsulated themselves in an almost entirely Jewish subculture. "In the place and time where Deborah was growing up, American Jews still fought the old battles that they had fled from in Europe only a few years earlier," Greenberg writes in the novel. And Deborah's friends were entirely Jewish: "I never knew anyone well who was not Jewish," she said, "and I never gave my last particle of trust to someone who wasn't Jewish."

What to do for Deborah? The mother had heard of psychoanalysis. She says to Deborah's psychiatrist at Chestnut Lodge: "They tell me that these illnesses are caused by a person's past and childhood. So all these days we've been thinking about the past. I've looked, and Jacob [her husband] has looked, and the whole family has thought and wondered. . . ." And they can't figure out what they might have done to cause Deborah's illness.

But the psychiatrist knows. The psychiatrist was in fact Frieda Reichmann. It was Deborah's mother's fault. Reichmann ("Dr. Fried") coaxes from Deborah a memory (or suggests her into one) in which the mother abandoned her at an early age. The memory comes tumbling forth. "The rush of words ended and Dr. Fried smiled. 'It is as big, then, as abandonment and the going away of all love.'"[176]

New York in the early 1940s: Within this encapsulated little subculture what other therapy could have seemed appropriate for Jews than psychoanalysis? The psychiatrists were mainly Jewish analysts. The expensive private clinics such as Chestnut Lodge catered to wealthy Jewish families. The subculture itself understood analysis to be the only thinkable option because it was a therapy that had come over from the sparkling Jewish intelligentsia of Europe. (Dr. Fried explains that one of her European patients had died in Dachau.)[177] Deborah, the Greenbergs, and the Jewish middle classes of the great American cities lived in a world permeated by psychoanalysis.

The breakout of the American Jews from this sequestered little existence occurred after the 1960s. Statistics on intermarriage are most revealing, because the chances of the children being raised as Jewish in a union where one partner is not Jewish are less than half as high as in unions where both partners are Jewish. Among Jews marrying before 1960, only 5 percent had chosen non-Jews; in 1960–1969, 12 percent; in 1970–1979, 19 percent; and in 1980–1989, 33 percent. The trend, in other words, was clearly toward intermarriage for young people. The same progression repeated itself on the basis of generation: For the first generation in the New World, intermarriage was 5 percent; for the 4th, 38 percent. Most unsettling of all, given the high levels of marital instability in the United States, was that in first marriages only 11 percent of the partners were non-Jewish; in second marriages 24 percent, and in third marriages 40 percent.[178] By 1990, as many as 52 percent of Jews were marrying outside the faith and fewer than half belonged to synagogues. The numbers offered a picture of a community in dissolution.[179]

This breakout from the Jewish subculture may have entailed the breakout from such former symbols of community solidarity as psychoanalysis. Recent data on the ethnicity of psychoanalytic patients are difficult to come by, yet one authority speculates that the percentage of Jews in the clientele of psychoanalysts has "probably declined."[180] If Jews were like everybody else, they could participate in the same kind of psychiatric treatment that everybody else was receiving, and after the 1970s, it was not psychoanalysis.

6

Alternatives

In the first half of the twentieth century, psychiatry was caught in a dilemma. On the one hand, psychiatrists could warehouse their patients in vast bins in the hopes that they might recover spontaneously. On the other, they had psychoanalysis, a therapy suitable for the needs of wealthy people desiring self-insight, but not for real psychiatric illness. Caught between these unappealing choices, psychiatrists sought alternatives. Some of these alternatives proved to be dead ends and were discarded; others became the basis of a new vision of psychotherapy; still others laid the groundwork for the revolution in drug therapy that would take place after World War II.

At the outset, however, all of these alternatives had an aura of desperateness about them, seemingly radical and possibly quite dangerous innovations. This desperateness must be understood in the context of the time. The asylums were filling, and psychiatry stood helpless in the face of disorders of the brain and mind. In these years, the profession reached the nadir of its descent from the therapeutic promises that had beckoned so brightly a century before. In the 1920s and 1930s, the center of gravity of psychiatry lay in the mental hospitals. In these snake pits, a bleakness prevailed that would have turned away any but the most resolute young medical graduate.

Bodies continued to pile in. Between 1903 and 1933, the number of patients confined in psychiatric institutions in the United States more than doubled, from 143,000 to 366,000. The vast majority were in institutions with more than a thousand beds.[1] There were psychiatric hospitals such as Georgia's notorious Milledgeville with more than eight thousand patients.

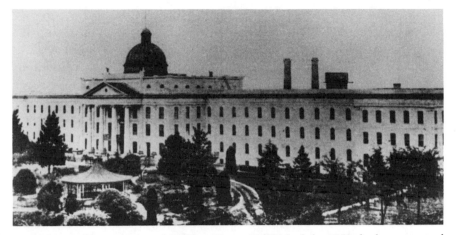

Georgia State Sanatorium at Milledgeville, at 10,000 beds by 1950 the largest mental hospital in the U.S., Home of the "Georgia Power Cocktail," a punitive form of electroconvulsive therapy (courtesy of Central State Hospital at Milledgeville).

Yet as mental hospitals grew in size, they fell in therapeutic power. In England, patients' rate of recovery dropped from 40 percent in the 1870s to 31 percent in the 1920s. At this point, even insiders began asking, "Has scientific psychiatry failed?"[2] Lothar Kalinowsky, a European refugee who in 1940 had joined the staff of the New York Psychiatric Institute, later reminisced, "Today's psychiatrists [1980] do not realize that those of us working in psychiatric hospitals before the 1930s could do little more for our patients than make them comfortable, maintain contact with their families, and in case of a spontaneous remission return them to the community."[3]

These mental hospitals, as asylums became called, seemed the very mirror of desolation. One English psychiatrist likened them to prisons, closed to outsiders and escape-proof. The doctors of course were uninformed in white coats, the nurses in regulation caps. The patients too were uniformed, in "coarse, ill-fitting suits" for the men and drab sacklike dresses for the women. Decorative schemes in the wards and corridors were "confined to variations on two colours—dark chocolate and oleaginous green." Walking through the wards, one would see the schizophrenics "who spent their entire day in assumed statuesque postures . . . or in rocking rhythmically and tirelessly backwards and forwards." In those days smearing with feces and open masturbation were still common.[4]

It had not been all downhill. These 1930-style asylums were considerably cleaner than half a century previously. Discharge rates for younger patients were actually quite high.[5] The horror of true lifelong incarceration was encountered in institutions for the mentally retarded and not in psychiatric hospitals. Yet from the viewpoint of physicians who had to practice in them, asylum psychiatry counted scarcely as a branch of medicine at all. One could cure nothing. There was little scientific understanding of mental illness. And one lived in rustication far from the medical centers with their state-of-the-art labs and great libraries. Younger, often idealistic psychiatrists bridled at this sterile incarceration and sought alternatives.

Fever Cure and Neurosyphilis

Most of the twentieth century has seen restless experimentation within psychiatry to find a cure for the chronic psychoses, mainly schizophrenia and manic-depressive illness. This long search was touched off by the surprising discovery in 1917 of a cure for neurosyphilis, the great middle-class bugbear of the nineteenth century. The story is indissolubly connected with the name of Viennese psychiatry professor Julius Wagner-Jauregg.

Wagner-Jauregg did not feel an inner calling to psychiatry, to say the least. Born in 1857 in the village of Wels—it was always said that he looked like an Upper Austrian woodcutter—he had graduated from Vienna in medicine in 1880. Like most Austrians of his day, he was a dyed-in-the-wool anti-Semite. When a Jewish colleague who had graduated three years previously received a residency with the famous internist Heinrich Bamberger that Wagner-Jauregg coveted, Wagner-Jauregg cursed the entire "Polish Club" and decided to try some other field of medicine.[6] He chanced upon psychiatry simply because the material circumstances of life in the Vienna Asylum were fairly comfortable.

Yet he soon found himself intellectually engaged with the organic side of the discipline. In 1883, during his residency at the asylum, Wagner-Jauregg noted that a female patient who had contracted erysipelas, a streptococcal infection, experienced a remission of her psychosis. This piqued his interest in the relationship between fever and madness, which long had been a subject of medical inquiry. In 1887, Wagner-Jauregg wrote an article speculating that it might be possible to treat psychosis through the use of fever. He mentioned neurosyphilis as being potentially treatable. Later in the article, without particular reference to neurosyphilis, he suggested that inoculating psychotic patients with blood from malarial patients might be attempted.[7] Fate, however, took a hand, for in 1890 the German microbiologist Robert Koch developed a vaccine, tuberculin, that was supposedly effective against tuberculosis. Wagner-Jauregg injected tuberculin into several patients whose psychotic symptoms were caused by neurosyphilis, with the aim of giving them a tuberculous fever. (It was thought that fever itself arrested the progress of neurosyphilis, on the grounds that the syphilis spirochetes are heat-sensitive.) By 1909, he was regularly obtaining long-term remissions of the symptoms of neurosyphilis through the use of tuberculin.[8] Yet he discontinued his experiments with tuberculin because it was considered to be toxic.

Wagner-Jauregg then returned to the possibility of giving paretics a fever with malaria, which, unlike other possible infections, had the advantage of being controllable with quinine. In June 1917, he learned that one of his patients, a soldier sent back from the Macedonian front with shellshock, seemed to have malaria. An assistant physician asked Wagner if the patient should be given quinine? No, said Wagner, who decided upon the spot to inject some of the soldier's blood into his neurosyphilitics.

In May 1917, a 37-year-old actor with the initials T. M. had been readmitted to the clinic with the now advanced symptoms of neurosyphilis,

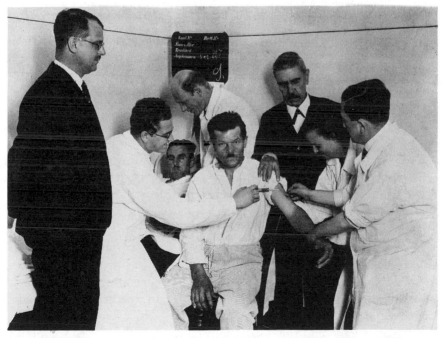

Julius von Wagner-Jauregg (on right), Viennese psychiatry professor, looks on as blood that has been taken from the arm of a patient with malaria is injected into the arm of a patient with neurosyphilis. This "malarial fever cure," discovered in 1917, was the first successful physical therapy in psychiatry. Photograph from 1934 (courtesy Institut für Geschichte der Medizin, Vienna).

including weakness of memory, fits, and pupils that were unequal in size and unresponsive to light, a clinical picture that customarily amounted to a death sentence. There being nothing to lose, on June 14, 1917, Wagner-Jauregg inoculated T. M. with malaria. Three weeks later, the patient had his first febrile attack, and after nine such attacks was given quinine. Astonishingly, after the sixth malaria attack, the syphilitic fits came to an end. "In the course of the following months, there was gradual improvement to the point of abolition of all of the patient's symptoms. From August until November, the patient, who at admission to the clinic had been incapable of working, was able to give weekly lectures and musical declamations to the patients of the head-wound clinic . . . drawing upon a great repertoire that he recited superbly by memory." T. M. was discharged apparently well on December 5, 1917. A year later Wagner-Jauregg gave the first report of this work, describing the effects of the malaria-cure upon a total of nine patients.[9] This was an epochal moment not just in the history of psychiatry but the entire history of medicine. Wagner-Jauregg's fever "cure" (it did not cure but it did restore an almost normal life to patients who otherwise would have died demented) broke the therapeutic nihilism that had dominated psychiatry in previous generations. If one could halt the neurosyphilitic psychoses, perhaps psychotic illness from other causes was treatable as well. Wagner-Jauregg received the Nobel Prize for this work in 1927.

Wagner-Jauregg's fever cure was tried on every condition imaginable within psychiatry, as for example on schizophrenia.[10] Alas, the fever cure did not turn out to be a panacea.[11] It also had powerful disadvantages. Although it was fairly effective in late-stage neurosyphilis, obtaining marked improvement in up to half of the cases, it was cumbersome, dangerous, and relied upon the availability of people of the same blood type as the paretic patient's. They also had to be infected with the right kind of malaria: tertian malaria producing chills every third day or so. Fever therapy was also very expensive.[12]

Yet Wagner-Jauregg's fever cure was a beginning, touching off other efforts to discover cures for psychosis. For decades to come, the search for physical therapies for the "functional" psychoses, meaning those in which no obvious lesion was present, was the main narrative strand in the history of major psychiatric illness.

Wagner-Jauregg and the Viennese organicists belonged to the grand Central European narrative of psychiatry's history, on par with Meynert, Griesinger, Freud, and other memorable names. But with the political turbulence of Nazism, efforts to find a cure for mental illness would shift to the New World. Just as the epicenter of psychoanalysis had gravitated to Central Park West, that of organic psychiatry too migrated westward, though not necessarily to New York.

This shift first occurred in efforts to improve on Wagner-Jauregg's fever cure. In 1910, the Berlin physician Paul Ehrlich had announced that the compound "Salvarsan" blocked the development of primary and secondary syphilis. It was an arsenical, a combination of arsenic and an organic substance, offering a way of stopping the spread of syphilis before it reached the central nervous system. Generations of American physicians remembered Ehrlich's discovery as arsphenamine, or "606," standing for the 606th compound that Ehrlich had tried. Yet the general jubilation that prevailed within the medicine about Salvarsan was moderated within psychiatry. To be effective in neurosyphilis, Salvarsan needed to be implemented early. The spirochete that causes neurosyphilis has, however, a long latency period in the central nervous system, and by the time that symptoms became clinically evident, it was often too late.

It was in peripheral American centers, precisely not in psychoanalytically dominated New York, that the definitive end to the neurosyphilis story was achieved with penicillin. The story began in 1929 at Oxford with Alexander Fleming's discovery that mold cultures of penicillin inhibited the growth of bacteria. At the beginning of World War II, Oxford researchers then recognized that penicillin was very useful against bacterial infection at the bedside. The problem was that so little of it was available, and what little could be produced was reserved for the needs of the military. Breaking this bottleneck was a "peripheral" American achievement, first attempted at Peoria, Illinois, and ultimately carried on at twenty-one different drug companies across the country (often using big fermentation vats first installed for making vitamin C to add to orange soda pop).[13]

Linking penicillin to neurosyphilis was very much an American accomplishment. In 1943, John Mahoney, a commissioned medical officer in the U.S. Public Health Service and head of the Venereal Disease Research Center at the service's marine hospital on Staten Island, obtained enough penicillin to be able to try it on primary syphilis, where it proved highly effective.[14] The Office of Scientific Research and Development of the U.S. government then organized a Penicillin Panel to investigate just what diseases penicillin was good for and how it should be administered. Clinics at eight different hospitals and universities were assigned to study penicillin in neurosyphilis. By August 1944, it was clear that penicillin was an overwhelming success.[15]

Penicillin was tried, for example, on a 34-year-old female paretic at Johns Hopkins Hospital. She had been experiencing auditory hallucinations, disorientation, tremor of her tongue, hands and mouth. By the

195

sixteenth day of her penicillin treatment, she had become completely oriented and was now free of tremor; her speech and writing had returned to normal; the hallucinations had vanished, and she was "satisfactorily performing housework including marketing . . . and driving car."[16] The handwriting of another patient, Helen M, had been reduced to a mere squiggle, so completely had she lost the use of her muscles. Penicillin treatment was started March 23, 1944. Helen M's handwriting reemerged like a bather from the depths steadily reacquiring its legibility. By May 13, it had become a proper signature.[17]

These were stunning stories. Neurosyphilis had once filled the asylums. Here was a definitive demonstration that one cause of insanity, at least, was curable.

Early Drugs

As psychotic illnesses go, neurosyphilis was an exception because its cause was clearly infectious. Penicillin would cure no other major psychiatric disorder because few others (aside from febrile delirium) are caused by a virus or bacterium. How about the so-called "functional psychoses" such as schizophrenia, where the cause was unknown? What did the new drug therapies before World War II have to offer these patients? Here the record is more unsettling.

The use of drugs in psychotic illness is almost as old as time. Administering laxatives to the mentally ill on the assumption that toxins bottled up in the colon were making them insane, reached back to the Middle Ages and before. Indeed laxative "cures" of mental illness would remain a constant theme in psychiatry throughout the nineteenth and into the twentieth century. "Diarrhoea very often proves a natural cure of insanity," opined Bedlam's John Haslam in 1809. Haslam called laxatives ("cathartics") "an indispensable remedy in cases of insanity."[18] As late as 1921, English psychiatrists were still expounding upon the virtues of croton oil (an oleaginous substance that irritated the bowels and caused diarrhea) "to abort or cut short a mental crisis."[19] Opium has a history in medicine as old as time and for centuries served the wealthy as a sedative. A young French demimondaine, unable to sleep for anxiety about her emotional life, wrote to her lover in 1773, "Suffering has softened my soul and I yield to it. At five in the morning I took two grains of opium. I obtained from it some calm that was better even than sleep."[20]

Yet if some themes in drug therapy have remained constant over the ages, other have waxed and waned. The early-modern period had its own therapeutic fancies, such as administering hellebore, or veratrum viride, a plant-derived drug that depresses the heart rate and causes vomiting. Hellebore had gone out by the beginning of the nineteenth century. Instead, two new trends in the pharmacotherapy of insanity established themselves: the widespread use of other kinds of alkaloids (plant-based drugs containing nitrogen); and the rise of compounds used mainly as sedatives and sleeping medications, synthesized in laboratories of the mainly German organic chemical industry.

The first of the new alkaloids to enter the asylum was morphine, isolated from opium in 1806. Like opium, morphine itself had been taken orally for many years. Samuel Kirkbride prescribed it in water for his patients.[21] A new phase began in 1855, when Alexander Wood, an Edinburgh physician, described the use of the hypodermic needle for injecting morphine directly into the circulation. He wrote thus of Miss X, an "old lady" with a long history of nervous symptoms, shoulder pain, and chronic insomnia (who had a history of fainting after taking opium orally): "On November 28, I visited her at 10 P.M. to give the opiate the benefit of the night. Having ascertained that the most tender spot was [in her shoulder], I inserted the syringe . . . and injected twenty drops of a solution of murate of morphia." Within ten minutes she began "to complain of giddiness and confusion of ideas." Half an hour later, her pain was gone. When he visited her again at 11 A.M. the following morning, "I was a little annoyed to find that she had never wakened; the breathing also was somewhat deep, and she was roused with difficulty." Her shoulder pain was gone, never again to return.[22] Here was clearly something new in sedation: an injectable drug that not only calmed patients (a sedative) but put them to sleep for long stretches (a hypnotic). Within asylum psychiatry in the second half of the nineteenth century, subcutaneous injections of morphine became an important means of subduing agitated patients, the practice finally fading when it was realized how addictive morphine was.[23]

The nineteenth century's second half was the "alkaloid period" of asylum treatment. Among numerous alkaloid sedatives, by far the most popular was hyoscyamus, a drug derived from the henbane species of the Solanaceae plant family, a family famous as a source of hallucinogens. Toward the end of the eighteenth century, various authorities had noted that henbane extracts calmed "maniacal delirium." In 1833, chemists isolated the alkaloid hyoscyamine from henbane and the Merck company in Darmstadt began marketing it for various nonpsychiatric indications. Finally in 1868, the Viennese pharmacologist Karl Schroff established that hyoscyamus acted as a sedative and hypnotic. Robert Lawson of the West Riding Asylum in Yorkshire began giving it to his patients around 1875.[24]

By the 1880s, hyoscyamine cocktails had come into wide use in institutions. This represented the true beginning of asylum psychopharmacology.

Yet the hyoscyamine story continued to evolve. In 1880, hyoscine, another drug that would later be extensively used in psychiatry (called in the United States scopolamine), was isolated from hyoscyamine.[25] It became an essential ingredient of the sedative "cocktails" used on manic patients, who otherwise would literally agitate themselves to death. As late as the 1930s, psychiatrists at places like the Bethlem Royal Hospital used hyoscine in dealing with "head-banging, rubbing, and pulling out of hair, relentless picking away at the skin causing sepsis. . . . In extreme form these symptoms, as well as excitement and aggression might be relieved for the time being by Hyoscine Co A, a potent compound of hyoscine, morphine, and atropine [a close relative of hyoscyamine]."[26] Well into the twentieth century, knowledge of these "cocktails" represented the basic lore of asylum psychopharmacology.

The story of hyoscyamine and its relatives shows the typical development of most drugs in psychiatry: They would be discovered and isolated by chemists and pharmacologists interested in other things entirely than disorders of the mind. An inventive psychiatrist would discover that the drug was good for X or Y; then a drug company would purify it and put it on the market so that it could be given to patients. This was drug discovery largely by serendipity, in contrast to the designed drug discovery of the second biological psychiatry.

During the long "alkaloid period," psychiatry never pretended to anything other than the momentary relief of symptoms with drugs. It is when we come to drugs synthesized in the laboratories of pharmaceutical houses that we encounter efforts, misguided or not, actually to cure patients who have psychotic illness. It is a story that begins largely in Central Europe—because of the enormous organic chemical industry in Germany—and ends in the United States, because of the emigration of Jewish scientists to the New World.

At the heart of this story is the torrent of sedatives that flowed from the workbenches of companies such as Bayer into the asylum. The first of these manufactured sedatives, chloral hydrate, was synthesized in 1832 by the Giessen chemistry professor Justus von Liebig. Liebig represented the first direct tie-in of psychiatry to industry. The founder of organic chemistry, he taught many of the chemists who ended up working for Bayer after it founded a pharmaceuticals division in 1888.[27]

Chloral became the first rehearsal of the "Prozac" scenario (see pp. 320–324) seen with drugs that acquire a great public following for the relief of common psychiatric symptoms. In 1869, Otto Liebreich, professor of pharmacology in Berlin, determined that chloral functioned as a hypnotic to relieve insomnia in anxious and depressed patients who were not insane. Plays and novels of the epoch often eased references to chloral into the plot, the heroine being drugged before being robbed of her virtue. Fans of detective stories recognized chloral as "knockout drops" and "Mickey Finns." Chloral trumped morphine and the Solanaceae alkaloids because it was reliable in strength from dose to dose and didn't need to be injected (although patients disliked its awful taste and characteristic afterodor on the breath). It remained for decades the workhorse of asylum pharmacology and enjoyed wide popularity—and abuse—as a drug that middle-class patients could take at home to avoid the asylum.

Women in particular often became chloral addicts for this reason, treated at home for psychotic symptoms because the family was too embarrassed to have them committed. Theodor Meynert referred a woman of 42 who had become addicted to chloral to a private medical clinic in Vienna for treatment. He thought that addiction was her main problem. But it was not, for when the clinic doctors took her off the chloral, a psychosis came to the surface. She had to be taken to a private asylum.[28] Virginia Woolf, with a long history of major depression and of treatment in private nervous clinics behind her, was taking chloral at home in the 1920s as she became involved in a sexual relationship with Vita Sackville-West. "Goodnight now," she wrote Vita in 1928. "I am so sleepy with chloral simmering in my spine that I can't write, nor yet stop writing—I feel like a moth, with heavy scarlet eyes and a soft cape of down—a moth about to settle in a sweet bush—Would it were—ah but that's improper."[29] Vienna and London: two typical trajectories in psychiatric home-care among the middle classes.

Other alkaloids would be almost comical, were the conditions they sought to ameliorate not so desperate. In mania, for example, patients would rage and agitate until they expired. Apomorphine, an artificial alkaloid of morphine that served as a powerful emetic (making patients vomit), came into the asylum after its discovery late in the nineteenth century. It acted against mania. At the Douglas Hospital in Montreal physicians mixed apomorphine with hyoscine, which calmed the patients by making them vomit.[30] At the asylum in Independence, Iowa, "in days gone by, patients who were bothered by mania and could not slow down were administered this drug. They were said to literally turn green and vomit for up to an hour. This would have a sapping effect and they would finally be able to get six hours or so of much needed rest."[31]

Chloral and apomorphine represented cures only in the sense of suppressing symptoms for a period. The first attempt to cure with drugs occurred in a rather bizarre setting: Shanghai at the end of the nineteenth century. It occurred quite by accident. This story involves the bromides, and requires a bit of background, for the element bromine, which occurs naturally in seawater and salt springs, was first isolated in 1826 from the ashes of seaweed by an apothecary in Montpellier. Believing it to be a substitute for iodine, French physicians began using it immediately on a variety of ailments, for all of which it was unsuitable. Bromine in its natural form is corrosive and had to be administered as a salt, combined with elements like potassium. The French noted that the salts of bromine often produced sedation, an *inrresse bromurique* such as the English novelist Evelyn Waugh described in *The Ordeal of Gilbert Pinfold,* a fictionalized autobiographical account of his own experience with bromism.[32]

Bromine entered mainstream medicine in 1857, when Charles Locock, a London internist with a tony Mayfair practice, was commenting on a paper about epilepsy at a medical meeting. Locock happened to mention that he had given 10 grains of potassium bromide three times a day over a period of two weeks to a patient with "hysterical epilepsy," suppressing the epilepsy. He had also given it "in cases of hysteria in young women, unaccompanied by epilepsy," finding it "of the greatest service."[33] He implied that it sedated them. Away bromium went on its career as a sedative.

The bromides spread rapidly within public asylums because they were cheaper than chloral. By 1891, the Paris asylums were using over a thousand kilos of potassium bromide a year.[34] Older asylum psychiatrists still remember giving "triple bromides . . . in liquid form to thousands of patients q. h. s. [at bedtime] and frequently p. r. n. [as needed] during the night."[35] The point is that when, around 1879, young Dr. Neil Macleod went out to Shanghai to practice medicine, he would have been thoroughly familiar with potassium bromide and perhaps already confident in its application.

Prolonged Sleep

Macleod, a recent Edinburgh medical graduate, quite unwittingly became the innovator of the first drug therapy in psychiatry that actually promised relief of psychotic illness.[36] Early in 1897, a married Englishwoman of 48, resident in Shanghai but staying in a hotel in Japan, "received by wire unexpected news of a family affliction, giving rise to a great nervous shock." The sounds of the other hotel guests soon began to drive her "frantic." She developed an attack of acute mania, and Macleod was summoned from Shanghai to bring her home. Not having skilled nurses available—but possessing considerable experience with weaning morphine and cocaine users from their addictions by putting them into prolonged bromide sleeps[37]—Macleod decided to try the same method on her that he had used on the addicts, even though her problem was psychosis. He gave her a large dose of bromide and then after she went into a deep sleep had her transported out in a hammock. After a 500-mile steamer trip and an odyssey lasting several days, she finally arrived back in Shanghai, awakening well without "a trace of mental disturbance."[38]

She remained well for two years, then relapsed in June 1899 after "another shock" that left her unable to ride to the hounds. She became irritable, then passed into "a state of incoherence, exaltation, and incessant speech activity with delusions of fear in the night and the desire to escape from the house, neither it nor its inmates being recognized." Macleod again diagnosed acute mania. In the absence of "a padded room" or "skilled attendants" within thousands of miles of Shanghai, he decided to treat her again with what he was now calling "the bromide sleep."

On the first day, Macleod gave her sodium bromide in two-dram doses (about a quarter of an ounce) starting at 8:30 in the morning and continuing for three more times that day. She wandered about the house for most of the day "talking nonsense nearly incessantly" and fell asleep about nine that evening. The second day, he gave her another ounce. By the end of this day, she was sleeping quite a bit and was "full of delusions expressed quite distinctly." At this point, he stopped the administration of the bromide. She had swallowed two full ounces. The third day, she could speak only with difficulty and could not walk without being supported. The fourth day, she could not be roused. Nor could she be roused for the next three days. On the ninth day, she began to surface, withdrawing her foot, for example, when tickled. Yet only on the twelfth day did she even begin to mutter, and not until another week had passed was Macleod able to assess her mental status: "Twenty-third day: A good night; the faintest trace of mental disturbance. From this day, no departure from the normal mental state could be detected; walking in the garden and downstairs, meals as usual."

Macleod treated eight other patients as well with his "bromide sleep." One died of pneumonia, the likely result of having aspirated vomitus while in a stupor. The others had either been cured of addiction or, like the preceding patient, of "acute mania." As Macleod described his newly discovered sleep, "the patient slept day and night for five to nine days, unable to "walk, stand, sit, speak, or carry on any of the higher cerebral functions." Every six hours, Macleod would put the patients on a commode, and every few hours give a tumblerful of milk. Upon awakening, the patients seemed actually to have recovered from their illnesses. It is unknown how many relapsed.[39]

The profound duration of torpor differentiated Macleod's deep-sleep therapy from previous psychiatric efforts to narcotize patients for brief periods.[40] For the first time in the history of psychiatry, a drug therapy had been described that seemed to alleviate major psychiatric illness with a physical procedure. Whether Macleod's bromide sleep really did cure patients is beside the point: A hint had been inserted into the profession's collective thinking that some kind of cure with drugs might be possible.

The bromide sleep cure was taken up briefly by other physicians, then abandoned.[41] Bromine itself was perhaps too toxic, or the whole notion too recklessly "heroic" to contemplate. The next step in the development of sleep cures would not occur under the aegis of bromine but of the barbiturates.

In 1903, the German chemist Emil Fischer and his collaborator Joseph von Mering modified a class of drugs originally synthesized in 1864 in a way that made them effective as sedatives and hypnotics.[42] The original inventor of the compounds had called them barbiturates, apparently after his girlfriend Barbara. Fischer and Mering realized that their new drug, "diethyl barbituric acid," or barbital, was a sedative. It improved vastly upon the congeries of previous sedatives by not tasting unpleasant, by having few side effects, and by acting at therapeutic levels far beneath the toxic dose (unlike potassium bromide, which tasted awful and had a therapeutic level close to the toxic dose). The Bayer company marketed Fischer's discovery as "Veronal," the Schering company as "Medinal." Both brand names would become household words.[43] The barbiturates were pricey. In Germany, one gram of Veronal cost 40 pfennigs, one gram of Trional, a competing nonbarbiturate sedative, 15 pfennigs.[44] Nonetheless Veronal and similar barbiturates caught on immediately. They calmed maniacal patients, restored the sleep of the melancholic, and were an effective hypnotic for insomniacs in general (and still are: the Lilly Company's short-acting Seconal, or secobarbital, is commonly used in North America today).

Veronal was first tried on patients in 1904 by Hermann von Husen, a young asylum psychiatrist who himself had problems sleeping. Among his other findings, he reported that one evening he had taken half a gram of Veronal, the next evening a gram. "In both cases after 10–15 minutes I felt an ever-growing weariness, which went over to deep sleep after half an hour. After half a gram of Veronal I slept 8 hours, after a gram around 9 hours. The first morning I awoke fresh and rested, the second morning after the higher dose I had trouble getting out of bed. . . ."[45] No other drug then available let people sleep deeply then wake up refreshed. The potential appeal of such a product was immense.

Veronal became the drug of choice in private nervous clinics (while the public asylums stayed with cheaper standbys such as bromium and chloral). Here is "Jane Hillyer," a young woman in the grip of manic-depressive illness, during one of her stays in a sanatorium:

> The sun was just beginning to sink behind the trees. . . . It would be hours before it was time for sleep—for Veronal. I continued my imperious demands. "Maybe they will break their old rules; maybe I can have it earlier if I make a fuss"; they did, a little. Yet long before the nurse stood before me with a glass of clear water and that magic white tablet—it always seemed the one cool, white thing in the world—long before then, I had heard my own voice, cracked and strange mingling with the unearthly cries of other patients. . . ."[46]

Dozens of other barbiturates came onto the market after the success of Veronal. In 1912, Bayer marketed Luminal (phenobarbital), a barbiturate still used for epilepsy. Because of its long-acting nature, "phenobarb" became a favorite drug in asylums well-off enough to afford it. "The prevailing anxiolytic," one elderly psychiatrist recalled, "was elixir phenobarbital. It was pink in color and many patients, most commonly female, carried their bottle of pink medicine with them and took a teaspoonful when necessary."[47] Not just in asylum psychiatry but within medicine as a whole, the barbiturates became widely used, the family doctor's familiar recourse in dealing with "a hysterical girl on her bridal night."[48] If a single class of drugs came to exemplify psychiatry before the advent of Valium (the class of benzodiazepines) in the 1960s, it was the barbiturates.

In this context of growing familiarity with barbiturates capable of inducing prolonged deep sleep, the first major attempts of the twentieth century to cure psychotic illness were launched. The actual priority for inducing prolonged sleep with barbiturates belongs to Giuseppe Epifanio in 1915, an assistant physician at the Turin university psychiatric clinic.[49] Yet his article about therapeutic success with deep sleep, appearing as it did in the middle of a war and in a language that few foreign psychiatrists read, made little impact. Prolonged sleep therapy, the first of the so-called physical therapies of the twentieth century, is associated with Swiss psychiatrist Jakob Klaesi, a staff physician at Zurich's university psychiatric clinic, the Burghölzli. In 1920, Klaesi began using an innovative combination of two barbiturates of the Swiss drug firm Hoffmann-La Roche marketed as Somnifen. It was Klaesi's aspiration to cure no less a disease than schizophrenia with prolonged narcosis (*Dauernarkose*).

Klaesi, then 37 and a private docent at the Burghölzli, was by no means a pill-grubbing biological type. He had always been enthusiastic about psychotherapy and indeed argued that deep sleep was a way of calming patients down to make them accessible to dialogue. But he was not known for good judgment—he became a Nazi-sympathizer in the 1930s—subject as he himself was to manic-depressive personality swings. He was also highly ambitious. All of these qualities made him perhaps overly receptive to the suggestion of the Zurich pharmacology professor Max Cloetta that Epifanio's deep-sleep therapy might be tackled again, this time with the aid of Somnifen.[50] "I decided upon introducing prolonged sleep, that is prolonged narcosis, into psychiatry," Klaesi rather grandly began his report, in an effort to "achieve an improved rapport between doctor and patient." Blocking out stimuli through sleep might help dig the schizophrenic patients out of their negativistic attitudes so that psychotherapy could begin. As Klaesi took over the ward for agitated females at the Burghölzli in April 1920, he encountered a 39-year-old woman who had been an "able businesswoman" until falling ill three years previously. She had become anxious, complained that someone wanted to kill her and her husband, had started hearing voices, and was put in a private nervous clinic. She improved, went home, became ill again, and was admitted this time to the Burghölzli in March 1919. She became so violent that the hospital had to put her in a special padded cell that had been unused for two decades.

Klaesi tried hard to establish a therapeutic rapport with her. On one occasion as she lay naked in her cell, Klaesi asked her, what are you "as an intelligent woman doing in such a hole."

"What do you want?" she asked him.

"To cure you at any cost so that you don't have such a horrible life," he replied. Thereupon she began to cry, then attempted to conceal her tears and got a runny nose. Klaesi handed her his handkerchief. Her face opened up. She looked at him smiling and said to the nurse standing by, "He's OK." Klaesi became intent upon establishing a psychological rapport with her.

At the end of April he decided to try and "dismantle her defenses" with a Somnifen course of deep sleep. He followed this by two further courses, each lasting typically five to six days. In October 1920, she was discharged as vastly improved. The husband later said he had never seen his wife "to be so industrious, circumspect and tender as she now is." The woman, however, just before discharge declared to Klaesi that her marriage was in trouble. She scorned her husband as a Caspar Milquetoast for permitting her to dominate over him—and expressed a desire for the husband to be like her doctors. Klaesi thoughtfully concluded, "Prolonged sleep and Somnifen had opened the way to a fruitful dialogue with the patient and to new insight."[51]

Of the 26 patients Klaesi treated with prolonged narcosis, about a quarter to a third improved so greatly that they could be discharged or transferred to wards for less agitated patients. On the face of it, this seemed to be a promising new therapy.[52] The problem was that three of the patients had died as a result of pneumonia or circulatory collapse. The Achilles' heel of prolonged sleep was its high risk. Several years later, Swiss psychiatrist Max Müller at the Münsingen asylum, determined to break out of "paralyzing therapeutic resignation toward my patients," did another study comparing two barbiturates, and found that prolonged sleep with Somnifen had a mortality of about 5 percent.[53] Klaesi had dismissed the deaths in his own study as owing to preexisting organic conditions, and never forgave Müller for having called attention to the potential lethality of the new treatment for schizophrenia that Klaesi had supposedly discovered.

In the following years, prolonged sleep with safer barbiturates than Somnifen became the first asylum therapy that offered any hope.[54] Deep sleep became widely adopted for affective, or mood, disorders, often by physicians who shared Klaesi's hope of somehow making these gravely ill patients accessible to psychotherapy.[55] Eliot Slater of the Maudsley Hospital called sleep therapy "the one treatment we had in the early thirties which was of any avail with acute psychotic illnesses." Maudsley doctors would have their patients sleep 12 to 16 hours a day, "with drowsy intervals in which the patient could be roused to eat and drink." Afterward, the patient would remember little of the psychotic episode and might expect early discharge from the hospital.[56]

The notion of addressing the brain with profound narcosis spread through psychiatry. German physicians in the early 1930s used it to withdraw addicted patients from morphine.[57] Washington psychoanalyst Harry Stack Sullivan would intoxicate his patients for "three to ten days" with alcohol in order to open them up to psychotherapy. ("Recourse is had to chemotherapeutic agencies, notably ethyl alcohol, which impair the highly discriminative action of the more lately acquired tendency systems . . .," Sullivan explained.)[58] Kalinowsky called Klaesi's prolonged sleep therapy "the first treatment with which at least transitory improvement was obtained in functional psychoses."[59] Thus prolonged sleep is partially exculpated from its condemnation at the hands

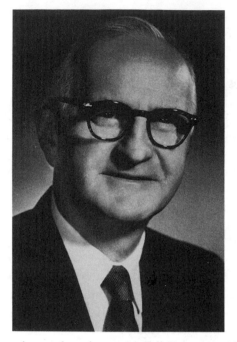

D. Ewen Cameron, professor of psychiatry, McGill University, 1943–1964, a distinguished North American psychiatrist of Scottish origin, whose work ran off the rails in the notorious "depatterning" experiments with sleep therapy and electroconvulsive therapy that he conducted in the 1950s (courtesy McGill University Archives).

psychoanalytically oriented historians of psychiatry. It gave new hope to physicians whose life mission was the care of patients with major psychiatric illnesses. After decades of warehousing patients, sleep therapy offered the prospect of cure.[60]

Yet this story has an unpleasant codicil. Just as most of the stories of the physical therapies began in the Old World and ended in the New, so did deep-sleep therapy begin in Zurich and end in Montreal, at the hands of Dr. D. Ewen Cameron. Cameron was born in 1901 in Scotland and graduated MB from Glasgow in 1924. Trained at the leading psychiatric centers of the day—Bleuler's Burghölzli and Meyer's Phipps Clinic—in 1929 he started working at an asylum in Canada's province of Manitoba, went on to several American posts, then in 1943 became the first director of Montreal's Allan Memorial Institute (which is the joint department of psychiatry of McGill University and the Royal Victoria Hospital, housed in a mansion next to the hospital belonging to the former shipping lord Sir Hugh Allan). By the early 1950s, Cameron had become a distinguished researcher, serving for example in 1952–1953 as president of the American Psychiatric Association.

An enemy of psychoanalysis, Cameron grasped at the new physical therapies. Having been in Zurich in the 1920s, what could be more natural for him than to apply in Montreal Klaesi's barbiturate narcosis. Yet Cameron added a twist, in the belief that forcing patients to listen to propagandistic messages ("brainwashing," he called it) during their prolonged sleep would somehow accelerate their recovery. He first attempted this "psychic driving" in 1953.[61] "The [tape] loop was broadcast from a speaker on the wall of the sleep room in a female and (he hoped) maternal voice," reports one writer. "At first [the young female patient from Bermuda] showed little response to the voice. Then, unexpectedly, she became as hostile as her condition would allow: 'at moments when she roused slightly from her sleep, [she] would crawl or stagger out of bed, and try to destroy the source of the voice.' The hostility peaked in about six days. By the end of ten days, 'she not only became quite undisturbed by the voice, but she slowly began to incorporate the content, saying, Yes, I want to go back to Bermuda; yes, my parents love me.' "[62]

This was Cameron's point of departure. In 1955, he began to put patients into deep sleeps, simultaneously giving them electroshock several times a day (passing electricity through the brain to induce therapeutic convulsions). He called this "depatterning," breaking down previous brain constellations that, he thought, had somehow produced psychosis.[63] Over the next decade, his therapeutic judgment clearly became unbalanced as he attempted this systematic depatterning of patients without their consent and without any pretense of applying the scientific method. In 1964 Cameron fled Montreal for a post at the Albany Medical School. He died, essentially in disgrace, three years later. (At his death the *New York Times* obituary headlined: "Led Research in Geriatrics at Hospital in Albany."[64]) With Cameron, sleep therapy died as well. By the 1960s, many safer and more effective treatments for psychotic illness had come along. Yet it had marked the beginning of a revolution in psychiatry.

Shock and Coma

Why shocking the brain to the point of eliciting convulsions makes psychotic patients better is unclear. But it does. So does the dangerous procedure of putting them into prolonged comas, as opposed to the stupors that bromide sleep elicited. So little understood is the relationship between brain and mind even now that the mechanism of these

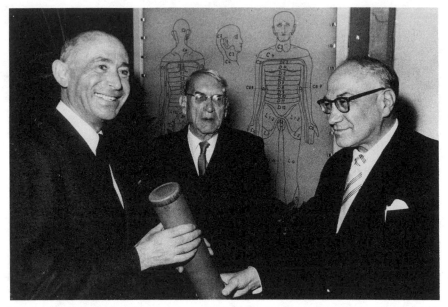

Manfred Sakel on left, discoverer in 1933 of insulin coma therapy. In the middle is Vienna psychiatry professor Otto Poetzl, in whose clinic Sakel did his early work; on the right is Hans Hoff, head of Vienna's university psychiatry clinic after World War II. Here Sakel is receiving an award in 1957, the year of his death (courtesy of AP/Wide World Photos).

treatments, which have helped retrieve many patients from the depths of profound illness, is not understood. Yet empirically, some of these therapies have proven themselves, so much so that electroconvulsive therapy, or ECT, is today the treatment of choice for major depression. Their advent in the 1930s, as clearly superior alternatives to either warehousing or to psychoanalysis, marked a great turning of the page in the history of psychiatry.

To this day, however, both coma and shock have remained controversial. The antipsychiatry movement has rejected them as a matter of principle, as have physicians who rely on psychotherapy to the exclusion of most else. The historical record, however, shows that coma and shock gave psychiatrists powerful new therapies in a field dominated for half a century by nihilistic hopelessness, and it is against that sense of despair that they must be set.[65]

This story begins in Berlin with a young medical graduate of the Vienna University named Manfred Sakel. Sakel was born in 1900 in Nadverna, Galicia (then part of Austria), of a pious Jewish family said to be descended from Maimonides. By the time of his graduation in

1925, so scorching had the blast of Austrian anti-Semitism become that he found a job in Berlin as assistant physician at Kurt Mendel's expensive suburban private clinic, the Lichterfelde Sanatorium. The clinic courted the actresses and physicians who typically were at risk of morphine addiction. Yet a cold-turkey withdrawal often entailed symptoms such as vomiting and diarrhea. In the late 1920s, Sakel discovered that such symptoms could be successfully managed by administering small doses of insulin, a hormone just discovered in 1922.[66]

Insulin had already been tried several times in psychiatry during the 1920s, as early as 1923, when the staff of the Psychopathic Hospital in Ann Arbor, Michigan, gained the impression that insulin relieved the depression of diabetic patients as well as their diabetes. In fact it did not.[67] Later in the 1920s, insulin was used on patients who had lost their appetites or refused to eat.[68] But it occurred to no one that a coma from insulin shock might be curative. (The hormone causes the muscles to take up glucose from the blood. If too much glucose is withdrawn, the patient will go into a hypoglycemic coma.)

Sakel was probably not aware of much of this previous writing in any event. Yet he did have to cope with the insulin comas that happened inadvertently to several of his own patients. He noted that after the comas were over the patients' desire for morphine had been abolished. In addition, these previously "restless and agitated" patients had become "tranquil and accessible." Sakel reported this finding in 1933.[69] At this point, he was clearly thinking that putting patients into an insulin coma might in and of itself be a cure for major psychiatric illness.

Evidently as a result of the Nazi takeover, Sakel returned to Vienna in 1933, getting a post at the university psychiatric clinic under Otto Poetzl, Wagner-Jauregg's successor as the professor of psychiatry. Sakel also became chief physician of a private clinic in a Viennese suburb. Sakel persuaded a reluctant Poetzl to try out the dangerous-sounding therapy, and in October 1933, Sakel began testing systematically at the university clinic his theory that insulin "shock" represented a cure for schizophrenia.

Colleagues at the clinic were astonished at the results. Said Karl Dussik: "As I worked from the first day in using this method in our clinic I can confirm its real effect. The personality of the patient can often be changed so entirely during the hypoglycemic reactions that it seems as though the glycopenic [low blood sugar] treatment has created a new being."[70] (Success in psychiatry often gives the impression of creating a new person, witness the huzzahs surrounding Prozac many years later, see pp. 320–324.)

In 1934, Sakel broadcast the first results of his study: Inducing hypoglycemia with insulin and putting patients into insulin comas were producing astonishing alleviations of symptoms.[71] Of his 50 patients experiencing their first episode of schizophrenia, he obtained a full remission in 70 percent and a "social remission" in a further 18 percent.[72] The first page of his clinical notebook in Vienna shows 8 of his 12 patients discharged to their homes as improved. A further patient died shortly after going home, three others were transferred to the Vienna city asylum at Steinhof.[73] These were recoveries in a patient population previously considered hopeless. One notes that at this stage the insulin "shock" did not include convulsions (or if they did, they were considered undesirable side effects).

Yet beyond the university clinic, Sakel's results were considered a joke, the man himself a charlatan, and Poetzl's patronage of him a mystery.[74] Sakel spent only three years in Vienna, traveling to the United States in 1936 to treat a wealthy private patient and staying on, first as a staff member of a New York State psychiatric hospital, then in private practice in Manhattan. It is incredible that the psychoanalytically dominated American Psychiatric Association at first refused his application for membership, admitting him only after the science writer of the *New York Times* called attention to the story.[75] Sakel died in 1957, having spent his life zealously defending his reputation and his priority.[76]

Rather than being adopted in Central Europe, insulin-coma therapy was taken up in Switzerland and in the Anglo-Saxon world. The Swiss private and public psychiatric hospitals were at the time probably the most progressive in the world, and it is no surprise that in 1937 the director of the Münsingen public asylum, Max Müller, arranged a world conference on new therapies for schizophrenia. Münsingen became the "world mecca" of insulin treatment. "People trust me, not Sakel," Müller boasted.[77]

As with all these new physical therapies, the diffusion of insulin-coma to the non-German-speaking world occurred within a web of personal to-ing and fro-ing. Herbert James Pullar-Strecker, who brought it to Britain, had been born in Würzburg of a German physician-father and a Scottish mother whose maiden name was Pullar. He emigrated to Britain in the 1920s and had just qualified in Glasgow as David Henderson put him in charge of the future insulin unit at the Royal Edinburgh Hospital for Mental Disorders. Pullar-Strecker initiated coma therapy there early in 1936.[78] Later that year Dr. Isabel Wilson of the mental-hospital Board of Control visited Vienna and Münsingen, returning to England with a positive report of the new therapy. She called the burden of schizophrenia "so heavy that it demands the full and careful trial of any therapeutic measure which claims to relieve or diminish it."[79]

For British psychiatrists, who had been suspicious of deep-sleep therapy, insulin coma came as heaven-sent. Eliot Slater had come to the Maudsley in 1931. He recalled the patients with chronic depression in the preinsulin days: "The involutional melancholic would be a thin, elderly man or woman, inert, with the head lifted up off the pillow. There were some sort of Parkinsonian-like qualities, mask-like face sunk deep in misery, and speaking in a retarded way. If you could get them to say anything, it would be something about how hopeless things were, how they were wicked, doomed to disease, death, and a terrible afterlife, if there was one." Insulin coma was the first therapy that actually permitted doctors at the Maudsley to help these patients.[80]

A sense of the enthusiasm of British hospital psychiatrists for insulin-coma therapy may be gleaned from the letters home of a young Canadian psychiatrist who was doing a "locum" in the summer of 1937 at the Warwickshire and Coventry Mental Hospital in Hatton near Warwick. Writing in July to his chief in Toronto, he said:

> [This] 1,400 bed hospital of block type [has a] staff of six physicians all under 35 and all keen. [The hospital employed a full-time pharmicist and (thank God, in the writer's view) no psychologist.] Our trust is not in extra staff but in drugs and the barbiturates in particular [for mania and depression]. . . . And now of course insulin shock for the schizophrenic group is giving us a chemical procedure for the other great biogenic group. How the heart of the "druggist" has been gladdened these past four years! Dr. D. N. Parfitt our chief spent six weeks in Vienna and we started in cases 5 weeks ago. Only 3 or 4 places in Great Britain have started and no literature of importance has appeared here. . . . I expect to spend August and September in the insulin shock clinic.[81]

The Warwickshire asylum was in the vanguard by only a bit. "By 1939 every self-respecting go-ahead hospital had its insulin unit," said one observer.[82] In William Sargant's and Eliot Slater's influential 1944 textbook of physical treatments, based on their experiences at the Maudsley Hospital, insulin-coma therapy was clearly the first choice.[83]

Not Sakel but a young American psychiatrist, who happened to be exposed to insulin therapy in 1934 while in analysis with Freud, introduced insulin coma therapy to the United States. Born in 1906, Joseph Wortis had graduated from the University of Vienna in 1932. He went to New York to intern and train in psychiatry at Bellevue Hospital with the recently arrived Viennese psychiatrist Paul Schilder. In the fall of 1934, in the context of his interest in human sexuality, Wortis underwent a kind of didactic analysis with Freud. During this analysis, in December 1934, he happened to visit Poetzl's psychiatric clinic at the Vienna General Hospital and saw Sakel administering insulin therapy. The enthusiastic young Wortis turned his back on psychoanalysis, returned to Bellevue and initiated insulin-coma therapy in the United States.[84] In November 1936, he gave a paper on the subject that later appeared in a neurology journal.[85] (The report was delayed 18 months, he said, because he could not persuade any of the psychoanalytically dominated psychiatry journals to publish it.[86]) Wortis translated Sakel's monograph into English.

Yet Sakel himself provided his own authoritative imprimatur to the introduction of his therapy in the United States, lecturing on it to a New York medical audience in January 1937.[87] The meeting was an American psychiatric microenvironment: Adolf Meyer was there and gave insulin coma "a verbose blessing," as he gave everything his blessing regardless how absurd. Unsurprisingly, Ewen Cameron made a "forceful contribution advocating insulin coma therapy." Psychoanalyst Smith Ely Jelliffe, in an involuntary caricature of Freudian thought, opined that insulin coma might work by "withdrawing the libido from the outside world and fusing it with the death impulse for the maintenance of the narcissistic ego."[88] Analysts like Jelliffe saw asylum psychiatrists as dim country cousins. Yet in the 1940s and 1950s, these country cousins nonetheless seized on insulin therapy to break out of the therapeutic impasse of custodialism and draw themselves closer to medicine. By the early 1960s, there were special insulin units in more than a hundred American mental hospitals.[89]

How was insulin-coma therapy administered? It was a dangerous procedure with a mortality of almost one in a hundred, and required a team of doctors and nurses in a special unit. There might be "twenty or more patients on the insulin ward all in coma at the same time," said Walter Freeman (the later devotee of lobotomy) of George Washington University. "There was no red flag waving on the brink [of hypoglycemic death]; and most therapists hesitated to approach it too closely."[90]

The therapy would begin in graded little steps. At the Maudsley Hospital said Slater, "Every day [the patient] received a dose of insulin, increasing until he started drifting off to sleep, insulin sopor, and then eventually from sleep into coma, deep unconsciousness." In coma, the patient was watched constantly and permitted to spend no more than twenty minutes in that condition before being brought round with a sugar solution. (At other hospitals two-hour comas and longer were not unusual.) "When he had had twenty comas or so one usually saw a remarkable improvement in the mental state, at first in the morning after treatment, and then

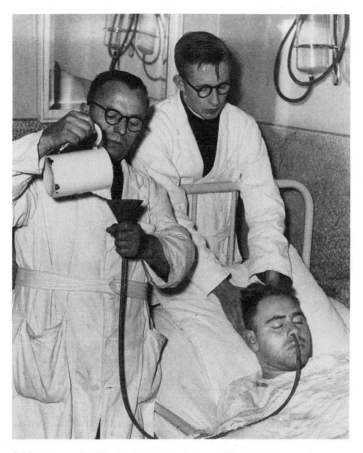

Brothers of Charity at the Dr. Guislain Asylum in Ghent, Belgium, bringing patient out of insulin coma therapy, c. late 1940s or early 1950s. The man with the rubber tube in his nose has been given a glucose (sugar) solution to bring him out of the coma. A strong concentration of glucose is poured directly into the stomach to prevent the coma from becoming lethal (courtesy of Museum Dr. Guislain, Ghent, which forms part of the present psychiatric centre Dr. Guislain).

persisting into the rest of the day, and finally persisting after the treatment had been tapered off." Insulin coma doubled the proportion of recoveries at the Maudsley, said Slater.[91] At Nova Scotia Hospital in Canada, where Charles Roberts ran the insulin unit around 1943, they would steadily increase the insulin doses over a period of 10 days or so until the patients reached the stage of deep coma with occasional convulsions. "On termination of coma, patients frequently had what was described as a 'lucid period' of varying duration during which conversations would be normal and delusions and hallucinations seemed to be absent."[92]

Is it any wonder that asylum psychiatrists became keen about insulin coma? It seemed to be a procedure that actually worked, at least for the short term, without the extreme dangerousness of sleep therapy. In the long term, it was discovered that insulin coma had about the same success rate as barbiturate-sleep therapy.[93] Both represented a substantial improvement on what was available before, which is to say, nothing.

Within months of the adoption of insulin coma, a second so-called shock therapy came along that marked the true beginning of convulsive therapy. The difference is an important one: this second therapy, with Metrazol, produced convulsions without coma. Shocking the brain to the point of eliciting a convulsion does seem to have a beneficial effect upon psychotic illness, particularly on major depression. The era of convulsive therapy began not with insulin (in which convulsions were undesired and incidental) but with a drug similar to camphor called by the trade name Metrazol (Cardiazol in Europe). Its discoverer was Ladislas von Meduna, a

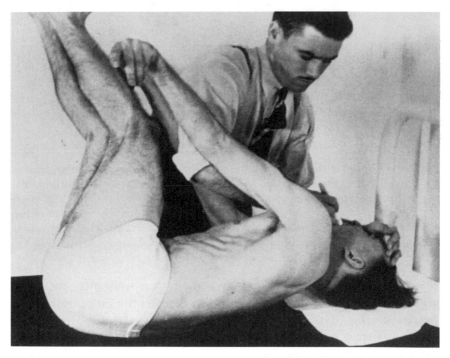

Patient in the midst of an unrestrained Metrazol convulsion in an American mental hospital, c. 1941. Discovered in 1934 by Ladislas von Meduna, Metrazol represented the first of the true convulsive therapies.

Source: American Journal of Psychiatry, 97 (1941), p. 1052, copyright 1941 American Psychiatric Association, reprinted by permission.

214

38-year-old Budapest psychiatrist who in 1934 proposed ameliorating the symptoms of schizophrenia by deliberately putting patients into a convulsive state.[94]

Meduna had trained as a neuropathologist between 1923 and 1926 at Budapest's Interacademic Institute for Brain Research, then followed his chief Karl Schaffer to the university department of psychiatry in Budapest where Schaffer had just been made professor. Here Meduna encountered clinical psychiatry for the first time. He became intrigued at the changes that his co-workers in the psychiatry department were finding at autopsy in the brains of schizophrenic patients who had died suddenly. As Meduna worked in the outpatient department, he discovered (or believed he discovered) that the brains of patients with epilepsy were quite different from the schizophrenic brains. Meduna pondered this. Then in 1929 other scholars reported that epileptic patients who developed schizophrenia seemed to experience less epilepsy. Meduna wondered if the relationship went the other way as well: Did schizophrenics improve after developing epilepsy? (The answer seemed to be yes.[95]) "I accepted the concept of a biological antagonism between the two diseases," said Meduna in his autobiography.[96] Could one therefore improve the symptoms of schizophrenia by giving the patients epileptic fits? Meduna selected camphor, a drug with a long history of causing seizures, as the drug of choice. Since the eighteenth century, camphor had been occasionally used in psychosis, though Meduna seemed to be unaware of this.[97] On November 23, 1933, the same day that Sakel gave his verbal report on insulin-coma therapy to the medical society in Vienna, Meduna began animal experiments with camphor. On January 23, 1934, Meduna gave camphor to the first patient.[98]

L. Z. was a 33-year-old man who had been admitted to the Budapest State Hospital in 1930 with the (delusional) belief that "people often wave at me." He heard voices in his ears and his stomach. The entire year 1933 he had spent under his bedcovers. By January 1934 he had stopped eating. On January 23, Meduna gave him the first injection of camphor. Forty-five minutes later, L. Z. had his first epileptic attack, his pupils dilated to the maximum. Over the next two weeks, he would have five more injections. "On the morning of February 10, the patient spontaneously arises from bed, is lively, speaks, and asks for something to eat. He is interested in everything going on about him, asks about his illness and realizes that he has been sick. He asks how long he has been in the hospital, and as we tell him that he has already been there four years he cannot believe it."[99]

That was the published version. In reality, the patient felt so good that he escaped from the institution, went home, "and found out that the cousin living with his wife was not a relation at all but his wife's lover. He beat up the cousin and kicked him out of the house; proceeded to beat up his wife and told her that he . . . preferred to live in the state mental hospital where there is peace and honesty."[100]

"From that time on," said Meduna later, "I considered this patient cured." The patient was still well at the time that Meduna left Europe five years later.

By January 1935, as Meduna submitted his first article on convulsive therapy for publication, he had treated 26 patients, ten of whom had improved dramatically.[101]

The problem with camphor was its unreliability in producing fits. Also, the patients hated the feeling of anxiety preceding the fit, the vomiting that camphor caused, and the pain in the muscles where it was injected. In 1934 the Budapest professor of pharmacology recommended to Meduna a drug that had been synthesized nine years previously and that was being sold under the name "Cardiazol" as a cardiac stimulant. Meduna began injecting his patients with Cardiazol and by 1936 had tried it on 110 of them, half of whom went into remission (mainly those who had fallen ill more recently).[102]

Cardiazol was never a big success, mainly because it too was unreliable in producing fits and was feared by the patients. Müller soon discarded it at Münsingen because of patients' "agonizing fears of dying and crumbling away. . . . It was no wonder that they often strongly resisted a repeat experience."[103] Indeed, during a Cardiazol fit they looked to be on the point of expiring. Said Müller: "The sight of the artificially produced attack of epilepsy, especially of the contorted blue faces, was so awful to me that I sought to get away from the room whenever I could. I realize now the inadequacy of my excuse that I could have achieved nothing with my presence and that my colleagues were more robust and not so squeamish. But it was my responsibility. . . ."[104] One psychiatrist at a mental hospital in Leicestershire recalled "the unseemly and tragic farce of an unwilling patient being pursued by a posse of nurses with me, a fully charged syringe in my hand, bringing up the rear."[105]

Walter Freeman had the colossal misjudgment of trying Meduna's therapy on a 70-year-old "disturbed" relative. He and his surgeon brother injected 6 cc. of Metrazol into one of her veins. "Within 10 seconds she began twitching, then opened her mouth widely, arched her back, stiffened out in a tonic [muscles rigid] convulsion that lasted about 20 seconds, followed by clonic movements [muscles flexing repeatedly] for

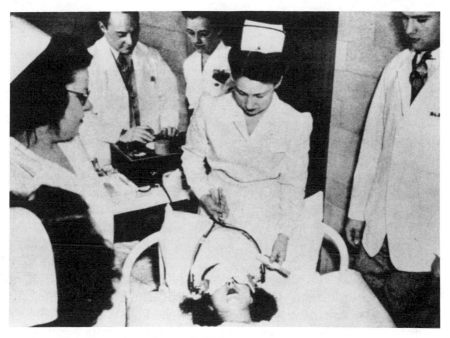

Applying electroconvulsive therapy (ECT).
Source: The History of Shock Treatment by Leonard Roy Frank (Ed.), 1978, p. 14.

another 25 seconds. Then she relaxed with no respiratory movements for many seconds. She became cyanotic. . . . Finally she gasped and then breathed heavily. Gradually, the color returned to her face—and also to my brother's."

"Jesus!" he said, wiping his brow.

Although the relative remembered Freeman in her will, she never forgave him.[106]

In 1939, Meduna migrated from Budapest to Chicago, where he became a professor first at Loyola University then at the University of Illinois Medical School, engaging in tenebrous experiments with carbon-dioxide therapy.[107] With the onset of war in Europe, Cardiazol therapy, like most of the other innovations in psychiatry, would become an American story. Institutions as disparate as the giant asylum at Milledgeville and the fashionable Sheppard private clinic experimented with Cardiazol (Metrazol) units in the late 1930s and early 1940s.[108] Then the hated Metrazol was pushed into the dustbin of history with the advent of a much less detested form of convulsive therapy, electro-convulsive therapy, or ECT.

Electroshock

It was now 1938. The air was full of talk about the new "physical therapies," as they had begun to be called, distinct from psychotherapy and psychoanalysis. Barbiturate narcosis, insulin coma, and Metrazol convulsion
had burst with full force into the life of the asylum, extending the promise
of lasting remissions and even cures. The next step was electroconvulsive
therapy, which Ugo Cerletti, professor of psychiatry in Rome, used for the
first time in April 1938. Although the history of psychiatry had known
many previous applications of electricity, Cerletti's historic innovation
was giving electric shock to the brain to achieve a convulsion.[109]

Cerletti was born in 1877 in the small manufacturing town of
Conegliano, about 80 miles from Venice, where his father founded the
first school of viticulture in Italy. He began medical studies in 1896 in
Turin, transferring two years later to Rome to work in the neuropathology
laboratory of Giovanni Mingazzini. While still a medical student, Cerletti
traveled to Heidelberg to study brain histology with Nissl. Finishing his
MD in 1901, Cerletti became an assistant physician of the psychiatric
clinic in Rome. Until World War I, he continued to do postgraduate work
in Germany and France, studying for example with Kraepelin at the university clinic in Munich. He soon established for himself a substantial reputation as an investigator of the architecture of the brain.[110] Up to this
point, little distinguished Cerletti from other typical representatives of the
first biological psychiatry in its dying days.

After World War I, Cerletti received a series of academic psychiatric
postings and had ample opportunity to experience clinical psychiatry
firsthand as a "funereal science."[111] In these years, particularly during his
stint in the early 1930s as director of the Neuropsychiatric Clinic in
Genoa, he did research on epilepsy. Was a lesion in a certain area of the
brain the cause or the result of an epileptic attack? To study the question,
Cerletti began inducing fits in dogs experimentally by applying electricity
to them.[112] Yet with one electrode placed in the animal's mouth, the other
in its anus, the results were intimidating: Half of the animals died as a result of shock stopping the action of the heart. In 1935, Cerletti received
the professorship of psychiatry in Rome, becoming simultaneously chief of
the Clinic for Nervous and Mental Diseases of the University of Rome.

In October 1936, he called together his three assistants, Ferdinando
Accornero, Lucio Bini, and Lamberto Longhi, themselves all young
MDs in their mid-20s and at the end of residencies.[113] Impressed by
Meduna's recent results with Cardiazol, Cerletti gave each of his assis-
tants an assignment: Accornero was to study insulin coma, Longhi was

to investigate Cardiazol, and Bini was to see if the dog experiments might be made applicable to humans. The three young psychiatrists were inseparable comrades, together day and night in the Rome clinic, and functioned more as a team than as individual researchers off in separate laboratories. It was, however, Bini who discovered that electric current could be delivered safely if the electrodes were placed on the dog's temples.[114] For a year, these dog experiments continued, the dog-catcher's wagon stopping weekly at the clinic, Accornero and Bini scrambling around the clock to perform the autopsies on the animals' brains and to get slides of brain sections under the microscope.

In 1937, Max Müller's big conference at Münsingen on new therapies in schizophrenia began to loom, and Accornero and Bini consulted with Cerletti about what they should present there. Accornero would offer the results of his insulin research and Bini would give a paper on the dog experiments. It was decided that Bini would casually mention that the dog experiments might be tried on humans. (He did mention it; the news was received at the conference with complete indifference.[115])

After the two had returned to Rome, Cerletti asked them to visit the city slaughterhouse, where, he had heard, pigs were being obtunded with electric current before being slaughtered. What could the researchers learn here about where to apply the electrodes, and about the margin between the convulsive dose and the lethal dose? Bini and Accornero then did systematic experiments at the slaughterhouse, discovering that placing the electrodes on the temples was practical, and that the margin between the convulsive and lethal doses was very wide.

Now all three young residents were keen to try electroshock on a patient. Still, Cerletti hesitated. Said Accornero later, "If the experiment on a human, for whatever unforeseen reason, had ended with the death of the subject, all the responsibility would have fallen on Cerletti. Our school, already considered to be highly interventionist, would have fallen into enormous discredit and its director would have suffered the consequences."[116] In the meantime, however, with the assistance of a technician, Bini had constructed a primitive apparatus that would permit application of 80 to 100 volts of electricity for a fraction of a second. Now the first patient arrived.

On April 15, 1938, the Rome commissariat of police referred to the clinic a 39-year-old engineer from Milan who had been arrested while wandering about the railroad station. "He does not appear to be in full possession of his mental faculties," said the commissar's note, "and I am sending him to your hospital to be kept there under observation." In clinic, the patient seemed lucid and knew where he was, but spoke in a kind of jargon and complained about being "telepathically influenced." He had hallucinations. His grooming was slovenly. "From a psychiatric viewpoint," said young resident Accornero, "the syndrome was clear, the disorder advanced, the presumed prognosis unfavorable."[117]

On the second floor (primo piano) of the clinic, there was an isolated equipment room. There Bini had set up his apparatus. On that morning of April 18, there were present in the room, in addition to the patient, Cerletti, Bini, Accornero, and two other assistant physicians, one assigned to keep watch on the corridor and make sure no one would intrude. The patient, his head shaved, seemed quite indifferent to what was going on. A nurse placed the electrodes on his temples while an orderly put a rubber tube between his teeth to prevent him from biting his tongue. Everything was ready. Bini looked at Cerletti, who nodded. There was a crack of electricity. The patient's muscles jolted once. Accornero put his stethoscope on the patient's chest. Heart rate up, everything else alright. Accornero was so excited he found himself unable to speak.

The patient said he had no memory of what had just happened. "We gave him 80 volts for a tenth of a second," said Bini. "He had an absence attack."

"Let's step it up to 90," said Cerletti.

Another electrical crack. Another spasm. The patient lay motionless for a minute, then began to sing.

"We'll try it one last time at a higher voltage," said Cerletti, "poi basta [and then enough]."

At this point, the patient said, in a perfectly calm and reasonable voice, as though answering an exam question, "Look out! The first is pestiferous, the second mortiferous." The residents looked at each other puzzled.

"Come on, let's go," said Cerletti.

Bini turned the apparatus up to the maximum. After this jolt, the patient went into a classic tonic-clonic epileptic fit, muscles contracting and relaxing rhythmically. His breathing stopped. He began turning blue, heart accelerating, corneal reflexes absent.

Bini began counting the seconds since the halting of respiration. At the forty-eighth second, the patient emitted a profound sigh. The doctors likewise. They had established that electrical current could safely produce convulsions in a human subject.

The patient sat up "calm and smiling, as though to inquire what we wanted of him," as Cerletti later remembered.

They asked, "What happened to you?"

He answered, "I don't know. Maybe I was asleep."

Thus ended the first application of electricity to produce a convulsion in a psychiatric patient.[118] Cerletti at once baptized it "electroshock."[119]

After eleven applications of ECT, the patient in fact did get well and was discharged from the clinic a month later "in good condition and well-oriented; ideation and memory perfect." He now realized that his previous notions of persecution and hallucinations were the result of illness. He returned to his job in Milan, and a year later was said still to be "perfectly well; but his wife reported that three months after his return home he resumed his jealous attitude toward her, and that sometimes during the night he would speak as though in answer to voices."[120]

Thus ECT was not a cure for schizophrenia. But it represented a great alleviation of the disabling symptoms of psychotic illness, and permitted individuals to function more or less normally. It spread with great rapidity within the world of psychiatry. Lothar Kalinowsky functioned as a kind of Johnny Appleseed. Born in Berlin with one Jewish parent, Kalinowsky earned an MD at the University of Berlin in 1922, then fled Germany in 1933 for Italy, where he acquired a second MD in Rome. He was present at the Cerletti clinic in the early days of ECT therapy. Leaving Rome in 1939 for Paris, he helped to introduce ECT at the Ste-Anne Hospital (obliging Bini to send instructions for building a machine). Arriving in England in July 1939, Kalinowsky helped Sanderson McGregor establish ECT at the Netherne Hospital at Coulsdon.[121] A German colleague at St. Bartholomew's Hospital asked Kalinowsky to attend rounds and had an apparatus constructed.[122] Thus Kalinowsky sowed ECT across the land.

In March 1940, Kalinowsky, an alien physician, reluctantly left England for the United States and by September 1940 got an ECT service going at the New York State Psychiatric Institute, which was part of Columbia University. They built their own machine.[123]

Everywhere the electroshock machine was introduced, it occasioned great enthusiasm among asylum psychiatrists. One no longer had to chase patients down to inject them with Metrazol. "ECT produced instant unconsciousness, no dread, no physical upset after the convulsion, no vomiting," said one Bethlem physician, who recalled the arrival of the ECT apparatus at that hospital. "It was the size of a small cinema organ, its top a rather bewildering array of dials and switches. Although the machine was fearsome to us nurses and doctors to begin with, the fears of patients about convulsion treatment became unusual and outright refusal rare."[124] As another veteran psychiatrist declared, "Without ECT I would not have lasted out in psychiatry, as I would not have been able to tolerate the sadness and hopelessness of most mental illnesses before the introduction of convulsive therapy."[125] By 1944 in England, ECT had supplanted Cardiazol in producing fits.[126]

The priority for bringing ECT to the United States belongs technically not to Kalinowsky—who did insert it in academic psychiatry—but to Renato Almansi, who had worked with Cerletti and who in 1939 imported a machine into the United States. Almansi collaborated with David Impastato, also Italian by origin but who had an American MD degree and who was on staff at the Columbus Hospital in New York. They first did experiments on dogs, then by February 1940 had begun applying ECT to patients at their office and at the hospital outpatient department.[127] Elsewhere in the country in these months, other attempts were simultaneously underway and no one person save Kalinowsky emerges as the godparent of American ECT.[128]

Yet ECT did not have a truly triumphal onmarch in the United States.[129] For one thing, the psychoanalysts were generally opposed to it, even though many of them conceded its usefulness in the treatment of major depression (where up to a quarter of all patients suicided). Washington psychoanalyst Harry Stack Sullivan had no more use for ECT than for any of the other physical therapies, based as they were (in his view) on the philosophy "that it is better to be a contented imbecile than a schizophrenic." Sullivan thought it better to leave schizophrenic patients untreated in the hope that these "extraordinarily gifted and, therefore, socially significant people" would experience a spontaneous recovery.[130] In 1947, the Group for the Advancement of Psychiatry bristled about the "promiscuous and indiscriminate use" of ECT while not condemning it outright.[131] (The organization later backpedaled somewhat to maintain they opposed only its "inappropriate" use.)[132] Throughout the American psychoanalytic literature ran a begrudging suspiciousness of electroshock. This was combined with an insistence that ECT's obvious utility must rest on some kind of psychodynamic basis rather than on brain biology.[133] For if the neurons of the brain itself were making people ill, the theoretical structure of psychoanalysis flew out the window.

Thus ECT posed psychoanalysis with a dilemma. The most effective means of treating major mental illness was theoretically unacceptable. As a resident, one would train either to be a psychotherapist, with a large and lucrative community practice, or a poorly paid mental-hospital psychiatrist who was able to do ECT.[134] When Arnold Rogow interviewed a cross-section of American psychiatrists and psychoanalysts in 1966, he found that a third of the psychiatrists used ECT but only one of the analysts.[135] The hesitant acceptance of ECT in the United States in the late 1940s and 1950s was thus partially due to ideological opposition from psychiatrists who found the physical therapies outside their worldview.

But it was also owing to real dangers in the use of ECT itself. As the patients thrashed upon the table, they were at risk of breaking limbs and fracturing vertebrae. At the Horton Hospital in England, the nurses would literally drape themselves on the patient to limit mobility, one holding the feet together, another pressing down on the pelvis, two more nurses on each side holding the patient's shoulders with one hand and the patient's hand with the other, and another nurse holding the patient's head and compressing the jaw.[136]

These dangers began to be mastered as a result of a chance encounter around 1939 between Walter Freeman and Omaha psychiatrist Abram Bennett. Bennett had been giving children with spastic paralyses small amounts of curare, attempting to relax their limbs by blocking the junction between muscle and nerve. He had also been conducting Metrazol shock therapy on depressed patients. Freeman suggested to Bennett that curare might solve the problem of fractured spinal vertebrae in shock therapy. Freeman knew a businessman with good curare connections in Ecuador, and so Bennett got a large supply of curare, which was standardized in the pharmacology laboratory of the University of Nebraska to make its effects consistent and predictable.[137] This represented curare's introduction into medicine.

In 1940, Bennett established that curare in fact briefly paralyzed the muscles of head and neck, preventing thrashing.[138] His discovery was soon applied to ECT, allowing the extension of electroshock to large numbers of patients with depression. Yet curare was a highly risky drug and could entail cardiac complications. A safer blocker of the nerve-muscle junction, succinylcholine, had been introduced into medicine in 1949 for short procedures such as inserting a tracheal tube. Starting in 1952, it was adopted in ECT units as a less risky means of preventing spinal fractures.[139] It would be used together with the ultrashort-acting barbiturate methohexital sodium (trademark "Brevital"), which served as a general anesthetic.

By 1959, ECT had become "the treatment of choice," as Kalinowsky put it, for manic-depressive illness and major depression.[140] It was more effective than any of the other physical therapies, acted swiftly, and was not unpopular with the patients. The year 1959 was a kind of golden year for psychiatry, when neither Kalinowsky nor anyone else knew that the antipsychiatry movement was about to bring ECT to an end.

In retrospect, the shock therapies represented a milestone in breaking psychiatry free from the tutelage of neurology. Until the 1930s, most of the psychiatric spectrum had been dominated by neurologists with their virtual monopoly on psychotherapy in private practice and their command of the few procedures, such as spa therapy for nerves, that seemed to do any good. Until then, psychiatry had been a poor Cinderella, eking out a paltry existence in the asylum. Malaria therapy, deep sleep, and the shock treatments represented the first independent therapies over which psychiatrists themselves disposed. Sakel, Meduna, and Cerletti succeeded in "shaking neurology from the saddle," as Louis Casamajor, a senior New York psychiatrist, put it in 1943. Added Casamajor tongue in cheek, "One may question whether shock treatments do any good to the patients but there can be no doubt that they have done an enormous amount of good to psychiatry."[141]

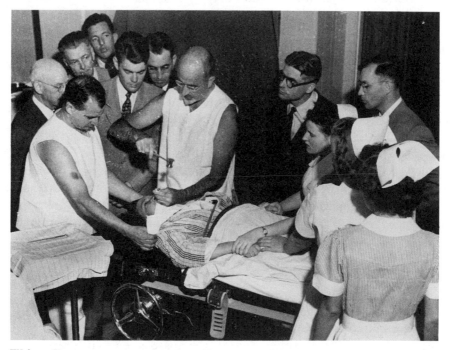

Walter Freeman, a neurologist at George Washington University Hospital in Washington D.C., who popularized lobotomy in the United States. Shown here in 1949 inserting a lobotomy instrument under the patient's eyelid in order to destroy tissue in the brain's frontal lobe (courtesy of UPI/Corbis-Bettmann).

The Lobotomy Adventure

The idea of operating on the brain to cure madness does not seem intrinsically unreasonable. Physicians have always intuited that a physical intervention in the brain, perhaps cutting some tract causing compulsive behavior or removing a center producing some malignant protein, might put an end to a pattern of psychosis. In the Middle Ages, doctors fantasized about cutting for the mythical "stone of madness." In our own time, there is evidence that the course of Parkinson's disease can be slowed by the transplantation of fetal dopamine-producing neurons.[142] It also seems to be the case that ablating the cingulate gyrus, in a cingulotomy, can relieve the symptoms of severe compulsive neurosis.[143] These are examples of successful psychosurgery.

The great wave of physical therapies of the 1930s included one unsuccessful example of psychosurgery: lobotomy, or destroying part of one of the brain's lobes. In the context of the apparent success of such physical interventions as barbiturate narcosis, insulin coma, Metrazol convulsion, and ECT, it began to seem reasonable that operating on the cerebral cortex itself might offer promise. And so psychosurgical notions last seen in the 1880s and 1890s began to resurface.

The modern history of psychosurgery begins with a Swiss asylum psychiatrist named Gottlieb Burckhardt, who earned his MD at Basel in 1860. After a lectureship at Basel, followed by a staff job at the Waldau public asylum, in 1882 Burckhardt became director of the private Préfargier Clinic in Marin near Neuchâtel.[144] Here he seems to have experimented widely with various new techniques such as hypnotism.[145] Untrained though he was in surgery, he also experimented rather clumsily with operations on various lobes of his patients' brains. Beginning in December, 1888, he performed psychosurgery on six patients with evident schizophrenia. The operations were not a big success. One of the patients died in convulsions, a second improved, a third and fourth experienced no change, and the last two became "quieter."[146] Burckhardt's report on his new procedure to the Berlin Medical Congress of 1890 produced disquiet. There was no discussion following the paper, and the participants agreed that complete silence was the best way to avoid attracting attention to the work.[147] Burckhardt's article the following year did occasion a brief flutter.[148] But the idea of intervening directly in the parenchyma of the brain was soon abandoned.

Yet a climate of meddlesomeness persisted. In the 1890s, there were efforts in England to relieve the symptoms of neurosyphilis by boring a burr hole (trepanation) in the cranium and incising the meninges to drain away pus or cerebrospinal fluid.[149] In unpublished work, the Breslau surgeon Johann Mikulicz attempted in the 1890s to remove the focus of epilepsy by scarifying a portion of the sensory-motor cortex.[150] Valentin Magnan, master of the Ste-Anne asylum in Paris, was enthusiastic about trepanation to forestall mental retardation in cases where the cranium was said to be too small. (He alluded to previous efforts along these lines, which he found "unencouraging.")[151] Thus there is no doubt that at the turn of the century a generalized willingness to meddle surgically with the brain and its casing was ticking away just beneath the surface of medicine. It required only a new finding, or pseudo-finding, to reactivate this meddlesomeness.

At this point, the Lisbon neurologist Egas Moniz walks on stage. Moniz had already earned himself a place in medical history by describing in 1927 cerebral angiography, a technique for visualizing the blood vessels of the brain radiographically. He had twice been nominated for a Nobel prize for this achievement and twice turned down. In this frame of mind of thirsting for greatness denied, Moniz attended the Second International Congress of Neurology held in London in 1935. Here he audited a full-day symposium on the frontal lobes of the brain, then an object of great interest among many scholars. Moniz heard Carlyle Jacobsen and John Fulton from Yale describe the emotional changes in a chimpanzee following the ablation of much of its frontal lobes: Prone to temper tantrums and wilfullness before the operation, the animal seemed to become almost cheery after it.

"Dr. Moniz arose and asked, if frontal lobe removal prevents the development of experimental neuroses in animals and eliminates frustrational behavior, why would it not be feasible to relieve anxiety states in man by surgical means?"[152]

The inspiration for lobotomy, or leucotomy as Moniz called it, had been planted. Between November 1935 and February 1936, Moniz prevailed upon neurosurgeon Almeida Lima to resect part of the prefrontal lobes of 20 patients transferred from the Bombarda asylum to the neurology service of the Santa Marta Hospital in Lisbon. Seven had been "cured," seven ameliorated, and in six there was no change.

Moniz provided little detail to support these claims.[153] In fact, this kind of grandiose communication characterized the first notice of almost all the physical therapies, their authors eager to ascertain their priority in history and unaffected as yet by the rigorous statistical tests and follow-up studies that would later be demanded. (Sakel's first report in the Vienna medical press did not even mention the number of patients receiving the insulin-coma therapy.) Yet with lobotomy, one was dealing with a savage mutilation of the human brain.

It was therefore most unfortunate that Washington neurologist Walter Freeman, who also had attended the London conference, fell upon Moniz's procedure with uncritical enthusiasm. For it was Freeman who, in collaboration with neurosurgeon James Watts, propagandized on behalf of lobotomy in the United States. (The term "lobotomy" is theirs.) In 1936, they did their first operation at the hospital of George Washington University in Washington, and in 1946 introduced the transorbital lobotomy, approaching the brain from the roof of the orbit, or eye socket.[154]

Freeman and Watts split in 1947 over the issue of making lobotomy an "office procedure," as Freeman wished it. Thereafter Freeman carried on alone. In the early 1950s, he popularized transorbital lobotomy in a kind of one-man medicine show traveling across the continent. In the summer of 1951, for example, he visited mental hospitals in 17 states as well as doing demonstrations in Canada, Puerto Rico, and Curaçao. In the words of Freeman's biographer Elliot Valenstein, "On one five-week summer trip that year, he drove 11,000 miles with a station wagon loaded, in addition to camping equipment, with an electroconvulsive shock box, a dictaphone, and a file cabinet filled with patient records, photographs, and correspondence; his surgical instruments were in his pocket."[155] The surgical instruments often included an ice pick.

Although lobotomy did tend to tranquilize the raving patients who were management problems, it generally deprived them of their judgment and social skills, making them tin-eared to social cues and inappropriately disinhibited. The authors of the standard textbook of physical therapies of the day wrote the following lines apologetically: "It is probable that every individual after the operation is happier than before, but this may be bought at too great a cost, not only to himself but to society. . . .

"The patient's temper becomes more hasty; he will be more easily irritable and will more easily give vent to his irritation, sometimes without adequate sense of its social consequences. He may become demanding in his desires and imperative in their expression."[156] What the authors did not say was that much of the patient's selfhood as well was given up with the physical loss of part of the brain's frontal lobes, producing, in the words of two of Freeman's opponents, "a defrontalized dement."[157]

There were two main forms of lobotomy. Moniz preferred prefrontal leucotomy, cutting the white matter in the oval center of the brain's two front lobes with a whisk-like leukotome through burr-holes cut in the top of the cranium. When stirred back and forth, the leukotome would destroy the nerve fibers. The version that Freeman propagated after 1946 was transorbital lobotomy, going via the orbital cavity.

Here Dr. Hatcher of the Milledgeville State Hospital describes the transorbital procedure on one February morning in 1952 to psychologist Peter Cranford:

DR. HATCHER:	"Peter, I'm doing transorbital lobotomies this morning. Come watch me."
CRANFORD:	"If I *saw* one, you'd have to do the next one on me."
DR. HATCHER:	"Nothing to it. I take a sort of medical icepick, hold it like this, bop it through the bones just above the eyeball, push it up into the brain, swiggle it around, cut the brain fibers like this, and that's it. The patient doesn't feel a thing."
CRANFORD:	"And neither do you. I *was* going to breakfast but I've changed my mind."
HATCHER (*laughing*):	"You can change your mind, but not like I can change it."[158]

In the 1950s, the world of American asylum psychiatry was Milledgeville writ large. Although only 684 lobotomies were conducted in the United States between 1940 and 1944, the propagandizing of Freeman and Watts helped the numbers soar in the late 1940s. In 1949, the peak year, 5,074 operations were carried out. "By 1951," writes historian Gerald Grob, "no fewer than 18,608 individuals had undergone psychosurgery since its introduction in 1936."[159] It was employed at more than half of the public mental hospitals in the country, and such prestigious institutions as the Boston Psychopathic Hospital counted as fortresses of lobotomy.

The procedure faded away in the early 1950s almost as abruptly as it had risen up, a blip in the history of psychiatry, though an illuminating one as a study in medical hubris. In Britain, the rate of lobotomies began to decline even before the introduction in the mid-1950s of the new antipsychotic drugs.[160] But in both Britain and the United States, it was unquestionably the advent of these drugs in the spring of 1954 that killed off lobotomy,[161] just as other physical therapies of the 1930s also died in the face of the new psychopharmacology.

In retrospect, frontal lobotomy was indefensible for ethical reasons. Yet it did have some success with agitated patients whom other physical therapies were unable to reach, or on whom they had not been tried. "After having personally performed perhaps 12 or 15 prefrontal lobotomies (all carefully selected and screened)," said one psychiatrist in 1987, "there were some gratifying results in people who had been institutionalized and uncontrollable for as long as 6 to 10 years. There were some dramatic responses, and some long-standing satisfactory responses—all better than the restraint of those same patients in back wards of mental institutions."[162] Follow-up studies found that about a third of all psychosurgical patients had been discharged from hospital and were living at home.[163] Yet many of these patients would sooner or later have recovered spontaneously. And the irreversible damage to their brain and spirit must be weighed against the extra months or years with which they would have encumbered the institutional system. "Not all so-called mental disorders were so severe that it was worth exchanging them for an organic brain syndrome," concluded one student.[164] True, lobotomy reached the most difficult of the difficult in the back wards. Yet unlike any of the other physical therapies, it caused deep uneasiness within the profession of psychiatry, and would be the first of these therapies to be abandoned as the new antipsychotic drugs came in.

Social and Community Psychiatry

These physical therapies represented a series of alternatives to the dilemma of custodialism versus psychoanalysis. Yet there was one further alternative. It concerned the milieu of therapy rather than a physical approach to the body. Social and community psychiatry insisted it was not the patients' genes nor early childhood that made them ill but the surrounding community. Psychiatric illness could thus best be addressed with therapies aimed at placing patients in a healing community environment. This tends to be an English story.

Each country has made its own distinctive contribution to the history of psychiatry. Germany offered the first biological psychiatry, France the therapeutic asylum. The United States contributed psychoanalysis in its fullest bloom and, latterly, much of the second biological psychiatry. The distinctive English contribution to the world narrative was the notion that at the bottom of mental illness lay poisoned human relationships. If psychosis and neurosis arose as a result of faulty human connectivity, illness could be treated by restoring healthy relationships to a person's life, principally in the form of group therapy.

The whole story of social and community psychiatry as a unified approach to mental illness is like a Lego, or Tinkertoy set, in that its various components, or pieces, had lain about the psychiatric landscape for many years. Only in Britain around the time of World War II did they come together in a single edifice.

One such piece was the open asylum. In an open asylum, voluntary patients could admit and discharge themselves at will, an essential concept if psychotic illness were to be destigmatized and neurotic illness made accessible to the psychiatrist. Germany had a long tradition of such institutions in the private sector, beginning with Otto Müller's Clinic for Nervous Patients, founded in 1861 in Helmstedt (and moved in 1865 to scenic Blankenburg in the Harz Mountains). As for the private asylum, in 1866 Adolf Albrecht Erlenmeyer established in his insane asylum in Bendorf-on-Rhine an open division that patients could enter and leave relatively at will.[165]

Another piece of the Lego set was discharging patients to some kind of family-based community care, not necessarily that of their own families. Putting patients in family care had been done for many years in the famous Belgian "colony for the insane" at Gheel, yet its example seems to have influenced few others. Scottish asylums were well-known for their policies of family care.[166] In the mid-nineteenth century, the Germans made extensive use of placing mental patients as boarders in the homes of nearby farm families eager to pick up a bit of spending money. From 1867 on, Caspar Max Brosius, director of a private asylum in Bendorf, started placing his wealthy patients under supervised care in private homes, thus avoiding administrative formalities and the ensuing stigma.[167] Ferdinand Wahrendorff later tried the same approach at a private asylum in Ilten near Hanover on a larger and more systematic scale.[168] By the turn of the century, "family care" (Familienpflege) had become common in Central Europe in both public and private sectors.

Outpatient clinics based in the asylum also increased the porousness of the mental hospital to the surrounding community. By the mid-1920s, most of the big Central European psychiatric hospitals had such outreach clinics. Charcot had founded an outpatient clinic at the Salpêtrière in Paris. By 1920, Massachusetts had 33 outpatient clinics, New York 25, and Pennsylvania 9.[169] Psychiatric outpatient clinics in general hospitals took this integration another step further. The first in Germany was created at Rostock in 1825.[170] Thus along an entire continuum of care, moves had been made before the 1930s to erase the boundary between the closed asylum and the community. The destruction of German psychiatry after 1933 erased the memory of most of these initiatives. In the two decades between 1930 and 1950, it was Britain that vaulted from international laggard to international leader.

Why this transformation took place is unclear, a mixture perhaps of burgeoning social democracy from below and the activism from above of socially committed elites. (One recalls how the Bloomsbury group flung themselves into psychoanalysis.) The transformation began in 1930 with the passage of a lunacy act of a decidedly different tenor. The Mental Treatment Act of 1930 began to open the asylum to the outside community, reversing completely the course set by the Lunacy Act of 1890, which sealed the "insane" in madhouses like dangerous beasts.[171] The new legislation made possible open-door policies in asylums, discarding locks and keys, and enabling patients on "outside parole" to stroll at will into town for a pint. (There were three other kinds of parole, which, rather than facilitating mass flight, had a tranquilizing influence on the inhabitants of the mental hospitals.[172]) Among the first to implement open-door policies was the "kind and benevolent Welshman" T. P. ("Percy") Rees, who on becoming superintendent in 1935 of Warlingham Park Hospital ordered that the gates be unlocked. All the ward doors in the hospital were unlocked too, including, to the horror of the staff, those of the "suicidal" patients.[173]

Yet the crucial event in the genesis of social and community psychiatry in Britain was not the 1930 Act but World War II. Following the Nazi invasion of Austria in 1938, Joshua Bierer, a 37-year-old Jewish physician and psychotherapist, fled from Vienna to London. Bierer had studied under Alfred Adler and had already acquired much psychotherapeutic experience in private practice and at the Steinhof mental hospital in Vienna. Once installed in 1938 at Runwell Hospital near London, an ultramodern facility organized on the "villa" system, he proceeded to set up a psychotherapy program. This was quite unusual in British mental hospitals then, few of which had full-time psychotherapists. Bierer asked his patients about their dreams and their earliest recollections from childhood.[174]

What was extraordinary however in the context of prewar psychiatry was group psychotherapy. In 1939, Bierer began to organize psychotherapy groups among Runwell inpatients, also for outpatients at two public general hospitals in London. In 1942, he extended group psychotherapy to the historic London teaching hospitals, Guy's and St. Bartholomew's.[175] Bierer thought that psychoanalysis prolonged the patients' problems by making them dependent on an analyst. Group psychotherapy by contrast let the patients become "independent, active and 'self-deciding,'" while at the same time helping them to achieve insight and work toward a cure.[176] This marks the first eruption of group psychotherapy in Britain and possibly on the continent of Europe.

How did these groups first assemble? "On December 8, 1939, 35 patients, neurotics and psychotics, met in 'Sunnyside House' [of Runwell Hospital] and formed a social club. The chair at the meeting was taken by a patient." The therapeutic group, or therapeutic community as it would soon be called, was in other words run by the patients themselves and not imposed on them top-down by the hospital staff. A staff member would be present at Social Club meetings, but otherwise the Club was "completely autonomous," the patients electing their own officers, publishing a magazine, and meeting three times weekly. A typical discussion question might be, "Why do we laugh about the downfall of others?"[177] "The discipline was left entirely in the hands of Club members," said Bierer. Thus Bierer had not merely facilitated group psychotherapy but established the principle that it be patient directed. He referred to the technique as "'community' treatment."[178]

Now the scene shifts from Bierer to a northern suburb of London, where at the outbreak of war the Ministry of Health set up the Mill Hill Emergency Hospital, a psychiatric center located on the site of a former public school, for the treatment of military and civilian shell-shock cases. It was staffed by members of the Maudsley Hospital and included an Effort Syndrome Unit, so named because much psychosomatic illness among troops presented itself in the form of shortness of breath and the like following exercise (so-called soldier's heart). Heading this 100-bed unit were a cardiologist and a psychiatry resident, Maxwell Jones, a young Scottish physician (born in South Africa) who had graduated several years previously from the University of Edinburgh and was at the Maudsley at the time the war broke out. It was under Jones at Mill Hill that the notion of "therapeutic community" truly germinated. And it germinated almost by accident. Many of the war nurses were not old-fashioned authoritarian ward sisters, but mature professional women who had chosen nursing as their war work. These women were accustomed to free communication, not to giving orders to patients and receiving them from doctors. A nurse might "frequently keep a ward log book," said Jones, "where the fourteen patients in her ward recorded some of the problems affecting the group, and described how these problems were met through discussion." So under these middle-class volunteer nurses some kind of group dynamic among the patients began to take form.

At the same time at Mill Hill, the doctors would bring the patients together in a group to explain, in a nice way, that what they really had was a form of hysteria. No particular therapeutic benefit was expected from this group congregation at first: It was merely an efficient way to communicate information without alienating the patients as a lecture might have. "It soon became evident," continued Jones, "that the discussion group was more than an educational meeting; it was affecting the whole social structure of the ward." Patients began raising problems arising from ward life. The atmosphere of the group would flux in unpredictable ways. The nurses who attended the meetings said the same process was occurring on their wards. Doctors and nurses at Mill Hill began to reflect on what these changes might mean. They began experimenting by raising social problems in the groups, or having the nurses act out little skits in front of the patients involving "the lives of a fictitious family comprising the parents (the 'normal' father and hysterical mother) and three daughters whose personalities tended to be schizoid, psychopathic, and hysterical respectively. This dramatic approach proved to be tremendously interesting to the patients and provoked a high degree of participation in the subsequent discussion." By January 1944, the patients themselves had begun to participate in the psychodramas, though as yet they did not use that word because they had not yet heard of Jacob Moreno, who first used psychodrama in an asylum.[179] Thus by 1944, Jones was toying with the possibilities of group interactions in and of themselves as a source of therapeutic benefit. He did not use the term group psychotherapy.

Early in 1945, the therapeutic community was field-tested on a larger scale. The Mill Hill group was asked to take over a unit at the Southern Hospital at Dartford in Kent for the treatment of returning prisoners of war with combat fatigue. Six psychiatrists, 50 nurses, and support staff from Mill Hill now applied their therapeutic model to this 300-bed service, helping the men find day-work in Dartford, to which they would commute from the hospital in three large Green Line buses. As Jones explained, "The men were housed in six 'cottages,' each with 50 beds. Each unit had a daily community meeting, along the lines we had developed at Mill Hill." In this kind of supportive atmosphere, the patients would discuss such matters as their fears about resuming sex with their wives, the children born while they were away, and their adequacy as husbands.[180]

Dartford led to a "considerable growth of interest in therapeutic communities," as Jones put it. Funded by various ministries, in April 1947 Jones opened what would become the most famous therapeutic community in the world, a 100-bed unit to study the problem of "the chronic unemployed neurotic" at the newly named Belmont Hospital, the dilapidated old wing of a London County Council asylum. (During the war many of the staff of the Maudsley Hospital who had not gone to Mill Hill set up a neurosis center at Belmont more oriented to the physical therapies than the psychological ones.[181]) Jones's new service was called the Industrial Neurosis Unit; it put into action all the concepts that he and his team had been developing. The patients' week was filled with group activity:

Monday: Unit conference, "when the patients air their grievances or make constructive suggestions."

Tuesday: Enlightening films.

Wednesday–Thursday: Unit staff member leads discussion groups.

Friday: Psychodrama. Also patients do occupational therapy from 10 to 12 and 2 to 4. Early Friday evening a pass outside, then at 7 P.M. an organized social program got up by the patients. "This is readily censured at the group discussions should it fail to cater for all needs."[182]

The Industrial Neurosis Unit became in 1954 the Social Rehabilitation Unit, later the Henderson Hospital (named after the Scottish psychiatrist David Henderson who had influenced many of these reformers), a premier center of social and community psychiatry.

The therapeutic community was an alternative to psychoanalysis on the one hand and custodialism on the other. It was not an alternative to the physical therapies, for even though the Industrial Neurosis Unit was not intended to accept psychotic patients, in fact it often did so. Jones and his staff would regularly do insulin coma treatment. They used sodium amytal, a barbiturate, for interviewing patients, and occasionally performed lobotomy on the premises.[183]

However, let's not get ahead of our story. Therapeutic communities became widely heralded during the war. Thomas Main, a former deputy superintendent of an asylum in Northumbria, set one up at the Northfield Military Hospital near Birmingham, emphasizing a kind of instantaneous emotional contact among staff themselves and between staff and patients. This became known as "the Second Northfield Experiment" and Main claimed credit for actually introducing the term "therapeutic community."[184] Northfield, said Main, was "a therapeutic setting with a spontaneous and emotionally structured (rather than medically dictated) organization in which all staff and patients engage."[185] "Sincerity," he explained, was the "basis for management."[186] Although Main's account of his activities was permeated with psychoanalytic jargon, it is interesting that at Northfield they gave barbiturate narcosis and ECT.[187]

The reason these progressive ideas disseminated so rapidly within the usually stodgy military medical bureaucracy was that they had some very powerful sponsors, far higher up the ladder than Jones and his associates. Main was one of what were known as the "Tavi brigadiers," a group of psychiatrists from the Tavistock Clinic in central London, who had taken charge of army psychiatry. The Tavistock Clinic had been founded in 1920 by Hugh Crichton-Miller and John Rawlings ("J. R.") Rees as an outpatient service having a quasi-psychoanalytic orientation for patients with nervous illnesses. In 1933, Rees became its medical director. At the outbreak of war in 1939, Rees became the director of army psychiatry. He brought with him into the military Research and Training Center a number of bright young psychoanalytically oriented psychiatrists, one of whom was Main. Another was John Bowlby, later noted for his work on attachment theory. As early as 1942, Rees was using the term "social psychiatry," a concept that had existed since Esquirol but a term that only at this point was gaining currency. From early in the war on, a number of seminars at the Tavistock dealt with social themes.[188]

Yet the therapeutic community needed a home. The doctrine emphasized the empowerment of patients and the normalizing of their lives, good community relations making well what bad human relations had caused.[189] The asylum therefore was not a perfect home for the group psychotherapy that was at the core of the therapeutic community. Where else then to situate it? Here was born the notion of the psychiatric day hospital, a kind of outpatient department attached to a mental hospital, a general hospital, or even free-standing, where patients could come for group sessions, counseling, occupational therapy and the other services that constituted a comprehensive approach to treatment. It was actually Ewen Cameron who established the first day hospital in 1946 at the Allan Memorial Institute in Montreal (introducing the term day hospital into psychiatry as well).[190] But Joshua Bierer was unaware of Cameron's efforts at the time, and in 1948 Bierer established the first day hospital in England.

Its home was the Social Psychiatry Centre that Bierer had founded in 1946 in two war-damaged houses in the London suburb of Hampstead. He and coworkers soon began discussing the outlines of a possible day hospital that would combine a patients' Social Club with psychodrama, group psychotherapy, ECT and insulin cure, and the other innovations that had established themselves within progressive British psychiatry.

235

Over the next 12 months, support for the concept welled among hospital administrators, psychiatrists in private practice, and family doctors. By October 1948, Bierer had lined up funding for eight psychiatrists on a part-time basis, two full-time psychiatrists, a part-time psychologist, a psychiatric social worker, an occupational therapist, a social therapist, and other staff.[191] This represented the apogee of British psychiatry's golden age, a tremendous marshaling of resources that was conceivable only in a social setting in which "social and community psychiatry" had become a watchword.

The day hospital caught on at once as a humane and inexpensive alternative to institutional care. Additional day hospitals were founded at Bristol in 1951, at the Maudsley in 1953, and so forth. By 1959, more than 38 such hospitals existed in Great Britain.[192] The movement incorporated Bierer's philosophy that, "Treatment must include the whole social environment of the patient and all his social relationships. He must be treated not only as a person but as part of a community."[193]

In retrospect, the day hospital movement is significant as the first effort to move the treatment of major psychiatric disorders from the asylum to the community. However naive this policy might seem with the benefit of hindsight, in the world of postwar Britain, Jones's therapeutic communities and Bierer's "social and community psychiatry" loomed as exciting prospects, true alternatives to the pessimism of the neurobiological approach on the one hand and to the esoteric rites of psychoanalysis on the other.

There was much less excitement in the United States. Although the Americans used such terms as social psychiatry, they usually meant some form of psychiatric epidemiology or study of human relations in the mental hospital rather than group psychotherapy, the core of social and community psychiatry in Britain.

Around the time of World War I, American psychiatry was hit by a strong activist impulse, trying to break the asylum stalemate and to see the patient and his illness in social terms. Among the first to use the term "social psychiatry" was Elmer Southard in 1917, director of the Boston Psychopathic Hospital, who understood a mixture of psychiatric social services and social psychology.[194] In the early 1920s, a string of speakers at annual meetings of the American Psychiatric Association, including two of the Association's presidents, gave impassioned addresses on the asylum's need to reach out to the community or to forestall mental illness through prevention in the community.[195] This kind of rhetoric was evidence of psychiatry's willingness to break out of the custodial mode (see pp. 67–68) and return to the mainstream of medicine. It fit with the American doctrine of "social medicine" in the 1920s, seeing medicine in part as social science and directing attention to "the whole man."[196] None of this had anything to do with group psychotherapy or community care.

Group psychotherapy made its initial eruption in the United States in 1934, as Paul Schilder at Bellevue in New York started bringing groups of two to seven patients in the outpatient department together for collective sessions once or twice a week. "In group psychotherapy," said Schilder, "a number of patients are seen simultaneously by the physician, and each patient is aware of the problems of the others." The patients, many of whom were quite disturbed, experienced relief at hearing they were not alone with their difficulties. "In one discussion, for example, a patient remembered an attempted sexual assault against his sister. It was astonishing how many members of the group recalled similar experiences in their own lives, so that a correct appreciation of such an event became possible."[197] The inventive Schilder, however, would soon be dead in an automobile accident. Unlike Britain, where the military establishment lay behind group psychotherapy, the movement did not take off in the United States. In the United States, psychoanalysts seized control of army psychiatry during World War II, and Freud's doctrines rather than patients' social clubs took pride of place.

The term social psychiatry thrived in the United States during the 1950s and 1960s, in the sense of large surveys of the mental health of the population such as the Midtown Manhattan Study, commissioned in 1950 by Thomas Rennie of Cornell Medical College.[198] Under "therapeutic communities," Americans understood mainly mental hospitals with open-door policies, a serious mistranslation of an Anglicism. And the American definition of social psychiatry was broad enough to encompass every influence imaginable on the patient's life: childhood, friends, social class, poverty, and the like. All of these elements helped give American psychiatry its stamp of social activism but bore little in common with what was understood in Britain under the term: group psychotherapy, day hospitals, and patient autonomy.

Later, therapeutic communities did flourish in the United States. "No progressive hospital worth its salt would be without the label of therapeutic community," said one observer in the early 1970s.[199] Yet these experiments were frequently deformed by the spirit of psychoanalysis with its emphasis on a one-to-one relationship between doctor and patient (to achieve "transference"). When the Americans did attempt to form a therapeutic community, they often produced a caricature of the British original. Witness the nightmare community that Ken Kesey described in

237

his novel, *One Flew Over the Cuckoo's Nest* (1962) (see p. 275). There was one day hospital in the United States: at the Menninger Clinic.[200]

American "community psychiatry" ended in tragedy, the massive disgorgement of disabled asylum patients to the rough care of the streets (see pp. 280–281). Little resembling the day care offered in Britain or on the Continent was available in the United States. The 1963 mental health act of John F. Kennedy's administration might be seen as an exception to this generalization. Yet the mental health centers the act made possible soon were given over to psychotherapy for middle-class neurotics rather than to the community care of patients with psychotic illness.[201] The subject of community psychiatry in the United States was, and remains, a kind of grotesque joke.

Yet for the grand narrative of psychiatry's history, the failure of communitarianism to gain headway in the United States did nudge events along. The absence of a sensible rival doctrine to psychoanalysis permitted biological psychiatry to overthrow the competition more easily than was the case in Europe, where community psychiatry offered tough resistance for decades to the biological approach.[202] But then, biological and social perspectives are not necessarily incompatible: Psychiatric illness is often triggered and molded by social stresses. Recognition of this gave social psychiatry a much more tenacious hold than the analysts possessed.

For half a century, the discipline of psychiatry stood trapped between the choices of custodial care and individual psychoanalysis. Forced to come up with alternatives, psychiatry cobbled together a band of options ranging from bromide sleep to ECT to social clubs. Among these alternative choices, there were no conflicting paradigms, no theoretical battles. A doctor might order psychodrama one day and ECT the next. So desperate were workaday psychiatrists to dodge the awful choice between custodialism (for the poor) and psychoanalysis (for the rich), that they were willing to try anything that held promise. Thus for half a century, the discipline of psychiatry averted choosing between the neurobiological paradigm on the one hand and the psychogenic paradigm on the other. After the 1960s, this kind of pragmatic eclecticism no longer became possible. The neurobiological paradigm came roaring back from the grave in which Kraepelin had interred it—with medications that truly worked and evidence that psychiatric illness represented a biological phenomenon far deeper than troubled human relations or a schizophrenogenic mother. The alternatives of the first half of the twentieth century were almost all wiped from the slate by the advent of the second biological psychiatry.

7

The Second
Biological Psychiatry

I n the 1970s, biological psychiatry came roaring back on stage, displacing psychoanalysis as the dominant paradigm and returning psychiatry to the fold of the other medical specialties. This triumph of the biological, the view that major psychiatric illness rested on a substrate of disordered brain chemistry and development, meant a return to themes that had last resounded in the nineteenth century at the time of the first biological psychiatry. It also entailed a repudiation of the psychoanalytic paradigm that saw psychiatric illness as psychogenic, arising in the mind as a result of faulty child rearing or environmental stress, curable through in-depth psychotherapy. There was room in the biological paradigm for psychotherapy, but it was the kind of informal psychotherapy inherent in the doctor-patient relationship and not the elaborate choreography of working through unconscious conflicts that psychoanalysis scripted.

Although the second biological psychiatry burst into the workaday world of clinical practice only in the 1970s, its views about genetics and brain development as causes, and its precepts about drugs and informal psychotherapy as remedies, germinated in the fading days of the first biological psychiatry. The immediate intellectual ancestor of the second biological psychiatry was the German Research Institute for Psychiatry in Munich that Emil Kraepelin, who wrote finis to the first biological psychiatry, had founded in 1917. Although Kraepelin himself was agnostic about causation—raising an eyebrow at the genetic and brain-biological views of his predecessors—he nonetheless surrounded himself with researchers such as Franz Nissl and Aloys Alzheimer who stressed the brain as the seat of psychiatric illness. Among these fellow researchers were several geneticists, who established at Kraepelin's institute a laboratory for the study of inheritance patterns in psychiatric illness. It was early in the history of this lab, itself so ill-fated under the Third Reich, that genetic patterns started to be traced establishing that the major psychiatric illnesses lay in the very substance of the brain itself and not in faulty patterns of mothering or an unhappy social environment.

The Genetic Strand

Among the most convincing kinds of evidence for a neural origin of major psychiatric illness would be genetic studies. A considerable portion of illness is noninheritable, the result of a developmental anomaly in the uterus or of environmental influences. Yet there is an inheritable, genetic portion as well, supporting the argument of biological psychiatry that nature plays at least something of a role.

The first biological psychiatry was mindful of this role, although its advocates, statistical naïfs, chose anecdotes rather than long series of patients balanced against control groups to support their case. It was also unhelpful to the historic reputation of the early biological psychiatrists that they cloaked their findings in the value-laden language of "degeneration." The precursors of the second biological psychiatry realized that to be convincing they would need quantitative data, comparing schizophrenic and depressed patients with controls. They also knew they must assemble data that would rule out the effect of family environment: It is always possible that children who become schizophrenic have somehow learned the behavior from sick relatives in the family environment rather than inheriting it.

That said, it is true that some of the first biological psychiatrists appreciated the importance of numbers. When Richard von Krafft-Ebing was still at Graz, he did a study of 19 psychotic female patients, of whom he found 12 to have some "neuropsychopathic family history."[1] As Emil Kraepelin reflected in 1913 on the charts of his Heidelberg patients, he noted that around 70 percent of those with schizophrenia had family histories of major psychiatric illness.[2] Thomas Clouston, master of the Edinburgh asylum, went about his task even more systematically. Whereas only 23 percent of all his patients had a family history of mental illness, 65 percent of those with "adolescent insanity" (his term for schizophrenia) did so.[3] Clouston was certain that these statistics embraced a genetic mechanism: "The . . . view of the individual as being organically one in structure and function with his ancestry and his posterity must always be kept in mind. They are not even links in a chain; links are separate from each other, and may have been forged from different pieces of iron; they are only one in function, whereas a man is just as much a part of his ancestry, and his posterity of him, as the root and stem are parts of one tree."[4]

The statistics of the nineteenth century all tended to confound genetic inheritance with family environment. To separate genes from environment, two approaches would be of service: twin studies and adoption studies. Not until the 1920s did the numerative skills of the international medical community achieve this level of sophistication.

The logic of a twin study is that identical, or monozygotic, twins develop from a single fertilized ovum and have a common set of genes. In the words of one British researcher, "This identical genetical inheritance must necessarily make them more alike, in all ways in which genes play a part, than are binovular [dizygotic] twins, who need resemble one another genetically no more than do ordinary brothers and sisters. Where differences do occur between the two members of an 'identical' twin pair it is the environment which is responsible."[5] But if there is a high degree of concordance, meaning a tendency for both of the identical twins to fall ill, it is likely that genetic influences are involved. This presumption of inheritance is even stronger if the concordance between the dizygotic twins is low. Studies from our own time show, for example, that the concordance between monozygotic twins in schizophrenia is about 50 percent, that for dizygotic twins about 15 percent.[6] This is one of the important pieces of evidence for the biological nature of schizophrenia. Francis Galton, who first proposed twin studies in 1875, called them an opportunity to "weigh in just scales the effects of nature and nurture."[7]

In 1928, Hans Luxenburger, a young Bavarian psychiatrist at the German Research Institute for Psychiatry in Munich, undertook the first large-scale survey of all twins born in a given area. He was trying to produce an unbiased series of twins rather than just concentrating on twins that happened to strike observers as curiosities. To establish the number of twin pairs in which one or both of the twins had a psychiatric illness, Luxenburger and colleagues asked all of Bavaria's mental hospitals to give them a list of patients present on a certain date. They then sent the list to all the local priests and pastors, asking if any of the listed individuals had been part of a twin birth. Among this series of 16,000 patients, the pastors were able to identify 211 as one of a twin pair. Going back to the patients' charts and doing further interviews of the hospitalized twin, the researchers made the diagnosis of schizophrenia in 106 cases. How often did the second twin have schizophrenia? The authors sought out the 65 second twins to have survived to adult life, interviewed them, and after much hemming and hawing about which twins were identical and which fraternal, found that in 7.6 percent of the monozygotic twin pairs both twins were ill, in none of the dizygotic.[8] This represented the first solid evidence that a major psychiatric illness—one considered "functional" by some (meaning cause unknown), psychogenic by others—had an organic substrate. Luxenburger, a staunch Catholic, was tarnished by association with his teacher and boss Ernst Rüdin, who later became a Nazi geneticist. Luxenburger himself served as an apologist for racist genetics for a few years under the Third Reich, then in 1941, as his criticisms of the regime endangered him, at Rüdin's suggestion he enlisted in the German Army, a place of relative safety from the Gestapo.[9]

Yet there was nothing intrinsically racist about the technique of twin studies in psychiatric genetics. Showing schizophrenia to be in part a genetic disease was really the high road of Central European scholarship. Manfred Bleuler, for example, who became professor of psychiatry in Zurich in 1942, was a mainstream scholar by any stretch. Yet when a visiting American researcher came calling at the door of the Bleuler home, Manfred met him waving "an old display case of butterflies" showing crosses and backcrosses in the wings. It has been Bleuler's high school science project. Bleuler told the visitor "that it had been his lifelong dream to discover the Mendelian basis of schizophrenia."[10]

So the undertaking was not Nazi-inspired. Indeed, the next major contributions to the field came from Jewish scholars. Aaron Rosanoff, born in Russia in 1879, came to the United States at the age of 13, graduated in medicine from Cornell University in 1901, then entered the New York State asylum system at King's Park State Hospital on Long Island. In a system known for attracting benchwarmers and time-servers, Rosanoff distinguished himself for his scientific curiosity, especially about medical genetics. After moving to Los Angeles in 1922 to open a private nervous clinic (the Alhambra Sanitarium), he resolved to undertake a large-scale twin study using data from state hospitals.[11] By the early 1930s, he had his numbers in place. Because the small number of twin pairs had been Luxenburger's Achilles' heel, Rosanoff compiled a list of 1,014 twin pairs in which one of the twins had a major mental disorder. Of these 1,014 pairs, schizophrenia was diagnosed in 142. Among the monozygotic twins, both twins developed schizophrenia in 68.3 percent of the cases, among the dizygotic, in 14.9 percent.[12] The difference was enormous. Rosanoff also looked at manic-depressive illness, where in 90 twin pairs at least one twin had the illness. The second twin got it as well in 69.6 percent of the monozygotic twin pairs, in only 16.4 percent of the dizygotic. Rosanoff concluded, "Hereditary or germinal factors play an important part in the etiology of manic-depressive syndromes."[13]

It must be emphasized that Rosanoff was not a marginal right-wing figure, as some historians of psychiatry have tried to characterize these early psychiatric geneticists.[14] After becoming director of the California mental-hospital system in 1939, he inaugurated a statewide program for the home-care of patients, and was instrumental in establishing a Maudsley-style research center in San Francisco, the Langley Porter Clinic. Rosanoff's twin studies arguably represent the major American contribution to international psychiatric literature in the years between the two world wars, yet the official histories of American psychiatry, dominated by psychoanalytically oriented writers, pass over his work in virtual silence.[15]

One of the coworkers in Ernst Rüdin's and Hans Luxenburger's genetics lab was the young Franz Kallmann. Born in Neumarkt, Silesia, in 1897, Kallmann earned his MD in 1919 at Breslau University, then trained in psychiatry at Kraepelin's research institute in Munich. In 1929, Kallmann became involved in the large-scale studies that Rüdin and Luxenburger were undertaking, and as an extension of that work moved to the Herzberge Mental Hospital in Berlin where he did a family study of all blood relatives of schizophrenics admitted to the hospital 30 years previously. The Nazi racial laws of 1935 obliged Kallmann to give up his post in Berlin, whereupon he took his notes across the Atlantic to the New York State Psychiatric Institute. In 1938, he published in English the results of the Berlin study (which did not include enough twins to make an interesting analysis).[16]

In the meantime, however, Kallmann had seen Rosanoff's work. In the early 1940s, Kallmann decided to apply his tremendous energy to a twin study of all patients in public asylums in New York State. Of the 73,000 patients in the system in 1945, Kallmann identified 691 schizophrenics with a traceable cotwin. For the monozygotic twins, the concordance rate was 85.8 percent, for the dizygotic 14.7.[17] Thus in identical twins there was an almost certain chance of the second twin developing the illness, in fraternal only a one in seven chance. These findings were such a solid index of organicity in schizophrenia that, when they were presented in 1950 at the First World Congress of Psychiatry in Paris, they caused a sensation. (Eliot Slater read Kallmann's paper.) Kallmann had written in an unvarnished manner about the Mendelian inheritance of schizophrenia (meaning a single locus in the DNA), and such was the storm of protest from delegates assembled from around the world that, to "de-dramatize" the discussion, the chairman refused to read from any of the written comments that had been sent in. Most opposed were the psychoanalysts, whom Kallmann had dubbed "a host of cynical armchair workers."[18]

Other large-scale twin studies were done after World War II[19], yet it was by now apparent that schizophrenia and manic-depressive illness were heavily genetic in nature. The closer the blood relationship, the higher the rate of schizophrenia in other family members.[20] Yet could the family environment play a role as well? After all, monozygotic twins grew up together. Perhaps living in a family environment that was "distorted"—in the phrase of the day—by mental illness made other family members ill. How much did environment contribute as opposed to heredity? How many patients had been brought low by a schizophrenogenic mother, a flawed family dynamic?

In 1959, Seymour Kety decided to look at children of schizophrenic mothers or fathers who had been raised in foster homes, thus eliminating the effect of growing up midst madness. Kety himself was one of the founders of biological psychiatry in the United States. Born in Philadelphia in 1915, he received his MD degree from the University of Pennsylvania in 1940, going on to do research at that university and teach the pharmacology and physiology of the brain. In 1951, Kety became the scientific director of the recently founded (in 1949) National Institute of Mental Health in Bethesda, shifting the institute's course from research on psychoanalysis to research into basic science. He remained at NIMH until becoming a professor at Harvard in 1967. After retiring from Harvard in 1983, Kety returned to Bethesda to continue directing one of the meatiest research projects in the history of psychiatry: the Danish adoption study. The state of Denmark has an exceptional capacity to follow its citizens through life. An adoption register of the state Department of Justice permits researchers to identify the biological relatives of children who are adopted; a population register makes it possible to locate adoptees and follow their trajectories through life. Thus in Denmark, one is able to study the biological background of adoptees as well as their fates in their new families. In 1968, Kety and collaborators published the results of their study of 5,483 adoptions in Copenhagen between 1924 and 1947. From this group, 507 adoptees were later admitted to a psychiatric hospital. Independent observers reviewed their case histories and identified 33 of them as schizophrenics. These patients and their families were then compared with an age-matched control group of adoptees never admitted to a psychiatric hospital. Within the biological families of the adopted schizophrenics, about 10 percent of the close relatives had schizophrenia, within the families of the control group there was very little schizophrenia. Nature and not just nurture had contributed to making these adopted children ill. Kety and colleagues concluded cautiously that "genetic factors are important in the transmission of schizophrenia." The mechanism must involve a number of genes rather than a single-gene Mendelian model as Kallmann had posited.[21]

By 1992, Kety had widened the study to include adoptees in all of Denmark, learning that almost half of the schizophrenic adoptees had a history of some form of the disease in their biological families, versus virtually none of the controls.[22] For all of Denmark, schizophrenia was 10 times more common in the biological relatives of the schizophrenic adoptees than in the biological relatives of the controls. It was also found more often in the brothers and sisters of the adoptees (12.5 percent) than in second-degree relatives (2.2 percent), which is "also consistent with genetic transmission," the authors noted.[23]

Kety's research on adoptees with schizophrenia unleashed an avalanche of genetic research involving family, twin, and adoption studies. In 1977, a Danish study of manic-depressive illness found concordances of 67 percent for monozygotic twins and 20 percent for dizygotic.[24] Twin studies in the 1980s implicated genetic factors in agoraphobia and panic disorder.[25] An adoption study of psychosomatic illness highlighted genetic factors: In families where the children of violent and alcoholic fathers were placed in foster homes, the boys tended to behave like their biological fathers (even though the father had no contact with them); the daughters of such biological fathers tended to display abnormal behavior also, the kind of chronic physical complaints of nonorganic origin that were once known as "hysteria."[26] Other kinds of research suggested that such hysteria is passed down in the female line at the same time as antisocial behavior in the male line.[27]

Twin studies soon began bearing fruit across the entire terrain of psychiatry. In such personality traits as hypochondriasis, hypomania, and depression, psychological testing unearthed significant differences between monozygotic and dizygotic twins—the litmus test of the genetic strand.[28] This was poaching on the classic terrain of psychogenesis: For a century, the doctrine had ruled that hysteria and the symptomatic psychoneuroses were the result of stress or dysfunctional family life. The genetic news implied that these illnesses must have a significant brain substrate, however much environmental circumstances might contribute to triggering them.

Yet what of the family? If overall, genetics accounted for about 50 percent of such "behavioral disorders" as schizophrenia, was the family responsible for the other half? Not at all. Studies of pairs of adopted children, themselves unrelated but raised in the same foster family, showed correlations close to zero. As one study put it, "the relevant environmental influences are not shared by children in the same family."[29] Whatever had made the one adopted child sick had no effect on the other. Thus the environmental influence could not have been family life itself.

In the 1970s and after, genetic psychiatry became even bolder in the search for causes, as molecular biology opened the possibility of identifying the actual genes involved. By 1995, the gene or genes causing schizophrenia had been tentatively placed somewhere on chromosome 6.[30] For manic-depressive illness, chromosomes number 18 and 21 had been implicated.[31] Psychiatric geneticists began to propose genetic anticipation, the tendency for some illness-causing genes to expand in size when passed from generation to generation, as the mechanism behind the increasing severity of schizophrenia or manic-depressive illness as handed down a family tree.[32] This was the exact equivalent of "degeneration" in the first biological psychiatry. The schizophrenogenic mother was truly dead.

The First Drug That Worked

The other wing that carried psychiatry into the biological era was drug therapy. Drugs had always been used in psychiatry, from the laxatives that were once administered to patients newly admitted to asylum—on the grounds that their problems might be caused by colonic autointoxication—to opium and its alkaloids for depression and mania: mildly successful but highly addictive. The modern era of drug therapy began with systematic experimentation into the chemistry of the brain. Brain chemistry means neurotransmitters, the chemicals that transmit the nerve impulse from one neuron to another across the synapse (the gap between the neurons). Although research on brain chemistry went back to turn-of-the-century English physiologists, it was only in the early 1920s that Otto Loewi, professor of pharmacology at the University of Graz, isolated the first neurotransmitter. On the basis of work he began in the winter of 1921, in 1926 he was able to say that the chemical acetylcholine mediated the transmission of the nerve impulse from one nerve to the next.[33]

The discovery of acetylcholine did not remain abstract knowledge but had rapid therapeutic consequences: In the 1930s, psychiatrists gave

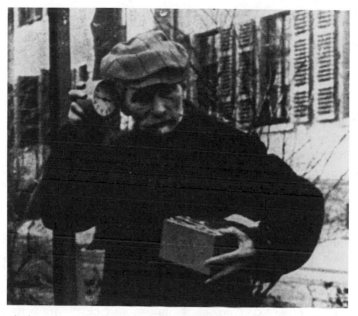

Psychosis before the introduction of chlorpromazine: Patient at a German mental hospital around 1900 listening to his wife's voice from an alarm clock (courtesy of the Universitätsbibliothek Leipzig).

acetylcholine to their patients in the hopes of relieving schizophrenia, although at this point they had no notion of the mechanism involved.[34]

Buoyed by the success of the physical therapies of the 1930s, many mental-hospital psychiatrists were open-minded toward the potential of drugs, and throughout the 1940s experimentation went on relentlessly in asylums to find agents that would improve on shock and coma therapies:

In 1937, Heinz Lehmann, a refugee psychiatrist from Berlin, had just arrived at Montreal's Verdun Protestant Hospital, where he was one of a few physicians for some 1,600 psychiatric patients. "It was pretty horrible to work under those conditions," Lehmann said. "So I did all kinds of things, always convinced that psychotic conditions and the major affective disorders . . . had some sort of a biological substrate. I kept experimenting with all kinds of drugs, for instance, large doses, very large doses of caffeine, I remember, in one or two stuporous catatonic schizophrenics—of course, with no results." He injected sulfur suspended in oil into his patients, "which was painful and caused a fever." He injected typhoid antitoxin to produce a fever analogous to the malaria therapy. "Nothing helped; I even injected turpentine into the abdominal muscles which produced—and was supposed to produce—a huge sterile abscess and

247

marked leucocytosis [raising the white count]. Of course, that abscess had to be opened in the operating room under sterile conditions. None of this had any effect, but all of this had been proposed in, mostly, European work as being of help in schizophrenia."[35]

The point is not that researchers such as Lehmann behaved inhumanely with their patients: They were searching in the best of faith for something better to offer them. It is rather that, by the time in 1951 that Henri Laborit, a surgeon in the French navy, began experimenting with a curious new "potentiator" of anesthetics, the ground had already been well prepared for the reception of new antipsychotic drugs.[36] Laborit himself was directly responsible for a drug that changed the face of psychiatry: chlorpromazine.

Stationed at the Maritime Hospital at Bizerte in Tunisia in 1949, Laborit was 35 when he began researching various synthetic antihistamines as a means of "potentiating" anesthetics. Operating on soldiers in shock has always been a big problem in military surgery, and Laborit's idea was that a potentiator could block the autonomic mechanisms involved in shock, increasing the chances of success of the operation. Among possible potentiators, Laborit was working with some recent antihistamines in the phenothiazine family synthesized by the Rhône-Poulenc drug company. Ever since the discovery of antihistamines in 1937, physicians had been experimenting with these drugs on psychotic patients, with little result. At this point, Laborit had no interest in psychosis, but he did note that some of his surgical patients became quite indifferent to the world about them (ataraxic was the term subsequently applied) after being given the phenothiazines. As he later said, "I asked an army psychiatrist to watch me operate on some of my tense, anxious Mediterranean-type patients. After surgery, he agreed with me that the patients were remarkably calm and relaxed. But I guess he didn't think any more about his observations, as they might apply to psychiatric patients."[37]

Early in 1951, Laborit was transferred from the marine hospital system, where interest in his work was virtually nonexistent, to the physiology laboratory of the Val-de-Grâce military hospital in Paris. Here, surrounded by inquiring minds and under the guidance of a benevolent lab chief, he pressed ahead with his work on shock. Because the previous antihistamines had not been ideal autonomic blockers, in June 1951 Laborit asked Rhône-Poulenc for a sample of a new phenothiazine that company chemist Paul Charpentier, a phenothiazine specialist, had recently synthesized, dubbed 4560 RP (for Rhône-Poulenc). Charpentier later called the compound "chlorpromazine." Even before Laborit's request, the company suspected that it might be a useful psychiatry drug but had not yet sent it to clinicians for trials.[38]

Laborit began using 4560 RP on surgical patients at Val-de-Grâce. He found that, in addition to doing what it was supposed to surgically, the drug produced a certain "uninterest" (*désintéressement*) on the part of the patient. In the tradition of antihistamine researchers who had tried to apply their compounds psychiatrically, Laborit decided to do so as well, and in November 1951 he tested it for toxicity on a colleague, a female psychiatrist, at the Villejuif Mental Hospital. Shortly after taking it intravenously she got up to go to the bathroom and fainted. The chief of the psychiatry service at Villejuif thereupon resolved to have nothing more to do with it.[39] So Laborit returned to Val-de-Grâce and, over lunch at the hospital canteen, finally persuaded three rather unenthusiastic psychiatrist colleagues to give it to their patients.[40] In early February 1952, Laborit reported to the medical press the results of his surgical work with 4560 RP, dropping out of the blue the suggestive line at the end of the article, "These findings allow one to anticipate certain indications for the use of this compound in psychiatry, possibly in connection with barbiturates in a deep-sleep cure."[41] Yet as he penned those lines, perhaps tongue in cheek, on January 19, 1952, the Val-de-Grâce psychiatrists were giving chlorpromazine to Jacques L., a 24-year-old patient with an attack of mania. "The patient is calm after the injection. He lies without moving, his eyes shut, responds when spoken to, with a maniacal look on his face; he closes an eye, pulls on his tongue, then sleep." He woke up manic again. Over the next three weeks he received chlorpromazine in combination with an analgesic, a barbiturate, and ECT. Finally by February 7, he was calm enough that he could play bridge and lead a normal life, though his attitudes remained somewhat "hypomanic."[42] What had moderated the patient's symptoms was not at all clear, but at least chlorpromazine hadn't harmed him, and in the meantime news was racing about the Paris grapevine that a big new psychiatry drug was in the works. Word of chlorpromazine reached the ears of two of the big guns in Parisian psychiatry, Jean Delay and Pierre Deniker at the Ste-Anne mental hospital, who began giving it to their patients in March 1952.[43] Delay, 45 at the time, was professor of psychiatry at the Sorbonne and director of the Ste-Anne. Deniker, 10 years younger, was on the hospital's medical staff. At the prestigious hundredth anniversary of the Medical Psychological Society in May 1952, they described briefly their work on chlorpromazine, omitting any reference to Laborit.[44] Then at the Society's June meeting, they delivered a fuller report on eight patients.[45] While it is true that they were the first to treat a series of patients exclusively with chlorpromazine, it is not true that they discovered the drug's psychiatric applications. And history has wrongly exalted Delay and Deniker in connection with opening this epochal new chapter in the annals of psychiatry, the advent of pharmacotherapy, while sliding in silence over that of Laborit.[46]

Nonetheless, by May 1952 it was evident that Delay's and Deniker's patients at the Ste-Anne had done well on chlorpromazine. Patient number one, Giovanni A., a 57-year-old laborer with a long history of mental illness, had been admitted most recently for "making improvised political speeches in cafés, becoming involved in fights with strangers, and for the last few days has been walking around the street with a pot of flowers on his head preaching his love of liberty." After nine days on chlorpromazine, he was able to have a normal conversation, after three weeks he had calmed and was about to be discharged. The results for the seven other patients were similar.[47] This was much better than ECT, insulin, and the rest of the physical therapies, much less dangerous, and easily tolerated by the patients.

Chlorpromazine spread at once through the French system. "By May 1953," writes one historian, "the atmosphere in the disturbed wards of mental hospitals in Paris was transformed: straitjackets, psychohydraulic packs and noise were things of the past! Once more, Paris psychiatrists who long ago unchained the chained, became pioneers in liberating their patients, this time from inner torments, and with a drug: chlorpromazine. It accomplished the pharmacologic revolution of psychiatry."[48]

The ultimate force behind the discovery and adoption of new drugs such as chlorpromazine was not academic scientists or clinicians such as Laborit and Delay but the drug companies. Although Rhône-Poulenc had not identified chlorpromazine as an antipsychotic, it was company scientists who had systematically designed the compound and tested it on animals.[49] The drug's discovery owed nothing to serendipity. As chlorpromazine made its way into the world, the driving force would be pharmaceutical executives and scientists, a point worth recalling because, in the decades that followed chlorpromazine, the race to discover new drugs would be dominated by the great pharmaceutical houses.

Clinicians brought chlorpromazine to North America but a drug house gained its acceptance. In 1952, young Dr. Ruth Koeppe-Kajander, who had earned her MD at Göttingen just after the war, was interning at the Oshawa (Ontario) General Hospital when she noted a staff anesthetist giving chlorpromazine (or Largactil, its trade name outside the United States) to potentiate the anesthesia. The anesthetist had received it on trial from Rhône-Poulenc. When Koeppe's internship ended in 1953, she began training in psychiatry at the mental hospital in London,

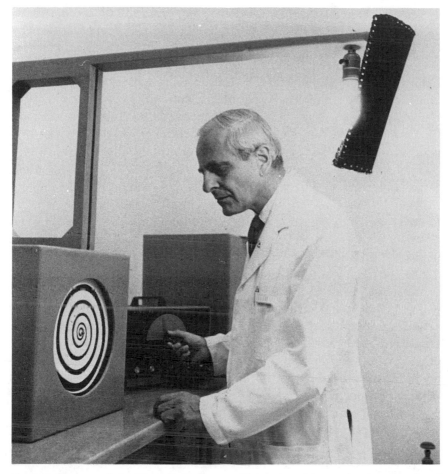

Heinz Lehmann of the Verdun Protestant Hospital in Montreal, who introduced chlorpromazine to North America in 1953. Here, in a photograph from the 1960s, Lehmann is using an Archimedes spiral to measure the effect of psychotropic drugs (courtesy McGill University Archives).

Ontario, and—as a first-year resident—gained permission to give the drug to 25 patients over a period of months. In November 1953, she reported "on the remarkable effects of this drug" at a psychiatric meeting near Toronto. "It calmed restless, excited or overactive patients without sedating them to the level where they could not function. Patients lost their agitation but not their consciousness. They could talk about themselves and eat and sleep without difficulty. Catatonic and other types of excitement were no longer life threatening."[50]

Yet the name associated with the introduction of chlorpromazine in North America is not Koeppe-Kajander but Heinz Lehmann at the Verdun Hospital in Montreal. French Canada was a logical beachhead because Rhône-Poulenc had an office in Montreal. "One day," recalled Lehmann, "there was a detail man [sales representative] from . . . Rhône-Poulenc, and he left all kinds of literature and samples. My secretary told him that I was much too busy to see him, but he said, 'It isn't necessary, I'll leave this here, this is something new and so good I don't have to explain it to him, he will certainly pay attention to it once he reads it.'"

Though Lehmann thought this rather arrogant, it did catch his attention. That Sunday as he lay in the bathtub he read several of Deniker's papers. Lehmann, a German, could read French easily because he had a French-Canadian wife and spoke French at home (the other hospital psychiatrists were all unilingual in English). At first, Lehmann thought it was just another sedative. "But there was a certain statement: it acted 'like a chemical lobotomy,' which puzzled me, and I said to myself, there is something more to it. Obviously these two, Delay and Deniker, are very sophisticated psychiatrists, they must know what they are talking about." Lehmann asked for several nurses to act as volunteers and gave them small oral doses, which made them drowsy but didn't alter any other intellectual functions, unlike the barbiturates. Lehmann got a supply of chlorpromazine from the company sufficient for 71 patients, and lined up a resident to help him.

The results astonished him. As he later said, "Two or three of the acute schizophrenics became symptom-free. Now I had never seen that before. I thought it was a fluke—something that would never happen again but anyway there they were. At the end of four or five weeks, there were a lot of symptom-free patients. By this, I mean that a lot of hallucinations, delusions and thought disorder had disappeared. In 1953 there just wasn't anything that ever produced something like this—a remission from schizophrenia in weeks."[51]

Between May and July 1953, he gave the patients the drug and recorded the results, writing up his findings as a "unique" new therapeutic agent.[52] The director of the asylum told him, "You never use the word 'unique' in anything that you publish, because you always regret it later on—there is no such thing as unique." Lehmann left the "unique" in.[53]

All kinds of things began happening. Said Lehmann, "Chronic schizophrenics who had been divorced because they had been psychotic for 10 years, now all of a sudden they were symptom-free and their husbands or their wives were married again. It was a very strange time."[54]

There was one more strange thing. As Lehmann and a colleague stood one day observing the patients, they noted that some "walked with a peculiarly stiff gait (they had that peculiar mask-like face) and we said that looks like Parkinsonism, but it did not seem possible because at that time there was no such thing as drug-induced Parkinsonism. . . . There were two of these patients, and then a couple of weeks later another two or three, and we then named these side effects extrapyramidal symptoms."[55] (The pyramidal tract in the spinal cord gives voluntary control of muscles; involuntary movements must be "extrapyramidal.") The symptoms would later be called tardive dyskinesia. What seemed in 1953 a rather innocuous side effect would turn out to be a massive social and medical problem, as patients from these mental hospitals were, in a few years time, discharged en masse to the streets: To avoid these and similar side effects they would stop taking their medication.

Yet in 1953, the issue of involuntary grimacing and embarrassing, uncontrollable bodily movements lay in the future. What counted was Lehmann's forceful presentation to an English-speaking audience of chlorpromazine as the first drug in psychiatry to abolish the symptoms of psychosis, though not necessarily to cure the underlying brain disorder. The images of rapturous release from illnesses such as mania were impossible to resist: "One manic patient stated after her recovery that with the drug she soon lost the feeling: 'I had to live my whole life in one day.'" Another patient suffering from anxiety said, "It was like a chairman taking control of a meeting where everybody had been shouting at once."[56] These arresting lines in a major medical journal guaranteed a continentwide hearing for the new drug.

The scene shifts to the United States, toughest market of all to crack because of the predominance of psychoanalysis and its predilection for getting to the "real" causes of the illness. Here an ambitious young drug house named Smith Kline & French enters the picture. The company was a maker of patent medicines, and its new president, Francis Boyer, wanted to upgrade it to a manufacturer of "ethicals," meaning drugs prescribed by the medical profession. Aware that Rhône-Poulenc had a hot new potentiator going—but unaware that it might have psychiatric uses—in the spring of 1952 Boyer went to France. Rhône-Poulenc was very close-mouthed. (The company had already tried unsuccessfully to interest several other big American firms.) When Boyer signed the licensing agreement, he thought he was buying an antiemetic (anti-vomiting drug). Having virtually no research budget, Smith Kline was not prepared to undertake extensive trials. Said Boyer, "Let's get this thing on the market as an antiemetic and we'll worry about the rest of that stuff later." The company brought it out as "Thorazine."

Many years later, this author interviewed John Young, who at the time was a 29-year-old member of Smith Kline's international division. When did Boyer realize that chlorpromazine was a major antipsychotic?

"Dr. Shorter, you're not old enough to remember that's a meaningless question because antipsychotics didn't exist. There were no drugs. Those cases were in the back wards and that was it. The notion that you could ever do anything about it hadn't occurred to anyone. These doctors and nurses who went into McLean [Hospital] at that time, their altruism was busted after six months. What this drug did was not to cure these patients but to tip the balance enough so that the doctor and the nurse in the hospital said, 'Hey, maybe we can do something for these people.'"[57]

The first psychiatrist to try Smith Kline's chlorpromazine on patients was William Long, the firm's medical director. One of his first five patients, all with mania, was a "severely disturbed nun," as Young recalled, "at the edge of violence and using extremely coarse language. He was very concerned about the patient. He gave her some of this stuff. The results? He couldn't believe it. She had been extraordinarily abusive with most un-nun-like behavior. In the afternoon she was calm. He described it at the table in the lunchroom. What he described was a typical chlorpromazine result."

It was important for Smith Kline to get outside psychiatrists to run drug trials, not an easy task given the prevailing climate of opinion in American psychiatry. In September 1953, psychiatrist Willis Bower at McLean began the trial that would prove most influential. He reported the drug to be "capable of strongly influencing the course of some psychiatric illnesses." There was no memory loss, as with ECT, and unlike the barbiturates it did not disinhibit patients nor sedate them. The study was published in the *New England Journal of Medicine*.[58]

Having ensured chlorpromazine's acceptance in academic medicine, Smith Kline formed a special chlorpromazine task force and proceeded to beat the bushes in the state asylums, the elective terrain of the drug. If the task force encountered a reluctant state hospital, it would point out to state legislators the money-saving aspects of using an antipsychotic drug.[59] Thus chlorpromazine, though scorned by analysts such as Jules Masserman as a "glorified sedative," became widely adopted in the red-brick state hospitals. *Time* magazine later mocked the Freudians for their airs: "The ivory-tower critics argue that the red-brick pragmatists are not getting to the patient's 'underlying psychopathology' and so there can be no cure. These doctors want to know whether he withdrew from the world because of unconscious conflict over incestuous urges or stealing from his brother's piggy bank at the age of five. In the world of red bricks, this is like arguing about the number of angels on the point of a pin."[60]

But it wasn't just in the snake pits that chlorpromazine found a use. It damped the delusions and hallucinations and calmed the agitation of patients in such expensive private-sector clinics as the Sheppard and Enoch Pratt Hospital in Baltimore. With chlorpromazine and other drugs, "the wild, screaming, unapproachable patients [became] a thing of the past," wrote one staffer. "Many more patients could go for drives in the country, visit Towson and Baltimore for shopping excursions, with or without attendants, go to the theatre, visit art museums, take in athletic contests, and go out with relatives for dinner. Life became more varied and interesting, and improvement was advanced."[61]

Chlorpromazine initiated a revolution in psychiatry, comparable to the introduction of penicillin in general medicine. While it did not cure the diseases causing psychosis, it did abolish their cardinal symptoms so that patients with underlying schizophrenia could lead relatively normal lives and not be confined to institutions. In 1955, Delay and Deniker proposed the term "neuroleptic" for drugs that diminished psychosis, though Americans preferred the term "antipsychotic."[62] English psychiatrist Henry Rollin, who had worked at the big asylum at Epsom, later said that chlorpromazine "tore through the civilized world like a whirlwind and engulfed the whole treatment spectrum of psychiatric disorders." It was the beginning of "the era of psychopharmacology."[63]

The Cornucopia

Following chlorpromazine, a veritable cornucopia of antipsychotic, antimanic, and antidepressant drugs poured forth, changing psychiatry from a branch of social work to a field that called for the most precise knowledge of pharmacology, the effect of drugs on the body. Of course, all that spilled from the cornucopia was not bounty. Some were me-too drugs, thrown onto the market for competitive reasons only; others were identified as toxic and soon withdrawn; still others lapped from psychiatry into the street as drugs of abuse. Yet on the whole the products of the cornucopia greatly ameliorated the lot of individuals with mental illness. It was with these psychiatric drugs that the journalist's cliched phrase "new hope" originated.

The story began in 1949 with John Cade, the 37-year-old superintendent of the Repatriation Mental Hospital in Bundoora, Australia. Cade, like Neil Macleod in late-nineteenth-century Shanghai, had not lost his scientific curiosity despite his provincial isolation. He was determined to see if the cause of mania was some toxic product manufactured by the body itself, analogous to thyrotoxicosis from the thyroid. Not having any idea what, exactly, he might be searching for, he began taking urine from his manic patients and, in a disused hospital kitchen, injecting it into the bellies of guinea pigs. Sure enough, the guinea pigs died, as they did when injected with the urine of controls. Cade began investigating the various components of urine—urea, uric acid and so forth—and realized that to make uric acid soluble for purposes of injection he would have to mix it with lithium, an element that had been used medically since the middle of the nineteenth century (in the mistaken belief that it could serve as a solvent of uric acid in the treatment of gout).

Then Cade, on a whim, tried injecting the guinea pigs with lithium alone, just to see what would happen. The guinea pigs became very lethargic. "Those who have experimented with guinea pigs," he wrote, "know to what degree a ready startle reaction is part of their makeup. It was thus even more startling to the experimenter to find that after the injection of a solution of lithium carbonate they could be turned on their backs and that, instead of their usual frantic righting reflex behavior, they merely lay there and gazed placidly back at him."

Cade had stumbled into a discovery of staggering importance, yet he was able to develop it only because of his resoluteness in taking the next step. He decided to inject manic patients with lithium. First he injected himself to see if repeated doses of lithium citrate and lithium carbonate would be harmful to him, which they were not. (Cade probably had a rather high tolerance of discomfort given that he had spent three years in a Japanese prisoner-of-war camp.) Then he injected 10 of his manic patients, 6 schizophrenics, and 3 chronic psychotic depressives. The lithium produced no impact on the depressed patients; it calmed somewhat the restlessness of the schizophrenics. But its effect on the manic patients was flamboyant: All 10 of them improved, though several discontinued the medication and were still in hospital at the time Cade wrote his article late in 1949. Five were discharged well, though on maintenance doses of lithium.[64]

Cade was lucky that he gave the lithium to patients with low-grade chronic mania rather than to those with full-blast mania, who are unresponsive to the drug. Yet not only was the serendipitous method of the discovery stunning, the results themselves were positive almost beyond belief. Consider patient number eight, a man of 50 years who had suffered recurrent mania attacks since the age of 20. "The present attack had lasted two months and showed no signs of abating. He was garrulous, euphoric, rest-less and unkempt when he started taking lithium citrate 20 grains three times a day on February 11, 1949." By the ninth day, he had commenced work in the garden. "By the end of two weeks, he was practically normal—quiet, tidy, rational, with insight into his previous condition. This was in marked contrast to his condition a fortnight before when he had to be locked in a single room at night with a regular nocturnal hypnotic and was too restless to eat in the dining room owing to his unsettling effect on the other patients."

The year 1949 was the worst possible time to bring out a paper on the benefits of lithium. In that year, the *Journal of the American Medical Association* published cases of two patients in congestive heart failure who died after being treated with lithium. The work of "an unknown psychi-atrist, working alone in a small chronic hospital with no research train-ing, primitive techniques and negligible equipment was hardly likely to be compellingly persuasive, especially in the United States," as Cade put it.[65] And so Cade's report on lithium, published in an obscure Australian medical weekly, slumbered on.

In 1952, Mogens Schou, a young Danish psychiatrist with a research post at the psychiatric hospital of Aarhus University, was searching for an appropriate biochemical subject on which to do research. The head of the hospital, psychiatry professor Erik Stromgren, drew Schou's attention to Cade's article and suggested that they try to verify the article's claims at Aarhus. Schou was particularly attracted to the theme given that manic-depressive illness ran in the Schou family and that his father, also a psy-chiatrist, had been most interested in the subject. Schou decided to carry out a placebo-controlled, double-blind trial, one of the first in psychiatry. (In such a trial, a control group receives a sugar pill; neither the patients, the controls, nor the assessing psychiatrists know who has received the lithium and who the placebo.) Schou's study confirmed Cade's claims: Lithium provided "symptomatic" relief of mania, meaning that when the treatment stopped, the patient relapsed.[66] Schou later said, "Perhaps more than most scientists I have been granted the privilege of reaping the fruits of my labor. A number of family members have been given lithium treat-ment with signal effect [Schou himself was among them]; they might have been hospitalized or dead today if prophylactic treatment had not come around."[67] Schou's study launched lithium into the international world of psychiatry.

Yet the launch was mightily protracted, for only in 1960 were the first North American studies of lithium conducted (one of them in Ewen Cameron's Allan Memorial Institute in Montreal).[68] The Food and Drug

Administration approved it in 1970 only after one Oregon psychiatrist threatened to practice civil disobedience and prescribe it anyway, saying that a doctor's duty to treat his patients responsibly took precedence over the government's power to regulate drugs.[69] Not until the 1970s, therefore, did lithium really take off in the United States.

Why a two-decade delay in the adoption of lithium? For one thing lithium was a plentiful natural substance and had no industry backer. Hence no drug company was rooting for it. It also had to confront entrenched therapeutic nihilism on the part of the analysts in the United States and at the Maudsley Hospital in London, the premier training center for British psychiatry. Both Aubrey Lewis, professor of psychiatry at the Maudsley until 1966, and the pioneering epidemiologist Michael Shepherd considered lithium to be "dangerous nonsense."[70] (The British resisted chlorpromazine less because the firm May and Baker was flogging it.) Thus for needless years, patients with mania languished.

Schizophrenia and mania affected at best 2 percent of the population. Depression, by contrast, was a massive illness affecting as many as one individual in four. A drug to treat depression successfully would have almost the same appeal as aspirin. In the history of the cornucopia, it was now depression's turn, and news of a drug called imipramine came soon after Cade's announcement of lithium. Imipramine was the first drug in the history of psychiatry to act specifically against depression.[71]

In 1950, the J. R. Geigy pharmaceutical firm in Basel asked staff physicians at the Münsterlingen asylum in Switzerland to see if an antihistamine that Geigy had developed might serve as a sleeping pill. The pharmacological air was thick with excitement about antihistamines at the time. The Münsingen psychiatrists found that the drug had few hypnotic qualities, yet in their reply to Geigy speculated that it might serve as an antipsychotic, a suggestion the firm ignored.

One of these staffers was Roland Kuhn, then 38, a tall, distinguished, and cultivated psychiatrist who combined an exceptional grasp of the humanities with a background in biochemistry. As part of his medical training in Berne, Kuhn had done an elective in organic chemistry. He had received his psychiatric training at the Waldau asylum under the tutelage of Jakob Klaesi (of the deep-sleep cure). Kuhn had pioneered in Switzerland the use of electroencephalography for studying the brain's electrical activity. Yet at the same time he was, in his early years, an adept of psychoanalysis. He had undergone a training analysis and was a good friend of Ludwig Binswanger at the nearby Bellevue private clinic in Kreuzlingen. Kuhn also attended meetings of Max Müller's "Psychology Club" at the asylum in Münsingen. For Switzerland, it was not a contradiction that someone like Müller could champion the early shock treatments and at the same time be interested in psychology. Switzerland was probably the world epicenter of both psychodynamics and organic psychiatry in the years between 1933 and the 1950s, and Kuhn was right at its heart.

Then Kuhn had one of those road-to-Damascus-type experiences. He had been treating with psychoanalysis a young woman whose complaints seemed to be of a "neurotic-hysterical" nature. He made great progress with psychodynamic therapy, "bringing out unconscious material that corresponded exactly to Freud's theories. Everything went beautifully and she was cured.

"A few days later she came to my office again, garishly made-up and perfumed, with costume jewellery hanging all over her, dressed in loud colors . . . and demonstrating irritable and euphoric mood changes, pressured speech and flight of ideas." Kuhn then realized he had made a mistake. The correct diagnosis was mania. He had falsely ascribed a spontaneous recovery to his psychoanalytic "cure." As so often happened in those days, Kuhn had also missed her earlier depression, giving her a misdiagnosis of "hysteria." For Kuhn, manic-depressive illness was an organic condition having little to do with Freud's ideas.

Yet as Kuhn fell away from psychoanalysis, he asked himself, what can we do to help patients like this? Admitting her to the mental hospital for ECT seemed a bit much. "How often I said to myself, 'We should improve the opium cure!' But how?"

Then in 1952, the discovery of chlorpromazine became known. Kuhn and his colleagues put depression and mania at the back of their minds for the moment. The Münsterlingen staff received free samples of chlorpromazine from Rhône-Poulenc for trials on their schizophrenic patients, but the asylum's limited budget made them unable to order large amounts for routine use. In February 1954, the Münsterlingen staff asked Geigy to send some of the previous antihistamine back for trials on their psychotic patients. The substance (G 22150) turned out to be of some benefit but had unacceptable side effects—and was useless on their depression patients—so they returned it.

At this point, Kuhn was heading up Münsterlingen hospital's pharmacological initiatives. (Only in 1971 did he become director of the hospital.) Kuhn asked Geigy—or Geigy asked Kuhn, according to some accounts—if the hospital might try another drug in the antihistamine series, one with a chemical side chain exactly identical to chlorpromazine's (G 22355 was Geigy's internal code for the drug). The staff tried it on patients with schizophrenia. It made many of them worse, converting quiet chronic patients into agitated whirlwinds of energy. Kuhn consulted with Geigy scientists on what the drug could possibly be doing to procure such bizarre effects, and sometime in 1955 the decision was made to give it to some depressed patients. The response was "absolutely incredible, so exciting," electrifying both the hospital staff and the Geigy scientists who had been following all this with bated breath. Kuhn and the Geigy people had obviously discovered a drug that could relieve depression.[72]

In the first 40 depressed patients who had received it, some of the recoveries were dramatic. Kuhn: "The patients become generally more lively; their low depressive voices sound stronger. The patients appear more communicative, the yammering and crying come to an end. If the depression had manifested itself in a dissatisfied, plaintive, or irritable mood, a friendly, contented, and accessible spirit comes to the fore. Hypochondriacal and neurasthenic complaints recede or disappear entirely." Kuhn told of patients who now were ready to jump out of bed in the morning, to socialize easily with fellow patients, "to amuse themselves

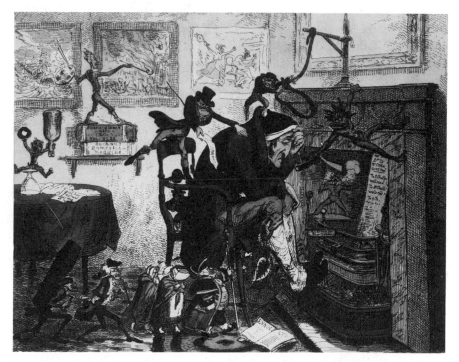

Depression before the introduction of imipramine (Tofranil) in 1958, the first drug specifically for the treatment of depression. Here George Cruickshank's 1823 caricature "The Blue Devils" (courtesy of The William L. Helfand Collection, Philadelphia Museum of Art).

and take part in the general life of the hospital, to write letters and interest themselves again in their family circumstances." At visiting hours, the
patients' relatives were astonished at the change, declaring, "We haven't
seen him this well for a long time." The patients themselves spoke of a
"miracle cure."[73]

The language in which Kuhn reported the transformation is interesting, because it illustrates how resurrectionlike the recovery from depression can be, a recovery that each new generation of antidepressent drugs
believes that it alone has achieved; witness the resurrectionist rhetoric
accompanying the introduction of the drug Prozac (see pp. 320–324).
Kuhn announced the drug at a meeting of the 2nd International Congress of Psychiatry in Zurich in September 1957. There were 12 people
in the audience.[74]

In the spring of 1958 Geigy named the compound imipramine
(Tofranil). Imipramine was the first of the "tricyclic" antidepressants, so
named because of their three-ring chemical structure (Chlorpromazine
has almost the same structure, differing only by two atoms). Given the
great utility of antidepressant drugs, rival tricyclics flooded the market,
the Merck Company, for example, bringing out amitryptiline (Elavil) in
1961. By 1980 American physicians were writing 10 million prescriptions
a year for antidepressants alone, the great majority of them tricyclics.
There would be several dozen brands to choose among.[75]

As the cornucopia opened its bounty, psychiatry acquired a new sense
of confidence. Psychiatrists were becoming actually able to make people
better. "With the introduction of modern treatments, it became relatively
easy to remove symptoms," said Felix Post, a veteran of the Maudsley who
specialized in geriatic psychiatry and was now thrilled that he could help
elderly patients with paranoid ideas or avoid institutionalizing those with
chronic depression (who formerly might have suicided if not admitted).
As Post put it, "In the past one had to carry psychiatric outpatients over
many months or years with bromides and very wearying supportive interviews: 'I.S.Q.' [In Status Quo] was usually the last or only entry in the
progress notes. Now most of these patients could be significantly improved. . . ." The availability of these new drugs had therefore transformed
the experience of psychiatry of Post's generation: "I started as a lone doctor," he said, "bewildered and frightened by the multitude of apparently
hopelessly ill and deteriorating patients. I end as a member of a professional team and with the certainty of being able to help to an important
extent almost all my patients."[76]

The discovery of the antipsychotics, antimanics, and antidepressants,
drugs that formed the pharmacological basis of the second biological

psychiatry, was owing to a mixture of scientific preparation and dumb luck. Yet the scientific interest they generated, and the profits that accrued from their sales, contributed to putting psychiatry on a much more solid scientific footing than it had previously been. This was a footing in the neurosciences.

Neuroscience

The neurosciences endeavor to make major psychiatric disorders understandable in terms of the chemistry and anatomic pathology of the brain. The conviction that this was feasible underlay the first biological psychiatry, although its representatives made little actual progress. As the young Heinrich Laehr, then an assistant physician at the asylum in Halle, said in 1852, "Insanity is nothing else than a disease, and only medical treatment can prevail against it." For Laehr, it was the chemistry of the brain that kept people in psychic equilibrium: "An extremely small chemical and physical change in the brain . . . will suffice to bring out a mental disorder."[77] This differs scarcely a whit from the explanation doctors would give patients 150 years later to the effect that, "You are suffering from an imbalance in brain chemistry." Yet Laehr and other psychiatrists, hunched over their microscopes for hours in the asylum, got nowhere. The task of understanding the brain was too vast for clinicians alone to undertake. In 1891, the Scottish psychiatrist Thomas Clouston adumbrated a grander vision of the neurosciences: "[Some day] it may be possible to take a larger, a more comprehensive, and a more physiological view of the whole subject of brain growth and development in its combined physiological and pathological aspects." Clouston even envisioned a neuroscience that could "classify the whole of the neuroses of development into one large and most interesting scheme—so giving a physiological coherence to what have been hitherto unrelated pathological facts."[78] By "neuroses of development" Clouston meant what would later be called schizophrenia and other disorders of brain growth. Yet for decades to come almost no progress was made on the difficult subject of brain chemistry in illness.[79]

The first comprehensive center for investigating the brain, mind, and their disorders was Kraepelin's Munich institute. Working alongside such researchers as the neuropathologist Walter Spielmeyer and the geneticist Hans Luxenburger, Felix Plaut took the first steps in the discipline of neuroimmunology, documenting the brain's immune reaction to syphilitic infiltration.[80] With the Nazi rise to power, this great institute lost its cutting edge. Plaut, for example, was driven in 1936 from his post as director of the Serology and Experimental Therapy laboratory to exile in London, where he suicided in 1940.[81]

After World War II, these threads were picked up again in other countries, so that by the time the first International Congress of Psychiatry met in Paris in 1950, there was a critical mass in the sciences underlying biological psychiatry. Each of the neurosciences on which the second biological psychiatry would later repose was present: Denis Hill, then a senior lecturer at the Institute of Psychiatry of the Maudsley Hospital, talked about the use of electroencephalography in psychiatry; he had pioneered the device in the study of schizophrenia.[82] The functional psychoses, he said, showed "a bewildering variety of anomalies and abnormalities" yet nothing specific for any given illness. (The technique would later be used for identifying developmental delay in child psychiatry.[83]) Max Reiss of Bristol, a refugee scientist from Prague and one of the founders of psychiatric endocrinology, talked about thyroid activity in psychiatric illness as measured with radioactive isotopes.[84] In 1950, Derek Richter had just arrived at Carshalton as the director of the Neuropsychiatric Research Centre and would go on to become a key figure in establishing the discipline of psychopharmacology in Britain. At the Paris conference, he described use of radiolabeled isotopes to follow metabolic activity in the brain.[85] Not all of these approaches would later turn out to be important in clinical psychiatry, but in Paris in 1950 pathways were sketched out that would permit the systematic investigation of the brain as the physical substrate of the disordered mind. The conference represented the true birth of clinical neuroscience as the term later became understood.

If any single individual should be considered the founder of biological psychiatry in the United States, it is probably Stanley Cobb, the Harvard neurologist who in 1934 founded a department of psychiatry at the Massachusetts General Hospital and therewith himself switched to the field of psychiatry. Cobb, who had extensive training in Europe, was interested in "psychobiology supported by the neurosciences." The words are those of neurosurgeon Wilder Penfield, and Penfield wrote about Cobb in the context of Penfield's wider interest in the life of Alan Gregg, the medical director of the Rockefeller Foundation, who from 1933 on funded research in the basic psychiatric sciences, especially neurophysiology and neurology. Gregg steered enough Rockefeller money to Cobb to permit him to do basic biological research at the Mass General for the next 20 years.[86] Out of Cobb's and Tracy Putnam's research came Dilantin, the first drug effective against epilepsy.[87] And out of Cobb's psychiatry department at the Mass General came a core of researchers such as Eli Robins (see p. 300) who would push forward biological thinking in psychiatry at a time when psychoanalysis was the order of the day.

In 1946, Cobb was part of a small group of researchers who met at the Fairmont Hotel in San Francisco. The meeting was organized by two California neurologists—Johannes ("J. M.") Nielsen and his student George Thompson (the following year they coauthored the first textbook of biological psychiatry in the United States[88]). From this gathering emerged the premier American organization in the biological field, the Society of Biological Psychiatry.[89] The founders saw themselves as continuing the first biological psychiatry. "The concept of the neuronal basis of psychiatry is not at all new," they noted, citing Meynert, Wernicke, and Flechsig. Yet since those days, the discipline had accumulated an "enormous superstructure of observations and interpretations." Now it was time to locate a brain substrate for all this clinical information about illness: "Those who seek to advance the biological concept wish only to build a foundation under that superstructure." "They wish . . . to trace the anatomical structures which make these concepts possible."[90] On both sides of the ocean, then, in the early 1950s small groups of researchers were determined to push the neuroscientific basis of biological psychiatry forward.

Perhaps the oldest component of the neurosciences was psychopharmacology, how drugs affect the brain and mind. The term goes back to a nonmedical usage in the late Renaissance, the cleric Urbanus Rhegius's *Psychopharmakon*, published posthumously in 1548.[91] The nineteenth century was dotted with efforts to use drugs as a means of studying the brain. In 1845, Jacques-Joseph Moreau (called "Moreau de Tours"), on staff at the private Parisian clinic of the recently deceased Esquirol, speculated that hashish could serve as a torchlight "in the mysteries of insanity, taking us back to the hidden source of these disorders that are so numerous, so variegated, and so strange." (Moreau himself took hashish for research purposes).[92] Two decades later, the great French physiologist Claude Bernard articulated the notion of using drugs to study the brain: "Poisons represent a means of analyzing the qualities of the nervous system, a kind of physiological scalpel, much more delicate and subtle than ordinary scalpels. . . ."[93] This was the gist of psychopharmacology: a scalpel with which to delineate and treat disorders of the mind and brain. Then in the 1880s, Kraepelin himself conducted the first systematic research on the effect of drugs upon the brain, coining the term "pharmacopsychology," though he saw no therapeutic application for the technique.[94]

264

Forty years later, things had changed very little. In 1920, the Johns Hopkins' pharmacologist David Macht, describing "the effect of drugs on psychological functions," said, "The number of contributions to the domain of what we may be permitted to call 'psychopharmacology' is certainly very meagre."[95]

The discovery of LSD in 1943 touched off another round of efforts to use drugs for chiseling out various psychological processes, in this case inducing psychosis experimentally.[96] Yet LSD became a street drug of abuse and this research led to no clinical payoffs.

With the discovery of chlorpromazine and the other early psychoactive drugs, the study of psychopharmacology came into its own. The physiological scalpel had been achieved. The new discipline set out to determine the mechanism of action of the various antipsychotic and antidepressant drugs. The first push in this direction came from Germany, a land effectively ostracized from the international psychiatric community until the mid-1950s. And this initial impetus itself represented a neat bridge between old and new. In 1956, Wolfgang de Boor, a professor at Cologne and graduate of Heidelberg, wrote a textbook of psychopharmacology.[97] This was the first in the world. At Heidelberg, de Boor had been a student of Kurt Schneider, one of the great modern investigators of schizophrenia. But it was at the urging not of Schneider but of Willy Hellpach that de Boor wrote the textbook. Hellpach had been one of Kraepelin's students at Heidelberg. Indeed, Kraepelin's textbook had inspired the young psychologist Hellpach to go into psychiatry. Now in the early 1950s, sick with revulsion at the recent Nazi past, Hellpach wanted to steer German psychiatry once again toward science. These men were academics.

Yet for the most part, the new psychopharmacology was driven by the drug industry and not by the academy. It was de Boor who in 1957 proposed founding the international college of neuropharmacology (CINP are its Latin initials), but Ernst Rothlin, director of the Sandoz Company, was its first president.[98] It was in the area of psychopharmacology that the private sector made a fundamental contribution to neuroscience. The drug industry funded research into such matters as chlorpromazine's action on the brain because only advances in basic science would permit the design of drugs specifically tailored to block whatever biochemical or anatomical pathways were causing psychotic illness. In fact, one could call psychopharmacology the creation of the drug industry, rather than of the academy or clinicians. In the 1960s and after, the discipline became big business in the United States and Britain, the two countries where it most flourished.

Dopamine and serotonin in particular would be the chief players in this psychopharmacological saga, and to find the origin of interest in them we return to 1952. In that year, Betty Twarog, a recent Harvard PhD working in the laboratory of Professor John Welsh, identified serotonin as a neurotransmitter (they worked with a small sample provided by Abbott Laboratories). A year later, she and Irvine Page of the Cleveland Clinic found serotonin in the mammalian brain.[99]

In 1957, pharmacologist Arvid Carlsson and coworkers of the University of Lund in Sweden discovered that dopamine was a neurotransmitter.[100] Carlsson's name recurs again and again in this story, and he is initially associated with establishing the presence of these chemicals in the brain. This was a first cut at applying neuroscience to psychiatry.

Did chlorpromazine and the other antipsychotics that were rapidly being developed work against dopamine? When Carlsson—now at the University of Göteborg—gave them to mice in 1963, dopamine levels in the mouse brain changed. He did not specifically implicate dopamine at that point, but he thought there was a strong possibility that the dopamine system was a site of action for these drugs.[101]

But what about humans with schizophrenia as opposed to well mice? The suspicion arose that dopamine itself made schizophrenia worse, or even caused schizophrenia. This suspicion was strengthened by the finding that amphetamines, which potentiated the action of dopamine, made the symptoms of schizophrenia worse.[102]

Meanwhile, serotonin became implicated in depression. In the mid-1950s, researchers at the National Institutes of Health—picking up on earlier English work—came to believe that imbalances in serotonin, or "5-HT" as psychopharmacologists still refer to it (5-hydroxytryptamine), were responsible for some psychiatric illnesses. It's worth following this particular powder trail because it ends with Prozac. Yet at the beginning, these researchers were not interested in serotonin because they thought it was involved in depression but rather in psychosis.

The trail was ignited in 1955 at Bernard ("Steve") Brodie's Laboratory of Chemical Pharmacology at the National Heart Institute. Brodie and team discovered that if one gave a compound called reserpine to animals, serotonin vanished from their tissues, including the brain.[103] This finding was the first hard-core link between biochemistry and behavior.[104]

This link began to be strengthened as various researchers discovered that the new psychiatric drugs changed the chemistry of the brain. When, for example, a group of English scientists gave imipramine to depressed patients in 1960, their blood levels of serotonin dropped way off. This was the beginning of the discovery of the "reuptake mechanism":

Antidepressant drugs caused serotonin to be sequestered somewhere in the body[105] (particularly, as it turned out, in the synapses between the neurons). Eight years later, Arvid Carlsson, who had worked in Brodie's lab in 1955, pinned this down in the chemistry of the brain itself rather than merely reasoning from what was happening in blood platelets, as the English had done: The tricyclic antidepressants prevented the neurons from taking back serotonin once they had released it into the synapse. The less the reuptake, the more remaining in the synapse, the more available to work against depression. Carlsson thus fortified a "serotonin hypothesis" of depression.[106]

While this research on brain chemicals, or neurotransmitters, was going on, the whole mechanism of neurotransmission itself, involving receptors for these chemicals at downstream neurons, was being uncovered. This first tapping toward a theory of neurotransmission was Arvid Carlsson's previously mentioned work in 1963: If drugs modified dopamine, maybe dopamine helped carry the nerve impulse about the brain. Then in 1974, Solomon Snyder of Johns Hopkins University noted that antipsychotics such as chlorpromazine attach themselves to the site of the dopamine receptor, preventing dopamine from acting.[107] The key to therapy therefore must lie in modifying the action of neurotransmitters at the receptor site.

Until the 1980s, research in the field tended to be organized along the lines of one-neurotransmitter, one-disease: the catecholamines, meaning such natural brain chemicals as noradrenalin, were assigned to mood disorders. This was called the "amine hypothesis of depression." It later included serotonin. Such neurotransmitters as dopamine were linked to psychosis; and acetylcholine was paired with dementia.[108]

The one-transmitter-one-disease hypothesis seemed so reasonable (and was, moreover, a perfect marketing concept for the drug companies). Yet correlation does not necessarily mean causation. The one-one paradigm tended to collapse in the 1980s. Highly effective antipsychotic drugs such as clozapine were discovered to have little impact on dopamine metabolism but instead affected serotonin. (Although clozapine was discovered in the mid-1970s, only after 1988 did the implications of it for the treatment of schizophrenia begin to sink in.) As more and more neurotransmitters were identified—over 40 by the mid-1990s—it became apparent that dopamine and serotonin were only two of many transmitters involved in these complex psychiatric disorders and probably did not play a master role.[109] Yet over the years, the one-transmitter-one-disease hypothesis proved highly fruitful in terms of stimulating research on basic brain mechanisms. Somehow these drugs did work, and their very efficacy opened up the domain of the neurosciences in a way that previous hypotheses had not.

Neuropathology—physical lesions in brain tissue—provided yet another leg of support for the neuroscientific interpretation of psychiatric illness. The anatomic study of schizophrenia had once been considered "the graveyard of neuropathologists."[110] Meynert had wrecked his health peering into his microscope, and subsequent generations of psychoanalytically oriented historians made merry of his attempts to identify an anatomic basis for the disease. But Meynert was right. Later neuropathologists, using sophisticated techniques of which he never dreamed, succeeded in discovering the lesions he was seeking. In the 1970s, it was neuropathology that began to discover the answer to one of the great riddles of schizophrenia: Why, if it was a genetic disease, did about half the people who got it come from families with no history of psychiatric illness? The answer turned out to be that nongenetic anomalies in the womb and obstetrical trauma could also damage the developing brain in a way that made it vulnerable to psychotic illness later in life.

This kind of research went back to the neuropathological work that Kraepelin and Spielmeyer had initiated in Munich and that Rosanoff had spark-plugged in the United States. In 1939, for example, Barney Katz, a student of Rosanoff's at the University of Southern California, compared obstetrical data on 100 male schizophrenics and 100 male controls: The patients with schizophrenia had experienced more obstetrical trauma. After World War II, this kind of histopathological research became taboo under the influence of psychodynamic psychiatry, to be relegitimated in the 1970s. At that point, many students of schizophrenia starting discovering problems in the wiring of the fetal brain during development. Joyce Kovelman and Arnold Scheibel of the University of California at Los Angeles, using techniques far more sophisticated than those available to Meynert, began doing autopsies on the brains of patients with schizophrenia who had died at a veterans' hospital in Los Angeles. Looking at a total of 13,680 neurons from 10 patients, they found that in certain brain areas the neurons of the schizophrenics were much more disorganized than those of controls, evidently a result of the failure of migrating fetal brain cells to link up to their targets. "It seems unlikely that the disorientation of cell-dendrite patterns which we have described can develop at any time except during embryogenesis," they noted.[111] Another group of scholars determined that individuals with schizophrenia had large numbers of abnormally sized neurons.[112] None of these events could possibly be a consequence of the disease because they occur during fetal development.

268

Viruses may disrupt fetal brain development. A cohort of Helsinki mothers had been exposed to a severe influenza epidemic in the second trimester of pregnancy (when brain development is most rapid). Twenty-six years later, their children turned out to have exceptional rates of schizophrenia.[113] A much larger survey of 40 years of influenza and schizophrenia among children born in Denmark in the years 1910 to 1950 came up with the same findings.[114]

The response of the brain to these inflammations and disruptions of neuron migration and connectivity is called gliosis: a proliferation of glial cells. As early as 1972, researchers began finding the kind of gliosis that is associated with fetal maldevelopment in adult schizophrenics at autopsy. In 1982, Janice Stevens at St. Elizabeths Hospital in Washington conducted a study of the brains of 25 schizophrenic patients who had died in the hospital, compared with a similar number of brains of non-schizophrenic patients at St. Elizabeths and of nonpsychiatric patients at a general hospital. She found substantial gliosis, particularly in those brain areas where other studies had showed changes in schizophrenia. The gliosis was not a result of ECT or drugs.[115]

Finally, what Meynert did not have at his disposal were the postmodern methods of brain imaging, particularly computed-tomography (CT), magnetic resonance (MR), and positron-emission-tomography (PET) which became available in the 1970s and after, permitting overviews of the brain of extraordinary clarity. In 1976, Eve Johnstone, Timothy Crow and other researchers at the Clinical Research Centre in London-Harrow did a CT study of 17 schizophrenic patients in the hospital, compared with a group of age-matched volunteers who worked at jobs similar to those of the patients before they fell ill. It became apparent at once that the brains of a number of the schizophrenics had a different topography than the non-schizophrenics. Particularly their cerebral ventricles, the reservoir of cerebrospinal fluid in the brain, were enlarged, the degree of enlargement directly proportional to the degree of impairment.[116] This enlargement was the result of the failure of the tissue around the ventricles to grow.[117] Meynert, laboring at his workbench on microscopic sections, had been unable to gain an overview of such structures as the ventricles. But the imaging techniques of the late twentieth century were able to open up the brain to an extent never before imaginable.

By the mid-1990s, the evidence of neuropathology pointed overwhelmingly to schizophrenia as an organic disease. As neuropharmacologist Floyd Bloom concluded in 1993 (he was at the time at the Scripps Research Institute in La Jolla, California, later editor-in-chief of *Science* magazine), "The wealth of evidence attesting to a substantial neuropathology in schizophrenia leaves few doubters."[118]

Kraepelin's "dementia praecox" had cast the net too widely. As an organic brain disease, schizophrenia seemed to have two faces. One face, neurodevelopmental in nature, affected males more than females in their teens and early twenties. The other face was probably not neurodevelopmental (the cause remaining uncertain) and struck at mid-life, affecting females more than males.

Yet the accent was on the growing brain. Early-onset schizophrenia seemed to occur in a kind of "two hit" model affecting the brains of fetuses and small children. The first "hit" was genetic, the second uterine trauma or even some later biological or psychosocial life event such as a difficult birth.[119] These events would leave behind physical and behavioral traces, such as smaller heads or the inability to play with other children, that represented fossilized evidence of pathology at the beginning of life.[120] In the mid-1990s, the causes of this failure of development were still unclear. It could be a virus, or genes switching off prematurely. Or, as Bloom put it, "the genome [genes] of a given family tree might 'simply' fail to maintain the expression of one or another of the genes required to complete the process of cortical neuronal migration."[121]

In the 1980s, brain imaging and other neuropathological techniques turned up an organic substrate in a number of psychiatric illnesses apart from schizophrenia. Enlarged ventricles also occurred in manic-depressive illness and were not unique to schizophrenia, suggesting that it too may arise during gestation.[122] From 1987 on, a string of researchers found anatomic and physiological changes in obsessive-compulsive disorder, an illness that psychoanalyst Otto Fenichel had explained in 1934 as "the ego hav[ing] already begun to adopt protective measures at the time of the original anal sadistic level of libido organization, so that the patient never reached the phallic oedipus complex."[123] It is hard to imagine more differing explanations.

Which was right? Was it the failure of the personality to evolve from the anal sadistic level or was it brain biology that caused obsessive-compulsive disorder? In 1987, one group of researchers attempted to sort this out with the use of positron emission tomography, in which a special camera followed the uptake in the brain of a radioactive isotope attached to glucose: Active parts of the brain would absorb this radiolabeled glucose. In these studies, patients with obsessive-compulsive disorder were given stimuli ("contaminants") that were known to set off a patient's ritualistic handwashing or some other form of behavior. A gamma camera then followed the isotope's pattern of uptake as the handwashing urge

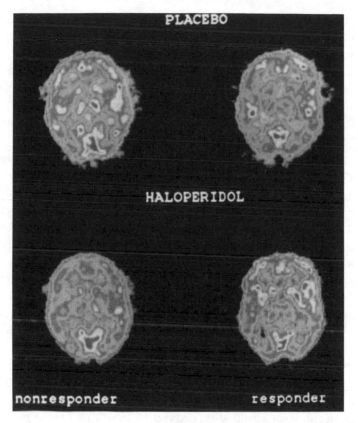

A PET scan (positron emission tomography) of the brains of two patients with schizophrenia on the left and right sides of the page respectively. The upper-right side shows one patient before treatment with the antipsychotic, or neuroleptic, drug haloperidol. (Before being given haloperidol, the patient had been receiving a placebo.) Before the real treatment began, this patient demonstrated quite a low level of metabolism in the deep structures of the brain called the basal ganglia. In the lower right photo, after receiving haloperidol the same patient's metabolic activity has clearly speeded up: The neurons have lighted up as they absorb a radiolabelled form of glucose.

The left side features a schizophrenic patient who did not respond to haloperidol. The pretreatment image of this patient (upper left) is similar to that of the patient who responded, with pretreatment metabolism being a bit higher. But after this patient is given the drug, he or she fails to respond: Glucose uptake in the basal ganglia does not increase: The neurons there do not light up.

The significance of this study is that patients who respond well to haloperidol tend to be those with low metabolism in their basal ganglia before treatment: Treatment seems to "normalize" metabolic activity.

Source: "Striatal Metabolic Rate and Clinical Response to Neuroleptics in Schizophrenia" by Monte S. Buchsbaum et al., *Archives of General Psychiatry,* 49 (1992), pp. 966–974, photo p. 969. Used by permission. Contrast in the original photo was enhanced because the PET computer prints images in color.

seized hold of the brain. (The patients were permitted to wash their hands between each scanning in order to return their symptoms to baseline level before receiving the next contaminant.)[124] By 1994, it had been established that a loop of electrical activity from the frontal lobe to the basal ganglia then back to the frontal lobe provided an important anatomic substrate of obsessive-compulsive disorder.[125] Such patients then improved (and blood-flow patterns changed) after the administration of a psychoactive drug (Prozac).[126]

Biological psychiatry thus became able to investigate the causes and treatments of psychiatric illness by using the scientific method, a method other psychiatrists had virtually abandoned for half a century. Only alliance with geneticists, pharmacologists, radiologists, biochemists, and pathologists made these kinds of advances possible. The Society for Neuroscience, formed of such disciplines, grew from 250 members at its founding in 1971 to more than 11,000 by the late 1980s. Their assignment: to investigate the thousands of gene products made by the brain.[127]

Yet psychiatrists are not really basic scientists; they are clinicians. Part of their mission is making patients feel good while helping them to feel better. They must buttress the human side of the doctor-patient relationship, which is after all an encounter between two human beings, while puzzling about the patient's genetic background, brain anatomy, and the most effective choice of drugs.

In the world of the clinic, it turned out to be unwise for the psychiatrist to take on the airs of a laboratory scientist, and those who did were rebuked in the massive outpouring of rage in the 1960s and after called the antipsychiatry movement. Antipsychiatry went hand in hand with the greatest debacle of twentieth-century psychiatry: the return of patients to "the community," sometimes known as deinstitutionalization. Both may only be understood as unwitting consequences of biological psychiatry.

Antipsychiatry

The history of medicine is full of ironies. One irony is that, in the 1960s and 1970s, the crown of victory was snatched from the physician's head at the very moment that he or she became able to cure organic disease in the body. In these years, primary care in general witnessed a new alienation in the doctor-patient relationship, a consequence of doctors, who knew that they could now cure patients with penicillin, neglecting the psychological side of their relationship with their patients.[128]

Similarly in psychiatry, the advent of effective new medications for psychosis and neurosis may have induced a certain insouciance toward the patients' need to feel cared for. A five-minute interview to check for drug side effects is not the same as the lengthy and persuasive expression of concern that psychotherapeutically oriented psychiatrists tended to display. It was the very aura of science, which the antipsychiatry movement would always put in mocking quotation marks, rather than custodialism as such that drew the protesters' rage: In the iconography of the movement the psychiatrist would be depicted with antennas on his head contemplating a naked female figure atop an oscilloscope, or wearing a space helmet and grimly proferring an outstretched hypodermic syringe.[129] Somehow, psychiatry's very real shift to science was associated with an imputed loss of caring.

Many other factors as well helped germinate the antipsychiatry movement, not merely changes within psychiatry itself. The whole social climate of the 1960s fostered hostility toward authority, medical and

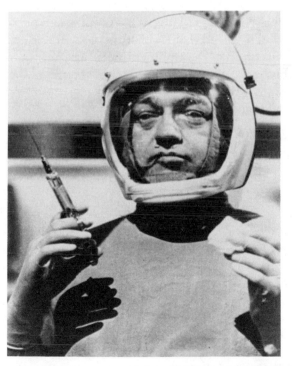

The antipsychiatry movement's image of biological psychiatrists.
Source: Madness Network News Reader, 1974, p. 91.

273

otherwise. Leftist writers saw in psychiatry the controlling arm of "the bourgeoisie," Karl Marx's term for the stock- and bond-holding upper middle classes. Early feminist writers saw in the male psychiatrist the comprador representative of the male gender, extending patriarchal power over women.

Yet a handful of intellectuals in particular became identified with the antipsychiatry movement.[130] And the force of their ideas brewed up a mass hostility to the advance of biological thinking within psychiatry. The movement's basic argument was that psychiatric illness is not medical in nature but social, political, and legal: Society defines what schizophrenia or depression is, and not nature. If psychiatric illness is thus socially constructed, it must be deconstructed in the interest of freeing deviants, free spirits, and exceptional creative people from the stigma of being "pathological."[131] In other words, there really was no such thing as psychiatric illness. It was a myth.

Although antipsychiatry movements had flourished throughout the nineteenth century, their late-twentieth-century rebirth began with the virtually simultaneous publication in the early 1960s of a series of exceptionally influential books on psychiatry. Most famous perhaps of these was Michel Foucault's *Madness and Civilization*, published in 1961 (see p. 276), which argued that the notion of mental illness was a social and cultural invention of the eighteenth century. Yet there were several other blockbusters, and collectively they became the intellectual springboard from which the theorists of deinstitutionalization of the late 1960s would launch themselves.

Earliest of the founding fathers—they were all men—was Thomas Szasz, a Budapest-born psychoanalyst, who had trained just after World War II in Chicago. When called to active service in the Navy in 1954, Szasz, who was then 34, used the time to put down on paper a notion that had long troubled him, that mental illness was in fact a "myth," a medical misapprehension foisted on individuals who had problems in living. In his 1960 book *The Myth of Mental Illness*, he called the whole notion of psychiatric illness "scientifically worthless and socially harmful."[132] The book enjoyed wide currency and the American intellectual class began asking, if there is no such thing as mental illness, how can we justify locking people up in asylums?

Sociologist Erving Goffman's work *Asylums*, published in 1961, had an even greater impact on intellectuals. In the context of a fellowship in 1955–1956 at the National Institute of Mental Health, he did field work at St. Elizabeths, an institution that, at the time, had over 6,000 patients. He didn't like what he saw, interpreting the asylum as a "total institution," or closed system that infantilized patients and restricted their lives. "Every social arrangement in a mental hospital seems to point to the profound difference between a staff doctor and a mental patient." On admission, said Goffman, "the recruit [the patient] begins a series of abasements, degradations, humiliations, and profanations of self." As with inmates in prisons, among psychiatric patients "there is a strong feeling that time spent in the establishment is time wasted or destroyed or taken from one's life; it is time that must be written off; it is something that must be 'done' or 'marked' or 'put in' or 'pulled.' . . . As a result, the inmate tends to feel that for the duration of his required stay—his sentence—he has been totally exiled from living." Although many of Goffman's criticisms were justified, again the underlying assumption was that there was no such thing as mental illness and that the pretension of professionals to treat it was nothing more than a shameless power-grab. As for psychiatric illnesses that might justify confining a patient, there were, thought Goffman, none.[133]

The works of Foucault, Szasz, and Goffman were influential among university elites, cultivating a rage against mental hospitals and the whole psychiatric enterprise. Yet the book that did most to inflame the public imagination against psychiatry was a novel written by Ken Kesey. Kesey had just finished taking a creative writing course at Stanford when he volunteered for government LSD experiments conducted at a veterans administration hospital at Menlo Park. He stayed on to take a job as an orderly at the hospital. Out of this experience came his 1962 novel *One Flew Over the Cuckoo's Nest*, a book that formed the image of psychiatry for an entire generation of university students. Kesey's notion of psychiatric illness was embodied in the novel's antihero, Randle McMurphy:

> [McMurphy] says he was just a wanderer and logging bum before the Army took him and taught him what his natural bent was . . . they taught him to play poker. Since then he's settled down and devoted himself to gambling on all levels. Just play poker and stay single and live where and how he wants to, if people would let him, he says, "but you know how society persecutes a dedicated man."

Indeed: Society persecuted McMurphy by locking him in jail a few times and then when he proved too troublesome, putting him in a psychiatric hospital.[134] The message: Psychiatric patients are not ill, they're merely deviant. In 1975, director Milos Forman made the novel into a movie that became United Artists' biggest-ever hit at the time. It swept the Academy Awards of that year by winning all five main Oscars.

In 1966, sociologist Thomas Scheff, at the University of California at Santa Barbara, determined that the real problem in so-called psychiatric illness was "labeling." "Most chronic mental illness is at least in part a social role," said Scheff. "The societal reaction is usually the most important determinant of entry into that role." Mental illness itself, which Scheff always put in ironical quotation marks, was nothing more than deviance. When society labels a rule-breaker as mentally ill, the effect is to stabilize the deviance, to let the "agents of social control" identify him or her as a target. A diagnosis of mental illness, therefore, said nothing about the person, it meant rather that the system was incapable of accommodating deviance.[135] (Of this entire approach, St. Louis psychiatrist Samuel Guze said, "Nearly all of us who spend our lives working with psychiatric patients and their families consider the 'labeling theory' fundamentally ludicrous."[136])

Among the earliest of the antipsychiatry writers in Britain was Ronald D. Laing, author in 1960 of *The Divided Self*. A Scot, Laing had trained in psychiatry at Glasgow and in psychoanalysis at the Tavistock Clinic in London. Like Szasz, he then turned on analysis. In his early work, he proposed a psychology of schizophrenia in which apparently gibberish speech was just designed "to throw dangerous people off the scent. . . . The schizophrenic is often making a fool of himself and the doctor. He is playing at being mad. . . ."[137] Laing later charged that sick families were the cause of schizophrenia and that the so-called illness in fact represented a gifted and creative state of consciousness, a sane response to a mad society. As he said in 1964, schizophrenics were off "explor[ing] the inner space and time of consciousness." "Perhaps we will learn to accord to so-called schizophrenics who have come back to us, perhaps after years, no less respect than the often no less lost explorers of the Renaissance." "Future generations," said Laing, "will see that what we call 'schizophrenia' was one of the forms in which, often through quite ordinary people, the light began to break through the cracks in our all-too-closed minds."[138] Incredibly, Laing became the chief investigator in the schizophrenia research unit at the Tavistock.

Foucault himself acquired official entree to progressive Anglo-Saxon circles with the publication in 1967 in the *New Statesman* of Laing's full-page review of the abridged English translation of Foucault's *Histoire de la Folie*, entitled *Madness and Civilization*.[139] At this point, Foucault became the chief authority on the wickedness of the psychiatric enterprise.

By the end of the 1960s, the antipsychiatric interpretation of "so-called psychiatric illness" had gained the catbird seat among intellectuals both in the United States and Europe. In these circles, a consensus had formed that the discipline of psychiatry was an illegitimate form of social control and that psychiatrists' power to lock people up must be abolished with the abolition of institutionalized psychiatric care, Pinel's therapeutic asylum.

Even though these interpretations were very popular among college students and intellectuals, actual patients found them less convincing. Joanne Greenberg, author as "Hannah Green" of *I Never Promised You a Rose Garden*, had a real psychiatric illness. She hated the Kesey book. She later said, "Creativity and mental illness are *opposites*, not complements. It's a confusion of mental illness with creativity. . . . Craziness is the opposite [of imagination]: it is a fort that's a prison."

"Some of the people at the [Chestnut] Lodge were people who were too soft on mental illness in that they thought it was creative and lovely or at least until they had seen enough of it. People would tell you what perceptive things a patient had said. The thing is I want to choose my perceptions. I don't want them to come out of some kind of unconscious soup. I want it to be something I choose to say, not something that says me."[140] Yet in the 1960s and 1970s, something that says me was still considered a positive experience, and persons undergoing it were to be sheltered from psychiatry. Above all, they were to be sheltered from the asylum.

Return to "the Community"

Long before the rise of the antipsychiatry movement, the destruction of the asylum had begun. Patients were to be returned to "the community." That the very phrase now turns to ashes in one's mouth is evidence of one of the greatest social debacles of our time.

Yet the pre-1960s asylum was not exactly a triumph of civilization. As early as World War II, the public began to learn from the negative reports of conscientious objectors doing service there that mental hospitals had become pretty desperate places. In 1946, crusading journalist Albert Deutsch, who had known Clifford Beers and had been active in the mental-hygiene movement, set out to investigate the state of the country's asylums. Taking a photographer with him, he toured mainly those "located in or near great centers of American wealth and culture." Deutsch's 1948 book *The Shame of the States* reflected the horrors of what he had seen. Gone was the sheltering environment that William White had evoked several decades previously, with its kindly but paternalistic superintendent and family-style staff.[141] Deutsch painted a picture of men and women who had been flung into misery and then seemingly forgotten. "One of the most poignant scenes in a mental hospital—one witnessed on every visit—is that of patients timidly pulling at a doctor's arm or coat as he rushed through the ward on rounds:

> "'Doctor, can I see you for just a minute?'
> "'Sorry, next time, next time,' is the invariable answer.
> "'What else can I do?' one doctor recently told me, despairingly. 'I know I should see many more patients individually. But how can I when I have five hundred patients under my care?'"

At the Philadelphia State Hospital for Mental Diseases—known to locals as "Byberry"—Deutsch saw "hundreds of patients sleeping in damp, bug-ridden basements. Noisy and violent patients made life intolerable in barnlike dayrooms because there weren't seclusion rooms where they might be isolated until calmed down." The hospital did not have enough personnel to administer insulin coma therapy. And the photographs Deutsch published of the male "incontinent ward" were truly hair-raising, like "a scene out of Dante's Inferno," as he put it. "Three hundred nude men stood, squatted and sprawled in this bare room, amid shrieks, groans, and unearthly laughter."[142]

The nation was appalled. Early in 1949, 20th Century-Fox released a movie of Mary Jane Ward's partly autobiographical novel about mental illness *The Snake Pit*, starring Olivia de Havilland. *Time* magazine previewed it in December 1948 with a smiling de Havilland on the cover, the face of madness just behind her. "When the superintendent of nurses at a California institution visited the set," *Time* revealed, "she looked at the sobbing, muttering, staring women and said, 'Why, they all look like my own girls.'"[143]

Midst this horrendous publicity for psychiatry, on which the antipsychiatric movement would later feed, several basic realities were obscured. One is that most patients younger than 65 were discharged relatively rapidly from mental hospitals: They did not experience prolonged stays to say nothing of lifelong incarceration. In the years 1946 to 1950 at Warren State Hospital in Warren, Pennsylvania, almost 80 percent of all patients under 65 were released within five years.[144] Second, much of the bizarre posturing and disordered movement that Deutsch and later antipsychiatric writers ascribed to "hospitalism," meaning the iatrogenic

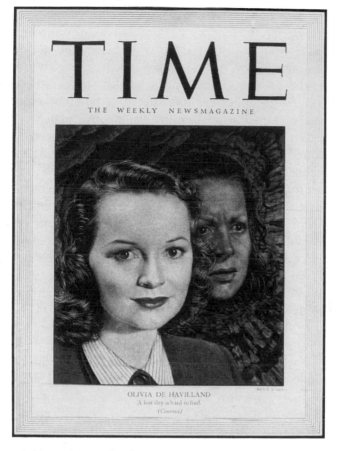

TIME

THE WEEKLY NEWSMAGAZINE

OLIVIA DE HAVILLAND
A lost day is hard to find.
(Cinema)

Time cover of Olivia de Havilland, starring in "The Snake Pit" released in 1949 (Copyright 1948 Time Inc., reprinted by permission).

results of institutionalization, turned out to be an inherent biological feature of such illnesses as schizophrenia that, in affecting the entire brain, affect the entire nervous system as well.[145] Third, even though conditions in mental hospitals were unsettling enough, there were worse alternatives. One was being tossed to the mercy of the streets.

What initiated the massive discharge of psychiatric patients to the "community," a process known as deinstitutionalization, was the introduction of antipsychotic drugs in 1954, the year the Food and Drug Administration licensed chlorpromazine.[146] Once it became possible to calm agitated patients and abolish psychosis with drugs, patients could in theory live quite easily in normal community settings until the psychosis finally just burned itself out. Henry Brill, assistant commissioner of mental hygiene in New York State, was among the earliest to initiate use of the new drugs. In January 1955, undertaking considerable risk to his own career from hostile Freudians, he began the use of chlorpromazine and reserpine in the New York public hospitals. Within the next 12 months, the decline in the state's resident psychiatric population began.[147] Similar declines were soon precipitated elsewhere. In a strict sense, therefore, deinstitutionalization was a consequence of the second biological psychiatry and not the antipsychiatry movement.

In the United States, the number of patients in state and county mental hospitals declined from its historic high of 559,000 in 1955 to 338,000 in 1970, further to 107,000 in 1988, representing a decrease over the 30 year period of more than 80 percent.[148] The red bricks lost four-fifths of their patients. In 1955, 77 percent of all psychiatric "patient care episodes" occurred in mental hospitals, in 1990 only 26 percent. Amplifying the shift was a fivefold expansion in the total volume of care in mental-health organizations over that period, from 1.7 million episodes in 1955 to 8.6 million in 1990.[149] This was a shift in the locus of care virtually without precedent in the history of medicine.

Yet if drug therapy kicked deinstitutionalization off, what kept it going, driving patients of all kinds into the community whether they were treatable with drugs or not? It was the combined pressure of the antipsychiatry movement outside of medicine and of the ideology of community psychiatry within medicine. The antipsychiatry movement preached that mental hospitals as such were wicked, given that there was no such thing as mental illness. And well-meaning psychiatrists who had absorbed the teachings of Joshua Bierer, Thomas Main and others, believed that "therapeutic communities" could be constituted out there in the cold streets of the big cities, a romanticized vision of welcoming friends and neighbors clasping the mentally ill to their bosoms. The National Institute for Mental Health, created by the Mental Health Act in 1946, was partly responsible for the propagation of this myth. The institute was supposed to administer the Community Mental Health Centers spawned by John F. Kennedy's 1963 legislation. But the CMHC's soon became diverted to psychotherapy sessions for the walking well, and in the first decades of deinstitutionalization no administrative arrangements were made to receive the actively ill patients who were simply being pushed out of the mental-hospital doors.[150]

Deinstitutionalization therefore became the true "shame of the states" in the United States. A third of the homeless were in fact mentally ill, unable to organize their lives and find shelter or work. Other discharged patients drifted into the criminal justice system, one study finding that

14 percent of county-jail inmates had had previous psychiatric treatment.[151] The community structures that were supposed to receive them turned out to be nursing homes and boarding houses.[152] And the antipsychotic medications that in hospital had provided such effective relief were often not taken once the patients were on the street because of tardive dyskinesia, the troublesome side effect that caused facial twitches and other involuntary movements.[153] "The street people, among the most helpless of adult human beings, are the natural prey of anyone looking for some loose change, a pack of cigarettes, a bottle," said one account. "They are rabbits forced to live in company with dogs."[154]

It was the politics of "discharge and be damned," said a British psychiatrist returning to the United States decades after having worked there in the early 1950s. "At least when I visited them [during my first trip] they had a home, inadequate as it was in many ways, and they were cared for, although the standard of care may not have been of the best. But despite all the shortcomings, life for those hapless, helpless, chronically sick people must be infinitely worse now that there is no alternative to the sidewalk, the doss-house, or the prison."[155]

In the 1980s, a backlash to these desperate conditions took place, as general hospitals and private psychiatric hospitals began admitting increasing numbers of psychiatric patients. The total number of private psychiatric hospitals in the United States increased from 150 in 1970 to 444 in 1988.[156] Of the 1.6 million Americans admitted to psychiatric institutions in 1994, 43 percent were in a general hospital, 35 percent in a state or county asylum, and 11 percent in a private mental hospital.[157] Ultimately therefore, the antipsychiatry movement failed. And community psychiatry though worthy in spirit became discredited as a practical means of treating serious psychiatric illnesses that, not having arisen in the community, could not be cured in it either.

The Battle over ECT

Before antipsychiatry faded, however, it left a last poisoned dart lying in the path: hostility to electroconvulsive therapy, or ECT. Throughout the 1950s, ECT had been regularly practiced. It counted merely as one psychiatric treatment among many and had no particular public profile. The *Reader's Guide to Periodical Literature*, for example, listed only one article on the subject in the entire decade, in *Science Digest* by journalist Lucy Freeman asserting that, "despite some amazing results . . . we're overdoing shock treatments."[158]

All this changed dramatically with the advent of the antipsychiatry movement in the early 1960s. The antipsychiatrists charged that ECT damaged the brain, that it was used as a form of discipline rather than therapy, and that it was therapeutically useless in any event. (It was in fact true that state asylums sometimes threatened patients with ECT to keep them in line, witness the "Georgia Power Cocktail" at Milledgeville.[159]) Yet since there was little evidence for the assertions about brain damage and therapeutic nullity, the ferocity of the opposition to ECT—for hostility to it became a kind of religious crusade—must have been based on something else. In retrospect, it was probably a cultural squeamishness about passing electricity into the body based on association with electrocution and the death penalty. There is no mistaking the hostility that ECT generated among the antipsychiatrists. Goffman, for example, referred to it scantingly in *Asylums*, where the sinister psychiatrists refused to show patients the ECT room in advance.[160]

Yet it was Kesey's book above all that identified ECT with psychiatric wickedness in the public mind, referring to "that filthy brain-murdering room that the black boys [the orderlies] call the 'Shock Shop.'" Here is what happened to poor "Ruckly" after they gave him ECT in the Cuckoo's Nest:

They brought him back to the ward two weeks later, bald and the front of his face an oily purple bruise and two little button-sized plugs stitched one above each eye. You can see by his eyes how they burned him out over there; his eyes are all smoked up and gray and deserted inside like blown fuses. All day now he won't do a thing but hold an old photograph up in front of that burned-out face, turning it over and over in his cold fingers, and the picture wore gray as his eyes on both sides with all his handling till you can't tell any more what it used to be.[161]

That this account had nothing to do with what actually happens in ECT was beside the point. It scared the wits out of a generation of readers: ECT must be stopped.

There was one more factor, too. ECT became an object of enmity in the eyes of the Scientology movement. L. Ron Hubbard, who launched "dianetics" in 1950 as an alternative to psychotherapy (Scientology was established as a "church" in 1954), opposed ECT from the very beginning. ECT, he felt, put new and poisonous "engrams" into the body, which it was the task of dianetics to remove if the brain had not been too badly damaged.[162] As the Scientology movement became wealthy and powerful,

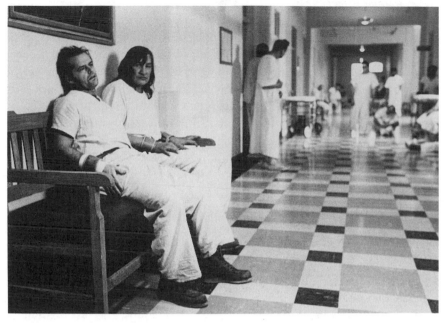

Randle P. McMurphy (Jack Nicholson) and Chief Bromden (Will Sampson) await a session in the "shock shop" in a scene from the 1975 film adaptation of *One Flew Over the Cuckoo's Nest*. The hit film's portrayal of ECT as a punishment for deviant behavior both reflected and contributed to the anti-ECT sentiments of the period.

Source: One Flew Over the Cuckoo's Nest. Directed by Milos Forman, produced by Saul Zaentz and Michael Douglas. Copyright © 1975 Fantasy Films. All rights reserved.

its Citizens Commission on Human Rights spearheaded campaigns to make ECT illegal. Thomas Szasz was the organization's first consulting psychiatrist.[163]

Responding to agitation by patients' rights groups, American state legislatures began regulating ECT. Utah in 1967 was first to pass such legislation, and by 1983, 26 states had passed some kind of statute, six others issued administrative regulations, and one state was operating under federal court orders.[164] In some jurisdictions, ECT was actually banned. In the fall of 1974, the California legislature passed a bill that was tantamount to prohibiting ECT, stipulating that, even when a patient volunteered for it, it could only be administered with the consent of a review panel appointed by community medical authorities, and only after all other psychiatric remedies had been exhausted. Violation could lead to revocation of a physician's license. Challenged in the courts, the legislation did not take effect.[165] In 1982, a Coalition to Stop Electroshock in the city of Berkeley gathered 1,400 signatures necessary to put a measure banning ECT on the ballot ("a misdemeanor punishable by a $500 fine or six months in jail"). It passed by a wide margin but again, the ban was overturned.[166] With the backing of the Scientologists, in 1995 legislation to ban ECT was introduced in the Texas legislature.[167] The bill did not pass but received wide press coverage. Given this kind of public alarm, it is little wonder that ECT virtually vanished from university training programs in the years from 1960 to 1980. Psychiatrists trained in this era tended to be unfamiliar with it. In Monroe County, New York, for example, the average annual incidence of first-time ECT dropped from 31 per 100,000 population in 1961 to 19 in 1975, a decline of 39 percent.[168]

The psychiatrists' counterattack began in Massachusetts in the early 1970s when the antipsychiatrists attempted to get the state legislature to ban ECT.[169] Early in 1972, Milton Greenblatt, the State Commissioner of Mental Health, convened a task force on "electroconvulsive therapy in Massachusetts," chaired by Fred Frankel of Harvard University. Frankel, whose research interests were in hypnosis and psychosomatic medicine, fell between the state's two warring camps, the psychoanalytically oriented psychiatrists in private practice and the institutional psychiatrists. The task force polled 650 psychiatrists in the state, of whom 66 responded, the balance of opinion being mildly favorable to the procedure. In their 1973 report, task force members betrayed a decided fondness for psychotherapy in any condition short of suicide. Yet they did manage to cough up a reserved approval for ECT in major depression and mania, though the hedges were high: How depressed did a patient have to be before qualifying for ECT? "The use of the term 'depressed' by the patient should not immediately be construed to imply the presence of an affective disorder." The principal advantage of shock therapy, they reasoned, lay in "help[ing] a patient re-establish lost control so that he can enter into a therapeutic relationship."[170]

In imitation of the Massachusetts task force, in the fall of 1974 the American Psychiatric Association decided to convoke its own task force on ECT and made Frankel the chair. The task force polled the APA membership, about a third of whose members were unfavorable to its use. Yet the Association's members who did use ECT reported the outcomes to be quite good. Moreover, 83 percent of the patients on whom these psychiatrists reported declared themselves satisfied with the results of treatment. As for the side effects, of which so much had been made, fewer than half the patients had experienced even temporary loss of memory of events surrounding the ECT, 13 percent "temporary loss of distant memories," and 1 percent "permanent loss of distant memories." How did ECT compare with drug treatment? In its 1978 report, the task force found the two treatments evenly balanced, preferring ECT for severely depressed and suicidal patients (given that antidepressants took about three weeks to act). Though hedged in the language of dubiety and caution, overall the report gave a green light to ECT in the major psychiatric disorders, particularly depression.[171]

The hedges began to come away in the early 1980s when Max Fink emerged as an energetic advocate of ECT. Fink, one of the early leaders in psychopharmacology while at Hillside Hospital in the 1950s, had later become professor of psychiatry at the Stony Brook campus of the State University of New York. He first encountered ECT as a resident at Bellevue in 1944 and had employed it ever since. In 1981, Fink argued that all available data made a "compelling" case for the superiority of ECT over antidepressant drugs. The main reason for not having recourse to ECT, he said, might be "the public image of its special hazards."[172] In other words, two decades of meddlesomeness by ECT's primarily lay opponents had resulted in scaring the public away from the treatment of choice in a major psychiatric disorder.

A full-scale effort to rehabilitate ECT now began. In the summer of 1985, the National Institutes of Health convoked a "consensus development conference," bringing together experts from all over the neurosciences to determine the benefits and dangers of ECT compared with other treatments. "Not a single controlled study has shown another form of treatment to be superior to ECT in the short-term management of severe depressions," the report concluded. And the risks? "Overall, the risk is not different from that associated with the use of short-acting barbiturate anesthetics." The commonest side effect was loss of memory for a few weeks surrounding the treatment. The report concluded that medical schools should restore training in ECT to the graduate curriculum in psychiatry.[173]

In the 1980s, psychiatric organizations in many countries began coming out in favor of ECT.[174] The begrudging document the American Psychiatric Association had issued in 1978 now sounded out of date, and in 1987 the APA constituted a new task force on electroconvulsive therapy. Their report appeared in 1990. No longer was ECT just for desperate cases on the verge of suicide. "ECT is an effective treatment for all subtypes of unipolar major depression," for manic-depressive illness (now called bipolar disorder), mania, and psychotic schizophrenia, the report concluded.[175] By 1994, psychiatry residents would be able to carry with them in the pockets of their white coats a compact guide listing the amount by which ECT improved on other treatments in depression: ECT versus simulated ECT, a 31 percent improvement; ECT versus placebo, 41 percent; ECT versus mainline antidepressants ("heterocyclic antidepressants"), 20 percent, and so on.[176]

The rehabilitation of ECT did not mean that it would be universally used in psychiatry but merely that it had ceased to be an object of horror. By 1988, according to one survey, fewer than one psychiatrist in ten had used it in the previous month.[177]

In the patients' culture, a pool of gentler anecdotes had started to fill, in contrast to scare stories about the cuckoo's nest. When psychologist Norman Endler was himself stricken by depression, he and his doctor tried everything in the book, to little effect. In the depths of the illness, Endler's behavior became "bizarre and paranoid," as he later put it after his recovery. There was the episode of the urine bottle: The doctor had requested a urine sample and Endler's wife, after searching the house, could find only an empty medicine bottle that had contained their daughter's antibiotic. "I was reluctant to use it because for some reason it was impossible to remove the label completely. It was possible, however, to remove all identifying information. This was not good enough for me. For some reason I was convinced, irrationally, that if I left a sample in that container Dr. P. would think that it was not my urine sample and would put me in the hospital for lying." Endler ran about the house refusing to leave the urine sample. "This upset everyone in the house and I remember my wife yelling at me."

Finally Endler's doctor recommended ECT. Endler, a psychologist, was at first horrified. He and his fellow psychologists had drunk deeply of the antipsychiatry lore of the 1960s. In the past, he had argued with psychiatric colleagues, showing them negative articles and accusing them "of getting a 'charge' out of it." "Most of my psychological colleagues had negative attitudes that were no different from mine. We were all biased and prejudiced and refused to accept the new techniques."

But now Endler was desperate. He said he would have walked naked down the city's main street if his psychiatrist told him that would help. That evening a fellow psychologist came over to remonstrate with him. "He wanted to know why I was willing to 'get half my brains burned out' and why I wasn't getting deep psychotherapy."

On Tuesday, August 30, 1977, Endler agreed to ECT as a course of treatment. He booked into the clinic that Friday morning, lay down on a cot and was wheeled into the ECT room. "A needle was injected into my arm and I was told to count back from 100. I got about as far as 91." The next thing Endler knew, he was awake and in the recovery room. "I was slightly groggy and tired but not confused. My memory was not impaired. I certainly knew where I was." He rested a bit, was given some cookies and coffee, and went home. Over the two weeks ahead, Endler received six more treatments. He felt better with each successive one. By September 15, he was able to resume the chairmanship of his department full-time. "A miracle had happened in two weeks," he said. "I had gone from feeling like an emotional cripple to feeling well."[178]

These are not trivial achievements. The ability of the new biological psychiatry to make individuals like Norman Endler better represents an accomplishment of historic dimensions. Yet it opened a schism within psychiatry between the "tough-headed" types, characterized by a fondness for medical models, organic explanations of illness, and pharmacotherapy, and "soft-headed" types, who invoked "psychosocial" models of illness, explained symptoms as the result of problems in living, and inclined to psychotherapy and family therapy. Whereas the soft-headed practitioners were represented by psychoanalytic, family, and existential schools of thought, the tough-headed identified with biological psychiatry.[179] "There is no such thing as a psychiatry that is too biological," said Samuel Guze, one of the toughest of the tough-headed.[180]

Yet is was not part of the biological brief to argue that all psychiatric illnesses are attributable to discreet, identifiable brain lesions. Social and psychological factors clearly play a role in the genesis of dysphoria, not merely by triggering an underlying genetic predisposition but by independently converting stress and despair into illness. As a leading biological psychiatrist said, "It would be clinical folly to underestimate the importance of psychological and social factors in the manifestations of mental illnesses or to overlook the psychological aspects of the . . . biological therapies."[181]

Yet in the 1950s, advocates of psychoanalysis and community psychiatry argued that biology played virtually no role, that it was all nurture and no nature. So the argument that nature and nurture stand in some kind of fifty-fifty relationship is already quite extreme from the viewpoint of 30 years ago. One need not be an organic absolutist to place organic factors in their proper perspective: Nature and nurture intertwine. But even winning for nature a place at the table has proven a capital achievement.

8

From Freud to Prozac

B iological thinking gave psychiatry at the end of the twentieth century the capacity to be as science-driven as the rest of medicine. But this promise has remained unfulfilled, a result of psychiatry's enmeshment in popular values, in corporate culture, and in a boggy swamp of diagnostic scientism. While the psychiatry of the major mental illnesses took the high road of the neurosciences in the 1970s and after, the psychiatry of everyday affliction has tended to lose its way.

Science wanders astray easily in the world of quotidian anxiety and sadness, in the obsessive traits of behavior and the misfiring personality types that are the lot of humankind. Here the genetic trail grows dim and the neurotransmitters evaporate. Biology counts for little, culture and socialization for lots. Perhaps there are many separate disorders in this domain of neurotic illness, perhaps only a few, or none. The edges of this kind of psychiatry are poorly delineated, the boundaries between pathology and eccentricity vague. Despite its anchoring in the rest of medicine, psychiatry could easily drift aimlessly here.

It was not all psychiatry's fault. At the end of the twentieth century, a capital problem for psychiatry lay in a new tendency for people to psychologize distress, rather than to medicalize it as in the nervous diseases of yore, or to socialize it by putting it in terms of social class or gender. In the 1970s and after, personal issues that might once have brought people to the neurologist for counseling tended to become defined in psychological terms, meaning that people believe their difficulties capable of resolution through nonmedical psychotherapy. Problems for which nineteenth-century Americans might have sought out Weir Mitchell or George Beard tended in the new era to escape the medical gaze in order to meld into the mainstream of North American trouble-talk. Hence psychiatry, an arm of medicine, lost out to nonmedical forms of counseling such as psychology and social work. As consciousness of the self in distress became part of society's general *Kulturgut*, the mission of psychiatry as the specialty of medicine best equipped to deal with such disorders became ever more threatened.

The pool of postmodern distress was enormous. By the early 1980s, the most recent period for which data are available, 22 million Americans a year were seeking help for mental problems.[1] Together, these individuals would make a third of a billion visits every year. By 1987, psychotherapy itself counted for 8 percent of all the nation's outpatient medical costs.[2] These are sizable figures. In a hundred years, psychotherapy had passed from an exotic procedure performed by neurologists to a virtual national pasttime: On a lifetime basis, more than a quarter of America's adult population would seek help from professional counselors of all descriptions.[3]

In this stunning rise in demand for psychological services, two developments were at work. One, the threshold of what people define as illness dropped sharply, increasing the overall volume of psychological complaints. Psychiatry itself had a clear role in lowering this threshold. Second, there was a tendency to seek therapy for nonillness, counseling for stress and for life's problems. This represented a psychologizing rather than a medicalizing of difficulties that previously might have been considered economic, social, or moral in nature and for which the help of the minister or a good neighbor might have been sought. These two events caused therapy for personal distress to flood way beyond psychiatry and out into the world of psychologists, psychiatric social workers, and other purveyors of what is termed generically "mental-health care." For psychiatrists whose income was based on office-practice psychotherapy, this outrush of potential business was alarming.

Maintaining Market Share

Reducing the threshold of what constitutes psychiatric illness was partially doctor-driven, partially patient-driven. Psychiatrists have an obvious self-interest in pathologizing human behavior and have been willing to draw the pathology line ever lower in their efforts to tear as much counseling as possible away from competing psychologists and social workers. Take, for example, the question of boyhood. Whereas once

Tom-Sawyer-esque enthusiasm was seen as part of the natural spirits of ladhood, in the 1960s and after, a whole series of psychological diagnoses arrived to define such behavior as pathological. The bidding opened high, with "minimal cerebral dysfunction,"[4] as it was called in the 1950s and 1960s. Tom Sawyer, in other words, had brain damage. When this diagnosis was discarded as obviously absurd, hyperactivity and inattentiveness were zeroed in on because boys can sometimes be exasperating to deal with in the classroom. Ignoring the perils of school-teacher psychiatry, educational professionals grasped gratefully for this new pathologizing of boyhood. In 1968, "hyperkinetic reaction of childhood (or adolescence)" entered the official nomenclature, supposedly manifest in restlessness and distractibility.[5] In 1980, this became officially known as "attention deficit disorder with hyperactivity."[6] It is still unclear whether there is some core group of those diagnosed as "ADD" who have a real organic disorder. The point, however, is that medical therapy for it could be done only by MDs, prescribing an amphetamine-like compound called "Ritalin" (methylphenidate). By 1995 doctors were writing 6 million prescriptions for Ritalin a year, and 2.5 million American children were on the drug.[7] This is one way of maintaining market share.

Since ancient times, both boys and girls have become anxious about scary stories. Yet it would have occurred to no one across the centuries to give psychiatric diagnoses to these anxieties about fantasms, not at least until the advent of "posttraumatic stress disorder" (PTSD), a syndrome initially associated with the trauma of combat (see pp. 304–305). Whether a distinctive veterans' psychiatric syndrome involving stress actually exists is unclear. But even if it exists, once PTSD became inserted into official psychiatric lingo, the popular culture grabbed it and hopelessly trivialized it as a way of psychologizing life experiences. By 1995, therapists were talking about "PTSD" in children exposed to movies like *Batman*. According to one authority, 80 percent of children who had watched media coverage of a crime hundreds of miles distant exhibited symptoms of "posttraumatic stress."[8] The anxieties of the children themselves were nothing new under the sun. New was psychiatry's willingness to persuade parents that the quotidian problems of maturation represent a distinct medical disorder.

The boundaries of what constitutes depression have been expanded relentlessly outward. Depression as a major psychiatric illness involving bleakness of mood, self-loathing, an inability to experience pleasure, and suicidal thoughts has been familiar for many centuries. The illness has a heavy biological component. Depression in the vocabulary of post-1960s American psychiatry has become tantamount to dysphoria, meaning unhappiness, in combination with loss of appetite and difficulty sleeping. Thus it comes as no surprise that the incidence of depression so defined has been rising steadily and occurring at ever younger ages.[9] In 1991, the National Institute of Mental Health began organizing a "National Depression Screening Day," in the context of its "Mental Illness Awareness Week." Such programs encourage family doctors to diagnose depression more often in their patients and refer them to psychiatrists. Although this is partly legitimate—a missed major depression may result in a patient's suicide—the ultimate effect is psychiatric empire-building against other kinds of care. Indeed, the American Psychiatric Association jubilates over "record numbers" each year.[10] As a consequence of this continual hammering of the depression theme, depression has become the single commonest disorder seen in psychiatric practice, accounting for 28 percent of all patient visits.[11] (The availability of drugs such as "Prozac," said to be specific for an entire "spectrum" of affective disorders [see pp. 323–324], has doubtless contributed as well to increasing the diagnosis of depression: Physicians prefer to diagnose conditions they can treat rather than those they can't.)

Personality disorders have become a whole sandbox for empire building. Although the concept of a disorder of the personality—in which everybody suffers but the patient—remains scientifically rather murky, in practice imputed personality disorders have taken off. Diagnoses such as antisocial personality disorder arose preferentially in private psychiatric practice and were virtually unknown in other medical settings.[12] Multiple personality disorder (MPD) roared in from obscurity to become epidemic in the 1980s.[13] Other so-called disorders of personality represented merely the exaggeration of familiar character traits. Yet the entire notion of giving patient-status to people because they are troublesome to others represented a pathologizing of essentially normal if irksome behavior. Thus these diagnoses of personality, as well as the other ballooned disease labels, dipped greatly the threshold at which individuals were said to be ill.

Lowering the threshold increased the patient base in a historically unprecedented manner. If in the nineteenth century, psychiatry had focused on psychotic inpatients, and in the early twentieth century on neurotic outpatients, at the end of the twentieth century psychiatry was increasingly interested in the kinds of patients previously seen by family doctors or not seen medically at all. Leaders in the field started speaking of "minor depression, mixed anxiety-depression, and mild neurocognitive disorder as . . . conditions that may deserve consideration as separate categories." The notion of "subthreshold symptoms" gained currency as a means of reaching out to "previously subthreshold patients."[14] This is the language of empire-building and market-conquest. The evidence that these conditions represent diseases, or disorders, in the sense that mumps and major depression are disorders, is extremely slim.

In insider discussions, psychiatrists were perfectly frank with one another about shifting the focus from disease to unhappiness. Said Robert Wallerstein, a senior figure in the profession, in 1991:

> Much of what we treat people for in intensive individual psychotherapy—gross dissatisfactions with the course of their life, difficulties in the area of interpersonal relationships or work adjustment . . . school or work inhibitions, and so on—are not considered by the third-party payers [insurance companies] to be formal diseases for which they should be expected to carry the treatment costs. After all, the inability of a graduate student to complete a doctoral thesis in comparative languages . . . is hardly considered a disease state for which an insurance program should provide treatment.

Wallerstein emphasized that the student might be disappointed and frustrated, and deserving of help.[15] Yet his problems were not psychiatric in the classic sense, rather of the subthreshold variety.

In many ways, therefore, psychiatry was pushing the envelope. In their struggle to maintain themselves against nonmedical competition, psychiatrists found irresistible the temptation to take familiar, real illnesses and expand their margins. This was not unlike the efforts of nineteenth-century neurologists to pathologize various internal sensations in women with the "hysteria" diagnosis and make hysteria virtually coterminous with femininity.[16] But now it was depression and the like that were being pumped up to give them uncommon currency. Memphis psychiatrist Hagop Akiskal slaked "the dilution of the concept of mental illness to such a degree that it is no longer meaningful." He cited "a pseudoepidemic of mental illness because of fashionable diagnoses like borderline schizophrenia."[17] In the continuum of symptoms that runs from major depression to sadness, or from schizophrenia to eccentricity, psychiatry pushed the boundary of pathology steadily to the right, away from the unwell and toward the commonplace. The message was that these ubiquitous features of the human condition represented billable psychiatric illnesses.

A Nation Hungers for Psychotherapy

Underlying this expansion of the envelope was psychiatry's determination not to be left behind in the public's rising clamor for psychotherapy. As psychiatry attempted to maintain its own market share, competition in the psychotherapy marketplace was booming. The earliest challenge had come from social work, which discovered psychotherapy in 1904 when Adolf Meyer's wife Mary Potter Brooks, who is considered the first American social worker, began visiting the families of patients on Ward's Island where Meyer was superintendent.[18] After World War I, social-work leaders began to shift the profession systematically from the provision of social services to psychotherapy. In 1920, at the National Conference of Social Work in New Orleans, Philadelphia's Jessie Taft termed social work "fundamentally psychological, or, if you please, psychiatric" in nature. And Mary Richmond, director of the charity division of the Russell Sage Foundation in New York, called for "social treatment" of families from the viewpoint of "small-group psychology."[19] The number of psychiatric social workers rose from around 2,000 in 1945 to almost 55,000 in 1985 (compared with 32,000 psychiatrists in 1985).[20] By 1990, there were 80,000 "clinical" social workers in the United States.[21] In that year a quarter of the members of the National Association of Social Work were in part- or full-time private practice.[22] The elective terrain of these social workers, in the words of Harry Specht, a senior professor of social work at Berkeley, was "'the worried well,' white middle class, 20–40-year-olds who are unhappy, unfulfilled, and unsatisfied."[23] This was exactly the client base of post-1970s psychiatry.

The psychologists, late in repositioning themselves from testing to psychotherapy, also offered massive competition. It was only with the publication of psychologist Carl Rogers' book *Client-Centered Therapy* in 1951 that psychologists jumped into the psychotherapy market. The "humanistically oriented psychotherapy" of Rogers did not require mastering some complicated therapeutic system like Freudian or Jungian analysis but rather feel-good beliefs about reconstructing the self. Rogers shunned systematic "methods" of psychotherapy. Being client-centered meant having "the faith or belief in the capacity of the individual to deal with his psychological situation and with himself."[24] It was, said Rogers, the idea "that the individual has within himself vast resources for self-understanding, for altering his self-concept, his attitudes, and his self-directed behavior—and that these resources can be tapped if only a definable climate of facilitative psychological attitudes can be provided," namely psychotherapy of the kind conducted by psychologists. "[My method] turned the field of counseling upside down," said Rogers later.[25] In the world of psychotherapy, his ideas became distilled as, in the words of a somewhat bilious Specht, "You can do it; you're wonderful and good, there is richness in you, if it feels good on you it's okay."[26]

Initially, the psychiatrists reacted sharply to the inroads of the psychologists, claiming they were practicing medicine without a license. At the University of Rochester, the psychiatry department tried to put Rogers' Guidance Center out of business. After Rogers moved to Chicago, only a sustained campaign on his part prevented the psychiatry department of the University of Chicago from closing his fledgling Counseling Center.[27] The psychologists finally prevailed. By 1996, the clinical psychology branch of the American Psychological Association had almost 7,000 members, to say nothing of other psychologists also offering psychotherapy.[28] By the 1990s, clinical psychologists and social workers together vastly outnumbered psychiatrists. "Psychotherapy . . . has become a predominantly nonmedical activity," mourned the Group for the Advancement of Psychiatry.[29]

Who was demanding the services of all these new mental-health professionals? Was it individuals with psychiatric illnesses, however broadly defined? No. To be sure, there was in American society a great volume of illness. By the estimate of the National Comorbidity Survey (NCS), a random sample of the American population conducted in the early 1990s, 48 percent of adult Americans would have a psychiatric or substance-abuse disorder over the course of the life cycle, and 30 percent had experienced such a disorder within the previous year of the survey. (The survey defined psychiatric in the widest possible terms, pushing the envelope truly to its outer limits.) These statistics, if accurate, made psychiatric problems among the commonest medical problems in American society, roughly of the same order of frequency as high blood pressure.[30]

Yet these individuals with psychiatric problems were not the main clients for psychotherapy. The NCS study found that only 21 percent of people with disorders were being treated.[31] The other four-fifths had no interest in psychotherapy or treatment and evidently were willing to coexist, happily or unhappily, with their problems.

Instead, the great demand for psychotherapy was coming from people unhappy with their lives but who were not experiencing the depression, anxiety, obsessive-compulsive behavior, and other symptoms characteristic of psychiatric illness. Various studies showed significant numbers of individuals in psychotherapy who had no psychiatric problems. For example, a survey of the Canadian province of Ontario conducted in 1990 found that "forty-two percent of those who have sought help in the past year apparently did not have a mental disorder during that time."[32] As Daniel Freedman, an influential biological psychiatrist at UCLA, put it, "Everyone has problems. But not everyone has symptoms, and fewer have a disorder."[33]

In the 1990s, psychiatry was being bent out of shape by a colossal kind of failure-to-fit. Psychiatrists had been trained for one thing and ended up treating another. They had trained as residents to treat the major psychiatric illnesses. But once in office practice, they gravitated to the commoner and more lucrative psychoneuroses. In doing so, they found themselves in direct competition with the social workers and psychologists. Rather than returning to the main psychiatric diseases, the terrain of choice of biological psychiatry, they went in the opposite direction, expanding the definition of illness to include behavior and symptoms previously reckoned as "subthreshold," and catering to the great American public's demand for psychotherapy in dealing with problems of living.

Even in terms of economic self-interest, remaining on the high road of science would have been preferable, for it was mastery of the neurosciences that distinguished psychiatry from its competitors. And the embarrassing jostling with nonmedical therapists for business could not help but drag down the reputation of psychiatry in the eyes of the public. In 1995, for example, the American Psychiatric Association lobbied the Congress fiercely to keep psychologists from prescribing drugs, humiliating psychiatry in full public view for its recourse to self-interest rather than to science.[34] Such episodes created the impression that psychiatrists were distancing themselves ever further from their scientific claims to be a medical specialty. In terms of diagnosis and therapy, therefore, American psychiatry had begun to lose its way.

Science versus Fashion in Diagnosis

The risk of wandering in the wilderness heightened as psychiatry took on the challenge of diagnosis and found it as much driven by politics as science. Diagnosis in medicine is important because it gives the key to therapy and prognosis, matters of vital significance to the patient. Compared with psychiatry, diagnosis in other medical specialties is relatively straightforward because the causes of most conditions are known: In pathology class, the medical students memorize the causes of disease in an organ system as: "traumatic, infectious, neoplastic, toxic, autoimmune . . ." and so on. The causes of most organic diseases are relatively limited in number and not a matter of great controversy. Just imagine a group of respirologists having heated battles over the cause of pneumonia, splitting into separate societies and founding their own journals over the issue. Not so in psychiatry where, genetics apart, the causes of few conditions are known. What is the cause of something like erotomania, the delusional belief that someone else is in love with you? Nobody knows. Psychiatric illness has tended therefore to be classified on the basis of symptoms rather than causes, which is where the rest of medicine was in the nineteenth century. Grouping the various symptoms into larger disease categories can thus be somewhat arbitrary: Is erotomania part of schizophrenia, part of delusional disorder, or a separate illness? And the groupings themselves have been historically highly controversial, with entire schools of psychiatry rising and falling over the issue of how to classify "hysteria." These considerations suggest that in classification it is very easy for psychiatry to lose its way.

Adding to the risk is the existence of various national traditions, so that a given patient might be diagnosed quite differently from one country to another. One thinks of "eruptive delusional disorder" (la bouffée délirante) in France, a diagnosis that has no counterpart elsewhere. "The English call almost any kind of emotional trouble 'neurosis,'" said Henri Ellenberger, the great historian of psychiatry, in the mid-1950s. "The French apply the diagnosis of feeblemindedness very liberally." As for the Swiss, "The French say that the Swiss diagnose schizophrenia in '90 percent of the psychotics and 50 percent of the normal.'"[35]

But nobody used the diagnosis of schizophrenia more often than the Americans. Schizophrenia was the great foible of American psychiatry. In the 1940s and 1950s American psychiatrists diagnosed it many times more frequently than their colleagues in Britain. In one study, 46 American psychiatrists and 205 British watched a videotape of "patient F," a young man from Brooklyn who had a hysterical paralysis of one arm and a history of mood fluctuations associated with alcohol abuse. Afterward, 69 percent of the Americans diagnosed "schizophrenia," 2 percent of the British.[36]

Such international differences were unscientific and embarrassing, for they suggested there was no science in psychiatry but simply the weight of national tradition, making the discipline a branch of folklore rather than of medicine.

Even worse, in the heyday of psychoanalysis many psychiatrists were simply indifferent to diagnosis, and believed that ascertaining the presumed psychodynamic cause was more important than classifying the presenting symptoms. Robert Spitzer, the Columbia psychiatrist who was the driving force behind the new system of classification introduced in American psychiatry in 1980, remembered attending annual meetings of the American Psychiatric Association in the 1960s: "The academic psychiatrists interested in presenting their work on descriptive diagnosis would be scheduled for the final day in the late afternoon. No one would attend. Psychiatrists simply were not interested in the issue of diagnosis."[37]

In the 1960s, the discipline began to wake up to the importance of getting the diagnosis right. A new generation determined that psychiatry should proceed as the rest of medicine did, establishing a differential diagnosis on the basis of the presenting symptoms, then conducting a proper investigation to come up with a clinical diagnosis, or "impression," at the end. The first wake-up call came from the Old World, or rather from the historic Viennese psychiatric tradition in exile. Erwin Stengel, born in Vienna in 1902, had studied medicine there. He knew Freud and Wagner-Jauregg, as well as being a classmate of Sakel. Yet even though Stengel had spent a year in analysis, he was not an adept of depth psychology but rather took a serious scholarly view of psychiatry as a whole. Forced to flee Vienna in 1938, Stengel landed first at the Maudsley Hospital, then in 1957 (driven, they said, from London by Aubrey Lewis) he founded the psychiatry department of the University of Sheffield.[38]

In 1959, Stengel published an influential critique of the lack of reliability in psychiatric diagnosis. He said that both the analysts and the American followers of Adolf Meyer "stress the uniqueness of the individual." "Such an approach," he noted drily, "has tended to discourage the categorization of mental disorders."[39] This was the opening cannon in the campaign to revive diagnosis.

Ten years later, in 1969, a large comparative study of diagnosis in the United States and the United Kingdom made it clear that the two countries were badly out of sync. Commenting on the results, Heinz Lehmann said that it was time for "a renaissance of psychiatric diagnosis, which in many quarters today has deteriorated . . . into an ill-regulated, superficial, unconvincing, and therefore often useless procedure."[40] Thus came from within the discipline an intellectual push for carving nature at the joints.

A second force pulling psychiatry toward a system of reliable diagnosis was the introduction of drug therapy. The availability of specific medications for psychosis and depression made diagnosis a practical matter. "With the availability of lithium and neuroleptic drugs," said Donald

Goodwin and Samuel Guze, authors of an influential textbook, "distinguishing between mania and schizophrenia—once an interesting academic exercise—might now determine how a patient was treated."[41]

These issues started to become acute in the 1970s. Previously, the tradition of diagnostic classification in American psychiatry—even outside psychoanalysis—had not been glorious. The alienists of the nineteenth century worked with a few obvious categories for the sake of their annual asylum statistics (melancholia, general paralysis of the insane, dementia, and the like). American psychiatry was pushed into greater reflectiveness only by the exigencies of the census. In 1908, the Bureau of the Census asked the American Medico-Psychological Association to organize a committee on disease nomenclature, or nosology, and by 1918 the association, in collaboration with the National Committee for Mental Hygiene, had finally put together the first American psychiatric nosology, the *Statistical Manual for the Use of Institutions for the Insane.*[42]

Until this point, American medicine in general had lacked a system of nomenclature of its own. In 1927, the New York Academy of Medicine took the initiative of organizing a nationally accepted "standard nomenclature of disease." The following year, it brought all the medical specialties together for a conference on the subject, out of which evolved the *Standard Classified Nomenclature of Disease*, published in 1933. The American Psychiatric Association had contributed the psychiatric part.[43]

At the outset of World War II, American psychiatry relied mainly on a naming system devised for patients in public asylums with major mental illnesses. Yet combat created psychiatric challenges quite different from insanity. Minor personality problems unremarkable in civilian life became of great importance in the military setting. But only such terms as "psychopathic personality" were available for understanding them.[44] Psychosomatic disorders were grouped in no single distinctive category, appearing under whatever term a gastroenterologist or cardiologist had devised (and there were many, such as "soldier's heart"). Psychological reactions to stress, combat fatigue: All demanded a new system of classification. And so new systems were devised. Psychiatric nosologies multiplied. By the late 1940s, there was chaos.

In 1948, the American Psychiatric Association's committee on naming went to work on a single national system of classification. A proposed draft was circulated to the membership, their suggestions were incorporated, and by 1952 the APA's first independent system of naming was published, the *Diagnostic and Statistical Manual [of] Mental Disorders*, known subsequently as *DSM-I*.

These details are important because a naming system incorporates the dominant philosophy of the day, and in 1952 analysts were heavily represented in the APA, on its naming committee as well as among the membership. Of the 28 current and past members in 1951 of the APA's Committee on Nomenclature and Statistics, at least 10 were members of psychoanalytic organizations or sympathetic to analysis on the basis of their writings.[45] *DSM-I* therefore codified much of their wisdom. "Psychoneurotic disorders," for example, received a straight Freudian analysis: "The chief characteristic of these disorders is anxiety which may be directly felt and expressed or which may be unconsciously and automatically controlled by the utilization of various psychological defense mechanisms (depression, conversion, displacement, etc.)."[46] More in a bow to Adolf Meyer than Freud, the term "reaction" was sprinkled liberally throughout, as in "schizophrenic reaction" or "antisocial reaction."

In the 1950s and early 1960s, psychoanalysis consolidated its hold over American psychiatry, and the second edition of the *Diagnostic and Statistical Manual* that appeared in 1968, *DSM-II*, reflected this sway.[47] Six of the ten members of the drafting committee were analysts or belonged to sympathetic organizations. The nomenclature mirrored this predominance: Psychoneurotic problems were no longer called "reactions" but "neuroses." The sturdy Freudian term "hysteria" appeared, replacing "conversion reaction" and "dissociative reaction." What was

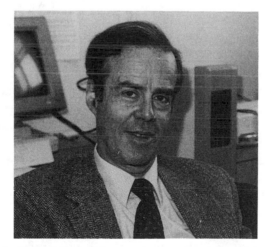

Robert Spitzer, the Columbia psychiatrist who was the main architect of "DSM-III," the diagnostic manual of the American psychiatric profession, introduced in 1980 (courtesy of Dr. Robert Spitzer).

hysteria? The term referred to symptoms associated with "emotionally charged situations" that are "symbolic of the underlying conflicts."[48] Descriptions of all disorders were brief and usually lacking in operational criteria for their application. Psychiatrists seeking guidance in differentiating, for example, schizophrenia from mania would find little to help them.

One of the members of the drafting committee was a sort of renegade analyst named Robert Spitzer. Born in 1932, Spitzer had graduated from New York University medical school, then trained at the New York State Psychiatric Institute, simultaneously qualifying as an analyst at Columbia's Psychoanalytic Clinic. Around 1959, however, he abandoned the analytic pathway to join the classifiers, and by 1968 he had become the head of the Evaluation Unit of the New York State Psychiatric Institute.

In these years, Spitzer decided to take psychiatric diagnosis in another direction entirely, making the diagnoses as precise as possible in order to correspond to what were presumably natural disease entities. This was known as "cutting nature at the joints," and was precisely what Kraepelin had set out to do many years previously. Yet where the joints lay exactly could only be determined by research. The best way to do research would be to devise operational criteria for determining exactly what symptoms must be present before a physician could make a given diagnosis.

Fortunately for Spitzer, elsewhere on the American psychiatric landscape other small groups of researchers were setting out to carve nature at the joints as well. In 1948, Eli Robins, a Texan with a Harvard MD who had trained at the Massachusetts General Hospital, accepted a fellowship in psychiatry in Washington University of St. Louis. As he arrived, he encountered two young residents, George Winokur and Samuel Guze, whose interests were very similar to his own: brain chemistry, biology, and classification—all at the time highly unfashionable subjects. The three of them became a nucleus from which a counterrevolution in psychiatry against psychoanalysis would ultimately emanate. Collectively, they became known as the "Neo-Kraepelinians,"[49] a not entirely accurate label given Kraepelin's uninterest in brain biology. In 1955, Guze became chair of the department and proceeded to give it an international reputation as a center of biological thinking, fostering such researchers as Paula Clayton (coauthor with Winokur of a textbook on psychiatry's medical basis[50]), John Feighner ("Finer," who became an important diagnostician), and Robert Woodruff (a student of the biology of "hysteria").

In 1972, the St. Louis group, led by Feighner, published the first set of rigorous criteria for making diagnoses, in which one would be guided not just by one's "best clinical judgment and experience" but by fixed conditions the patient had to meet. Was the patient depressed? He or she would have to have (a) a dysphoric mood; (b) at least five of a list of eight criteria, including poor appetite, feelings of guilt, and so forth; (c) a psychiatric illness that had gone on for at least a month before seeking help. Similar sets of criteria were spelled out for the entire gamut of psychiatric disorders.[51] The "Feighner criteria," or "Research Diagnostic Criteria" as Spitzer refined them,[52] were revolutionary in permitting the standardization of diagnosis from clinician to clinician, university to university, country to country.

Meanwhile, the American Psychiatric Association was under pressure to revise *DSM-II*. Gay groups were unhappy that homosexuality had been included as a disorder.[53] Insurance companies wanted more precise diagnoses if they were going to pay for long-term psychotherapy. Many clinicians were becoming disaffected from psychoanalysis and wanted diagnoses based on symptoms rather than on dubious theories about underlying causes. Early in 1973, Walter Barton, medical director of the APA, initiated a task force "to revise *DSM-II* and prepare *DSM-III* within the next two years."[54] Melvin Sabshin, a Young Turk, then succeeded Barton as medical director. Sabshin realized that if the group who had designed *DSM-II* were to take on the revision, *DSM-III* would become just "a minor variant" of its predecessor. What was needed was something completely different. In April 1974, Sabshin summoned Spitzer and Theodore Millon, another Young Turk who was a PhD psychologist at the Neuropsychiatric Institute of the University of Illinois Medical Center in Chicago, for an all-day conference.[55] Out of this conference came the leadership team that would drive forward *DSM-III*, published in 1980.

Spitzer headed the task force. Also serving on it were Clayton and Woodruff from the Guze group (a third of the task force had trained at Washington University); Donald Goodwin at the University of Kansas who had studied with Guze was on it, as was Z. J. ("Bish") Lipowski, a specialist in delirium, which is an organic psychiatric condition. There was Donald Klein, a psychopharmacologist and psychiatrist who in 1978 became professor of psychiatry at Columbia, as well as 13 other members. Just as previous *DSM* task forces had been weighted in favor of psychoanalysis, this one was weighted against it and toward biological psychiatry, though the members did not use that then inflammatory term. As Spitzer later said, "With its intellectual roots in St. Louis instead of Vienna, and with its intellectual inspiration derived from Kraepelin, not Freud, the task force was viewed from the outset as unsympathetic to the interests of those whose theory and practice derived from the psychoanalytic tradition."[56]

There is no doubt that the task force intended to produce a science-driven document. As Spitzer said in the introduction to *DSM-III*, "In attempting to resolve various diagnostic issues, the Task Force relied, as much as possible, on research evidence relevant to various kinds of diagnostic validity." Between 1977 and 1979 the National Institute of Mental Health sponsored a field trial in which 500 psychiatrists from many different centers used drafts of *DSM-III* in diagnosing over 12,000 patients. Around 300 psychiatrists were paired, their evaluations then compared for consistency.[57] Whereas *DSM-II* contained 134 pages, *DSM-III* ran on to almost 500 pages, each page containing long lists of criteria that had to be met before a given diagnosis could be made.

So the spirit of science was there. It was on the basis of Kety's Copenhagen adoption study, for example, that Spitzer proposed the diagnosis "schizotypal personality disorder," a certain type of personality occurring in individuals with a family history of full-blown schizophrenia.[58] Harvard psychiatrist Gerald Klerman called *DSM-III* "a victory" for science.[59] Indeed, on the basis of the presumed scientific underpinning of *DSM-III*, American psychiatry returned to the world of medicine, applying the medical model in diagnosis and downplaying the vague "biopsychosocial model" under which so much mischief had occurred. In the judgment of one historian of psychiatry, *DSM-III* became "the centerpiece of the knowledge base of the profession."[60]

This repositioning of American psychiatry had a great impact on events elsewhere. By the early 1990s, *DSM-III*, or the revised version of it that appeared in 1987 (*DSM-III-R*), had been translated into over 20 languages. French psychiatry residents, initially taken with antipsychiatry and the doctrines of Jacques Lacan and Michel Foucault, began memorizing the 4 criteria (and the 18 possible symptoms, 6 of which must be present) for anxiety disorder.[61] In Germany, the translation of *DSM-III-R* reawakened Kraepelinian memories of psychiatric "diseases" (*Krankheiten*) and not just "disorders."[62] The appearance of *DSM-III* was thus an event of capital importance not just for American but for world psychiatry, a turning of the page on psychodynamics, a redirection of the discipline toward a scientific course, a reembrace of the positivistic principles of the nineteenth century, a denial of the antipsychiatric doctrine of the myth of psychiatric illness.

Yet there were nagging worries. Rather than heading off into the brave new world of science, DSM-style psychiatry seemed in some ways to be heading out into the desert. For one thing, with each successive edition of the *DSM* series, the number of discrete disorders kept growing. *DSM-III* listed 265 different disorders, up one third from the 180 in *DSM-II*. *DSM-III-R* had 292 and *DSM-IV*, published in 1994, 297 disorders.[63] Did nature really have 297 joints? Even though the drafters shunned the Kraepelinian label "disease," at bottom identifying distinct "disorders" meant distinct disease entities.[64] One would not expect to find so many different diseases in nephrology or cardiology. Of course the brain is more complex, but even so, Pinel had managed to reduce the number of psychiatric disorders from "an indefinite number of varieties" to four.[65] Psychiatry had a tradition of intellectual compactness, of lumping rather than splitting. One of the *DSM-III* drafters justified wide inclusiveness on the grounds of wanting to "embrace as many conditions as are commonly seen by practicing clinicians," in order to let future researchers judge the validity of those conditions as "a valid syndromal entity."[66] Yet the sheer endlessness of the syndrome parade caused an uneasy feeling that the process might somehow be out of control.

DSM-III also seemed highly ethnocentric, a major flaw in a discipline that presumes to universality. Many of its disorders, such as anorexia nervosa, were simply unknown in other parts of the world. One can be sure that, if *DSM-III* had been drafted in India, it would have included a big section on demonic possession.[67] Was it possible that the brave new world of psychiatry was bogging down in "borderline personality disorder" and the like—read "Woody Allen syndromes"—generated by very specific East-Coast cultural pathology? As one critic said, "Borderline and narcissistic personalities are rarely seen in Iowa City or in Mobile; certainly, they are not recognized in Tangiers or Bucharest."[68] For two centuries, culture had proven to be a swamp for psychiatry; witness the "ovarian hysteria" of the nineteenth century, the "colonic autointoxication"—born of an urban middle class's bowel obsessions—of the early twentieth. If supposedly scientific psychiatry was merely trying to classify the cultural preoccupations of the North American middle class, its naming manuals would soon be as outdated as the etiquette guides for Victorian ladies.

Politics represented a final pothole on the high road of science for the *DSM-III* drafters. Even though they were struggling to cling to "the data," they were buffeted by ideological lobbies and forced to make a series of concessions. All this negotiating left the impression that what the drafters had created was as much a political document as a scientific one. First, there was the squabble about removing homosexuality from the illness list. (*DSM-II* had called homosexuality a "sexual deviation."[69]) A subcommittee of the *DSM-III* task force deliberated about calling it "homodysphilia, dyshomophilia, homosexual conflict disorder, amorous relationship disorder . . . and finally, ego-dystonic homosexuality." Unable to agree, the subcommittee kicked it upstairs to the task force members, who decided to delete it entirely.[70] A referendum of the APA membership confirmed the decision in 1974. At a stroke, what had been considered for a century or more a grave psychiatric disorder ceased to exist.

The political power of the psychoanalysts also shaped the structure of *DSM-III*. The analysts were outraged when they saw in the task force's first draft, completed in 1975, that disorders were to be based on cause "when known," avoiding "unproven etiologic concepts." The analysts argued that decades of experience in analytic practice constituted proof of Freudian-style psychogenesis. Nor were they pleased that "neurosis" had vanished from the task force's draft. Faced with the analysts' threat to derail the entire enterprise at the meeting of the APA's Board in May 1979, the task force pulled back and restored "neurosis" in parentheses after the word disorder.[71] The drafters somewhat lamely explained in the introduction that they meant neurosis "only descriptively," without implying a "neurotic process."[72] This clearly political sop to a major interest group had nothing to do with science.

In the years after 1971, the Vietnam veterans represented a powerful interest group. They believed that their difficulties in reentering American society were psychiatric in nature and could only be explained as a result of the trauma of the war. In language that anticipated the "struggle for recognition" of numerous later illness attributions, such as repressed memory syndrome, the veterans and their psychiatrists argued that "delayed massive trauma" could produce subsequent "guilt, rage, the feeling of being scapegoated, psychic numbing, and alienation." In early 1973, the National Council of Churches organized a First National Conference on the Emotional Needs of Vietnam-Era Veterans. Out of this grew a nationwide campaign to persuade the recalcitrant psychiatric establishment to recognize the new disease. Once it became known how easily the APA's Nomenclature Committee had given way on homosexuality, it was clear that the psychiatrists could be rolled. A "working group" of psychiatric advocates of the veterans' cause suggested the diagnosis "post-combat disorder," and as the working group began meeting with Spitzer and a task force subcommittee on "reactive disorders" that he had appointed, it became inevitable that there would be agreement: In 1978, the committee on reactive disorders recommended to the task force the inclusion of a diagnosis of "post traumatic stress disorder," or PTSD, in the new manual. One student of this campaign concluded, "PTSD is in *DSM-III* because a core of psychiatrists and veterans worked consciously and de-liberately for years to put it there. They ultimately succeeded because they were better organized, more politically active, and enjoyed more lucky breaks than their opposition."[73]

The experiences of the homosexuals and the Vietnam veterans made it evident that psychiatric diagnosis was up for grabs. The next group to pressure the naming committee was the feminists, unhappy that *DSM-III-R*, published in 1987, contained listings such as "self-defeating personality disorder," said to be commoner in females than males by a ratio of two-to-one. The committee put this in a category of new disor-ders "needing further study." Nor were feminists enchanted by "late luteal phase dysphoric disorder," also in the category of "needing further study."[74] It was not as a result of further study but of political pressure that self-defeating personality was dropped from *DSM-IV*, published in 1994. Menstrual problems continued on the list for study as "premen-strual dysphoric disorder."[75]

Given such antics, it would be difficult to take seriously any official psychiatric pronouncement about problems surrounding sexual orienta-tion, the psychiatry of stress, or women and the menses. These matters could all apparently be pathologized and depathologized at the will of the majority, or following campaigns of insistent pressure groups. The under-lying failure to let science point the way emphasized the extent to which *DSM-III* and its successors, designed to lead psychiatry from the swamp of psychoanalysis, was in fact guiding it into the wilderness.

The Decline of Psychoanalysis

In the background of the evolution of the *DSM* series lay the ongoing decline of psychoanalysis. *DSM-IV* dropped the term neurosis because the new task force realized that it now had enough votes to get away with it. As psychiatric historian Mitchell Wilson said of the psychoanalysts in the 1970s, "The balance of power within American psychiatry had been shifting under their very feet. What had been the new, modern psychia-try only two decades earlier had become . . . an encumbrance too un-wieldy for [1970s psychiatry] to bear."[76]

Yet ironically, the fall from grace of psychoanalysis contributed to fur-ther disorientation and confusion with psychiatry rather than freeing it up for a walk toward science in the way that the decline of humoral theories in the early nineteenth century had freed up pathology for such a grand promenade. With the transformation of psychoanalysis into yet another postmodern form of "discourse," competing psychotherapies mushroomed, so that by the 1970s one could count at least 130 different versions.[77] In the psychotherapeutic jungle that arose, any therapy was considered valid no matter how bizarre, from "therapeutic touching" to practicing being born again midst the sofa cushions on the living-room rug. For psychiatrists, touching these was like touching a coiling mass of serpents.

The decline of psychoanalysis had a disorienting effect in particular on the "biopsychosocial" wing of psychiatry, which hitherto had depended on Freud's ideas for most of its psychological understanding. If not Freud, then what do we offer for psychotherapy? The alternative psychotherapies all had similar success rates. It really didn't seem to matter whether one chose interpersonal therapy, group therapy, family therapy, psychodrama, hypnosis, or narcosynthesis. The patient's chances of recovery were mostly the same.[78] Even more unnerving, as psychologist Hans Eysenck pointed out, was that statistical studies suggested none of these therapies improved significantly on chance.[79] Is it any wonder therefore that in the 1970s and beyond, the psychotherapeutic side of psychiatry began wandering in the wilderness, a paradoxical result of the decline of psychoanalysis, the one psychotherapy that had formerly given therapists great certainty.

Old hands were shocked at the changes. When Robert Wallerstein was a resident at the Veterans Administration Hospital in Topeka, Kansas (then under the sway of the Menninger Clinic), psychoanalysis was "*the* road to the treatment of mental disorder." His residency training consisted mainly of sessions in depth psychotherapy. In a resident's average workweek of 40 hours, 20 would be given to "individual psychotherapeutic work with patients." Twenty hours a week times 50 weeks times three years equaled "3,000 hours of psychotherapy during the residency training period."

Since 1949, noted Wallerstein, there had been vast changes in the training of young psychiatrists. In a typical four-year residency today, the major rotations are "no longer psychotherapy focused but rather are drug-management focused." Because the patients rarely stay longer than a month, the residents have no opportunity to try out long-term psychotherapy. Today's psychiatric resident has to attend clinics at community mental health centers, eating disorder clinics, sexual disorder clinics, drug maintenance clinics, "all with their drug treatment and behavior treatment focus." All of this training is taken from the time once allotted depth psychotherapy, so that today's resident would typically log about 200 hours of practice in psychotherapy. "Given that the total 4-year residency program constitutes up to 8,000 scheduled hours, and that the 200 psychotherapy experience hours constitute only 2 and one-half percent of that time, one can well ask. . . ."[80] Although Wallerstein left the question dangling, the implications were clear. In the passage of psychoanalytically oriented psychotherapy from 50 percent to 2.5 percent of the graduate curriculum may be traced the decline and virtual demise of psychoanalysis within psychiatry.

The analysts lost control of the great bastions of psychiatric training. In 1945, said Bertram Brown, director of the National Institute of Mental Health, "it was nearly impossible for a nonpsychoanalyst to become chairman of a department or professor of psychiatry." By the mid-1970s dedicated analysts were rarely being selected as department chairs.[81] By 1990, more than 100 of the 163 residency training programs for psychiatry in the United States had abandoned instruction in intensive psychotherapy. "More than 60 percent of the psychiatrists now in training," said one observer, "may complete their training without ever seeing a patient in twice-a-week or more intensive psychotherapy."[82]

With the decline of analysis, the whole social experience of becoming a psychiatrist changed, from preparation for a white middle-class society practice to preparation for the real world. The programs of the 1940s and 1950s were dedicated to training "cream puff" psychiatrists, as Paul Hoch, the tough-minded senior research scientist at the New York State Psychiatric Institute, put it: "men and women oblivious to the harsh realities facing millions of Americans . . . content to live out their professional lives dedicated to the welfare of a thin layer of well-heeled patients at the top of the economic heap."[83] When in 1955 the Institute's new director Lawrence Kolb decided to stop admitting only "interesting" patients, meaning those suitable for psychoanalysis, and to open the doors of the hospital to the local population of Manhattan's Washington Heights district, a dramatic change occurred in the patients, who went from being white and Jewish to black and Protestant.[84]

As the academic training programs lost their following, the supply of psychiatrists interested in becoming psychoanalysts dwindled. The percentage of psychiatrists who were also analysts declined from around 10 percent in the 1950s to 2.7 percent by 1988.[85]

Simultaneously, psychoanalysis was losing its grip in the world of psychiatric practice. When Fritz Redlich and coworkers surveyed psychiatric practice in New Haven in 1950, they found psychoanalysis everywhere in ascendancy, used on 32 percent of all patients and an object of "universal acclaim" among the residents at Yale. When Redlich went back 25 years later, psychiatrists who did not prescribe drugs "had become the exception," and group and family therapies had outdistanced

307

depth psychotherapy. "The major emphasis was on symptom relief . . . rather than on achievement of personality insight or change," said Redlich.[86] At the Menninger Clinic in Kansas—once a bastion of psychoanalysis—by 1965 only one patient in 209 had been referred for psychoanalysis and only 23 percent were participating in any kind of psychotherapy (down from 62 percent receiving psychoanalysis or psychotherapy in 1945).[87]

Former chieftains such as Ludwig Binswanger, Freud's Swiss disciple, began falling away: A relative of Binswanger's with a psychiatric illness was successfully treated by a young, pharmacologically oriented German psychiatrist named Fritz Flügel. At the end of the treatment, Binswanger told Flügel, "Fritz, with two pills, you destroyed a psychodynamic castle that took me 50 years to build."[88] The Binswanger clinic at Kreuzlingen, once a fortress of Binswanger's own depth "existential analysis," closed its doors in 1980.

Sniffing calamity, in 1974 the American Psychoanalytic Association polled its membership to see what was happening on the ground. Alternative psychotherapies, such as group and family therapy and the "human potential movement" were tearing away at the patient base. "Self-help measures such as biofeedback, meditation, autohypnosis, imagery, and alternative styles of life are held to promise great benefits to their users. In short, two decades ago when one was dissatisfied with his life, he had a limited choice as to what to do about it. Now he can turn in many directions, only one of which is psychoanalytic therapy." Three-fifths of the Association's members had started prescribing medications, a further third were offering marital therapy or some variant. "There are fewer good classical neurotics," the report lamented. Along with the schizophrenogenic mother, the housebound, neurotic, frustrated female who had been the darling of the couch was also vanishing, replaced by "women patients with achievement conflicts."[89]

Finally, even the patients themselves lost faith. The American Psychoanalytic Association's 1974 poll of its membership showed significant declines in the number of patients seeking full-blown analytic treatment compared with the period 1962–1967: Earlier, almost half of the association's members were treating four to seven analytic patients per week; by 1976 this was down considerably. Previously, a third of the members were treating eight or more patients per week. Now, complained the authors, "only one-fifth of our members had such thriving analytic practices last year."[90] The reluctance of Health Maintenance Organizations, or HMOs, the new wave in American health care, to pay for long-term therapy helped account for part of the decline, but only part: The demand for analysis was receding.

In cinema, images of psychoanalysis went from the idolatrous, such as John Huston's *Freud* (1962) or *Captain Newman MD* (1963, a film about Los Angeles analyst Ralph Greenson, who later treated Marilyn Monroe) to films depicting analysts as sex-mad letches (*The Girl in the Freudian Slip*) or domestic stumblebums (*The Impossible Years*, a 1968 film starring David Niven and Ozzie Nelson). It was joked that in the movies "bad psychiatrists have sex with their patients and then murder them while good psychiatrists simply have sex with them."[91] A 1993 *Time* cover story on psychoanalysis showed Freud with his cranium crumbling into pieces of a picture puzzle; an inside photograph had an analytic couch flying out the window. "What if Freud was wrong?" the magazine asked a presumably unsettled readership.[92] Unlike the sleek Berliners of the 1920s discussing their "Minko's," the American middle classes of the 1990s had moved onto other themes. The "P" word was no longer psychoanalysis. It was Prozac.

A 1980s court case represented a final humiliation for analysis as a medical therapy. The widely followed case pitted a depressed patient, Rafael Osheroff, against the psychoanalytically oriented Chestnut Lodge private hospital. In 1979, Osheroff, a 42-year-old physician from Alexandria, Virginia, was admitted to Chestnut Lodge with the symptoms of psychotic depression. In the course of his seven-month stay at "the Lodge" he was treated with four sessions in intensive psychotherapy a week and denied medication despite his own requests, on the apparent grounds that his clinicians wanted him to regress back to the point in childhood at which the initial trauma occurred and then "build" from there.[93] Dr. Osheroff, by contrast, merely wanted to get better and finally obtained a transfer to another private clinic, the Silver Hill Foundation in Connecticut, where he was treated with phenothiazines and antidepressants. Within three months, he was discharged and able to return to normal life. On returning home, Osheroff found that his world had disintegrated, his wife having left him, his hospital accreditation gone, and his partner (the man who had driven him to Chestnut Lodge) having ousted him from their joint practice.

In 1982 Osheroff sued Chestnut Lodge for malpractice on the grounds that he should have been given state-of-the-art treatment with medications of demonstrated efficacy rather than left to vegetate for seven months. An arbitration panel awarded him $250,000. Both the Lodge and Osheroff appealed, and in 1987 the case was settled out of court for an undisclosed sum just before coming to trial. Did psychoanalysis meet "accepted standards of care"? Gerald Klerman, an influential psychiatrist then at Harvard who had testified on Osheroff's behalf, made the point that the efficacy of intensive psychotherapy had never been established with controlled trials, whereas that of medication had, and that controlled trials were the ultimate standard of science.[94] The case left the strong impression that treating major psychiatric illnesses with psychoanalysis alone constituted malpractice.

The Osheroff case set the leaves to rustling. Even though a court had not definitively ruled that biological and behavioral treatments constituted the new gold standard of care, any clinician who henceforth treated patients as Chestnut Lodge had Dr. Osheroff ran the risk of incurring heavy penalties.

Thus psychoanalysis began to demedicalize itself. As medicine lost confidence in it, nonphysicians began filling the vacancies in the analytic training programs. For many years, American psychoanalysts had strenuously resisted accepting non-MDs in psychoanalytic training. In 1985, four psychologists filed a class-action suit against the American Psychoanalytic Association, arguing that its training monopoly violated federal antitrust law. In 1988, the various institutes agreed to begin admitting nonmedical candidates. At this point, social workers and psychologists began to pour into psychoanalytic training programs: By 1991, 21 percent of the training candidates were nonmedical.[95]

And why not? Increasingly, the view became accepted that psychoanalysis was not for illness but for the interior voyage. While insisting that psychoanalysis was still valid therapy for "the major psychoses," analyst Robert Michels decided to take a more embracing stance: The discipline was ideal for "the optimalization of experience and the enhancement of sensitivity."[96] Indeed, said critic Adolf Grünbaum, picking up on comments that Michels had made elsewhere, analysis was most akin to "an edifying experience of the kind provided by, say, a season ticket to the opera."[97]

From *Studies in Hysteria* in 1895 to a ticket to the opera in 1994: what an odyssey! By the mid-1990s, psychoanalysis had by no means gone out of fashion among intellectuals, and it was a rage in many departments of languages and sociology. In 1994, the University of Dublin began offering an undergraduate arts degree in psychoanalysis.[98] The late-twentieth-century trajectory of psychoanalysis had carried it beyond the discipline of psychiatry and into the ether of arts and letters where, however it fared, it would no longer be identified as a privileged treatment for psychiatric illness.

What had gone wrong for psychoanalysis? There were external factors, such as the changing demographics of part of its social base (see pp. 307–308). But internal ones mattered as well. The demise of psychoanalysis was in large measure a result of its own lack of flexibility, its resistance to incorporating new findings from the neurosciences. And this reluctance was directly related to the analysts' fear of being proven wrong.

American psychoanalysis had always exhibited strenuous resistance to the collection of data on the outcome of therapy. In 1948, the American Psychoanalytic Association set up a committee to evaluate psychoanalytic therapy. The committee met with "insuperable resistance among the membership," and the idea was permitted to lapse.[99] At the Association's May meeting in 1952, President Robert Knight decided to try again: "The highly individualistic nature of psychoanalytic practice . . . [has] made the gathering of statistical data from psychoanalytic experience exceedingly difficult in the past. Analysts have tended to hide behind the curtain of professional secrecy and have been loath to participate in sufficient numbers . . . ," particularly in research on the "outcome of therapy of patients under psychoanalytic treatment." But Knight was determined to turn this around, and in 1953 he and Lawrence Kubie prompted the Association to organize a Central Fact Gathering Agency.[100] The committee worked in secretiveness, and was instructed that before any information could be presented "to any group outside of the Association" the executive council must first approve.[101] By the time that Kubie reported on the committee's progress in April 1956, the grumblings had grown loud indeed: The committee's statistical categories were, it appeared, much too coarse "to express the shadings, degrees, and grades of thinking relative to mental illness." Kubie urged the members to be patient: "Nothing which the American Psychoanalytic Association had ever undertaken as an association had aroused as much enthusiasm among outsiders interested in medical and psychiatric education as this research project of the Central Fact-Gathering Committee. The project may be expected to elicit financial backing from foundations. . . ."[102] It is clear, therefore, that the ultimate rejection of psychoanalysis by researchers interested in scientific standards did not happen without a long period of suspending disbelief, indeed of benevolent encouragement.

And yet the committee brought it to nothing. In December 1957, chair Harry Weinstock told the annual meeting that the committee had encountered great difficulties. Only a few results would be circulated. "Because of . . . the potentially misleading nature of the statistics it is recommended that members keep this report confidential." The committee was disbanded.[103] What then happened was even more piteous: The 3,000 reports from members plus follow-up data on outcomes of their analyses were sent to IBM for keypunching. The original data were lost. Some of the codes permitting the interpretation of the punchcards were lost. Some of the punchcards themselves were lost. Much later, in 1967, the Association managed to stagger together a few anodyne factoids and the whole project of "evaluating" the results of psychoanalysis was abandoned.[104] The entire fiasco was a monument to the psychoanalysts' fears of statistical verification.

With good cause. The few statistics that outsiders had managed to assemble spoke quite negatively of the effectiveness of psychoanalysis compared with other psychotherapies. In 1952, Hans Eysenck, director of the psychological department of the Maudsley Hospital, became the first to compare the outcomes of psychoanalysis with other "eclectic" therapies. Pointing out that two-thirds of all neurosis patients recover spontaneously within two years, Eysenck found that only 44 percent of psychoanalytic patients had improved by the end of their analysis, compared with 64 percent of those treated with eclectic therapies.[105] Even the eclectic therapies had not improved on chance, whereas psychoanalysis had, if anything, impeded the recovery of its clients.

In the coming decades, expressions of scientific disbelief in psychoanalysis mounted. A 1954 textbook by William Mayer-Gross, a Heidelberg psychiatrist (and Nissl student) who had found refuge in England, charged that "Freud's superficially rational appeal, made under the cloak of science, is probably the most effective form of faith-healing today."[106] Although Mayer-Gross had scorned the Americans for their curious obeisance to Freudianism, it was above all in the United States that the hammer blows against analysis began to ring out.

An example: In 1959 Donald Klein was still at the Hillside Hospital. He had a group of very anxious, panicky patients whom he put on the new drug chlorpromazine. Nothing happened. Wait a minute, Klein reasoned. American psychoanalytic theory said that psychic problems were caused by anxiety, itself the result of intrapsychic conflicts. Schizophrenics, who often were very anxious, did get better on chlorpromazine. But anxiety patients did not. Hence, it was probably not true that simple anxiety was just a few degrees down the anxiety scale from schizophrenia. "The continuity theory, which held that psychosis was simply a quantitative spilling over of the same anxiety suffered by people with more moderate disorders, could not be correct. If anything, the situation implied a physiological discontinuity, as with pneumonia and colds." Penicillin worked for pneumonia but not for colds. "This fact alone should lead one to guess that pneumonia and colds are not simply quantitative variants of the same theme, but are qualitatively distinct illnesses."[107] There must, in other words, be separate disease entities in psychiatry, not just a sliding scale from wellness to neurosis, to psychosis.

How about the psychoanalytic approach to schizophrenia? In the early 1960s, two researchers at the Camarillo State Hospital in California compared the length of stay of various groups of first-episode schizophrenics. One group was treated with psychoanalytic-style psychotherapy, another with drugs, still others with various combinations of therapy, or—the control group—with nothing. Those who received psychotherapy alone did least well (an average stay of 191 days). In fact, they did worse than the control group who received no treatment. Those who received the antipsychotic drug Stelazine (trifluoperazine) with no psychotherapy were out in 151 days.[108] For followers of Harry Stack Sullivan and Frieda Fromm-Reichmann, these were not encouraging results.

In the 1970s and after, the retreat of psychoanalysis turned into a rout. Concluded psychologists Seymour Fisher and Roger Greenberg in 1977, "There is virtually no evidence that therapies labeled 'psychoanalysis' result in longer-lasting or more profound positive changes than approaches that are given other labels and that are much less time-consuming and costly."[109] In two large tomes published in 1984 and 1993, philosopher Adolf Grünbaum of the University of Pittsburgh exposed the nullity of such notions as "transference," the core therapeutic concept in analysis.[110] Scholar after scholar scored the analysts for substituting essays and anecdotes for clinical data capable of scientific validation. One 1995 opus with 75 pages of footnotes gently explained *Why Freud Was Wrong*.[111] The Oedipal complex, infantile sexuality, the nature of dreams, women's special sexual attributes: All simply became objects of disbelief, not so much disproven—for they were incapable of disproof—but relegated to the same scientific status as astrology. Mainline psychiatry and psychology lost interest in psychoanalysis, stopped citing contributions in psychoanalytic journals, and pressed on in the study of thinking, memory, perception, and dysfunction as processes driven by a genetic program rather than by "the pressure of instinctual drive gratification invoked by Freud," as Grünbaum put it.[112]

"All sciences have to pass through an ordeal by quackery," observed Eysenck in 1985. "Chemistry had to slough off the fetters of alchemy. The brain sciences had to disengage themselves from the tenets of phrenology . . . Psychology and psychiatry, too will have to abandon the pseudo-science of psychoanalysis . . . and undertake the arduous task of transforming their discipline into a genuine science."[113]

Cosmetic Psychopharmacology

When Peter Kramer, a psychiatrist at Brown University, coined the delicious phrase "cosmetic psychopharmacology" in 1990,[114] he was applying it to a new antidepressive drug the Eli Lilly Company had developed called Prozac (fluoxetine). Kramer came in for much scorn in hyping a drug that, he claimed, made patients feel "better than well."[115]

Yet the symptoms of depression and anxiety that Prozac and similar drugs treated were not trivial affairs. The NCS study found that within the previous 12 months, 10.3 percent of all Americans had a major depressive episode, and that on a lifetime basis 19 percent of the population—1 person in 5—would undergo an often-disabling mood disorder. Almost 20 percent of the entire population had experienced a phobic disorder such as agoraphobia, fear of open spaces, within the previous 12 months; and almost 1 in 20 would feel a generalized kind of anxiety.[116] Such conditions were, in other words, extremely common, and those suffering from them were entitled to help rather than ridicule for their failure to pull up their socks.

There is no doubt that psychotherapy helped patients feel more comfortable with their psychiatrists, in contrast to the old-style alienists with their lack of interest in the complexities of the human spirit. Yet lifting symptoms rather than cultivating a sympathetic rapport in the office remained the ultimate therapeutic objective. And problems that had their origins in the brain would find their remedy in drugs that acted on the brain's chemical receptors. This was the good news for psychiatry: that a new panoply of drugs made it possible to help people with garden-variety anxiety and dysphoria, as opposed to the major psychiatric illnesses for which the antipsychotics, tricyclic antidepressants, and antimanic drugs stood ready.

The bad news was that by the end of the twentieth century these drugs had acquired such currency that, much as in the eighteenth century, patients began to view physicians as mere conduits to fabled new products rather than as counselors capable of using the doctor-patient relationship itself therapeutically. With the introduction of cosmetic psychopharmacology, medicine had come full circle. In olden times, patients had often been impatient with physicians, seeing them mainly as boil-lancers and enema-givers whose main resource lay in being able to write a prescription for a very powerful laxative, the kind of therapy that traditional patients coveted. In the world of postmodern medicine as well, patients often resented doctors for their real or imagined shortcomings, and saw the consultation mainly as a way of getting a prescription for drugs that they, the patients, had already predetermined were the answer to their problems. Physicians in primary care experienced this drug-seeking around requests for penicillin and other antibiotics.[117] In psychiatry it was experienced as patients' demands for Valium and Prozac.

Psychoactive drugs have always been available in one form or another to help people deal with depression and anxiety. Alcohol, which acts initially as a stimulant then a depressant, is as old as time. Opium achieved currency in the eighteenth century, and its alkaloids were used medically for depression in the nineteenth. The barbiturate sedatives had been available since the turn of our own century. Yet all had disadvantages in terms of addiction, daytime sedation, and inability to lift the core symptoms of psychiatric disorder.

The story of cosmetic psychopharmacology, the use of drugs with relatively few side effects to lift quotidian anxiety and depression, began with the advent of Miltown. Frank Berger, a Jewish refugee from Hitler, was the architect of this tale. Berger was born in Pilsen, Czechoslovakia, in 1913 and graduated in medicine from Prague in 1937. He fled to England and tossed about during the war as a bacteriologist, going to work in 1945 for the firm British Drug House. There he did some work with a muscle-relaxant called mephenesin, thinking that it might help patients with Parkinsonism. It did not, but Berger noted that it reduced anxiety for very short periods. "I was interested in the neuropharmacological basis of mental disturbances," said Berger later. "The phenomenon that interested me most was the physiological basis of nervousness. Most people get nervous and irritable for no good reason. They flair up, do not differentiate between serious problems and inconsequential ones, and somehow manage to get excited needlessly. These people are not insane; they simply are over-excitable and irritable, and create crisis situations over things that are unimportant. What is the physiological basis of this overexcitability?"[118] That turned out to be the billion-dollar question.

In 1947, Berger emigrated to the States, becoming assistant professor of pediatrics at the University of Rochester, and consulting for a small drug house named Carter Products whose chief previous claim to fame had been "Carter's Little Liver Pills." Carter wanted Berger to develop a mephenesin-like product for anxiety, and the firm instructed their crackerjack organic chemist, Bernie Ludwig, to synthesize some new compounds. In May 1950, he produced one that was later given the generic name meprobamate. Yet Carter lost interest in the drug after polling a sample of physicians and asking them if they would use a drug that acted against anxiety. Most said no. Meanwhile, in 1949 Berger had joined Carter's subsidiary Wallace Laboratories in Wallace, New Jersey. Berger had confidence in meprobamate and, with his executive authority at Wallace, went through all the steps of working meprobamate up, arranging trials for a thousand patients, giving it to pregnant animals to see if it caused birth defects, even making a movie to show how meprobamate calmed Rhesus monkeys, who usually are very angry about being in captivity.

Some people from Wyeth Laboratories saw the movie, expressed their interest to Berger, and learned that Carter Products wanted to sell the license. In 1955, Wallace began marketing meprobamate as "Miltown," Wyeth as "Equanil."[119] Both names went on to have enormous resonance in American cultural history in the 1950s as "tranquilizers."

Within psychiatry, there was intense excitement about Miltown. At the May 1955 meeting of the American Psychiatric Association, a "whispering campaign" went on, possibly instigated by Wallace Labs. "Have you heard of Miltown? I hear it's terrific." As veteran psychopharmacologist Frank Ayd recalled, "Few psychiatrists or science writers returned home from the 1955 APA meeting unaware of the existence of meprobamate."

In the following months, the demand for Miltown and Equanil was far greater than for any drug ever marketed in the United States. The supply in drugstores soon ran out and pharmacists would put signs in the window reading "out of Miltown" or "Miltown available tomorrow."[120] Miltown became a household word when television-host Milton Berle started humorously referring to himself as "Miltown" Berle. The title of S. J. Perelman's 1957 book *The Road to Miltown* made the drug common coinage among the Book-of-the-Month set.[121] *Look, Christian Century, Today's Health,* and *Time* ran stories about "Happy Pills," "Happiness Pills," "Peace of Mind Drugs," and "Happiness by Prescription."[122] By 1956, one American in twenty was taking tranquilizers within a given month.[123] Miltown was thus the first psychiatry drug to become the object of a popular frenzy.

Valium was the next frenzy.[124] Competing pharmaceutical houses had been observing intently the emergence of chlorpromazine and Miltown. In 1954, Hoffmann-La Roche, a Swiss-based drug house with a large American office in Nutley, New Jersey, instructed its organic chemists to develop a "psychosedative drug."

Interestingly, neither university scientists nor government grants were involved in any of this: It was all driven by the profit motive. As Irvin Cohen, one of the psychiatrists who first tested Valium's sister-drug Librium later reflected, "The benzodiazepine [Valium etc.] story is essentially a model of how a therapeutic agent is conceived and brought forth by an enterprising pharmaceutical manufacturer who simply seeks to find a drug superior to others already in the marketplace."[125] Thus Roche was merely hoping that its organic chemists would bring it abreast of the game.

One of Roche's chemists was a refugee named Leo Sternbach, who had received his PhD in organic chemistry in 1931 from Krakow's Jagiellonian University. Sternbach went on to do postgraduate research in Zurich, then in 1940 was hired by Roche in Basel. In 1940, the Swiss were highly fearful that the Germans were about to invade them. Roche decided to send its Jewish scientists to safety, and in 1941 Sternbach was transferred to the Nutley branch plant.

When Sternbach received this directive from on high in 1954, he thought about a class of dyes that he had worked with in Krakow in the mid-1930s. He set to work synthesizing a series of new dye-type products (benzheptoxdiazines) but got nowhere. All were inert in pharmacological testing on animals. Finally, the Roche management asked him to discontinue the research. In April 1957, as he was clearing his cluttered lab bench, he noticed that one of the compounds he had synthesized in 1955 had developed crystals at the bottom. With typical Central-European thoroughness, he decided to send it for testing, promising management that "this would be his last product of this series."[126]

A few days later Sternbach got a phone call from Lowell Randall, Roche's director of pharmacology. This last compound in the series, later called chlordiazepoxide (Librium), had proven very interesting indeed. They were particularly impressed with its "taming effect" in a colony of imputedly vicious monkeys, at doses that did not otherwise affect the monkeys' alertness. Also, "Librium causes a mouse to hang limply when held by one ear; but [unlike meprobamate] it is able to walk when prodded."[127] The drug did seem to have extraordinary qualities. Roche applied for a patent in May 1958.

In January 1959, Roche's medical director persuaded a few psychiatrists to try chlordiazepoxide on some of their office-practice patients. The patients did very well, becoming much less anxious and tense, and sleeping better.[128] Emboldened by the enthusiasm of the psychiatrists, Roche marketed chlordiazepoxide in February 1960 under the trade name Librium. It was the first of the benzodiazepines, or "benzos," and during the 1960s was the number one prescription drug in the United States. Ultimately, there would be more than a thousand kinds of benzos on world markets.[129]

Yet Librium had a number of side effects and could cause fits if suddenly discontinued.[130] Roche felt the series Sternbach was working on

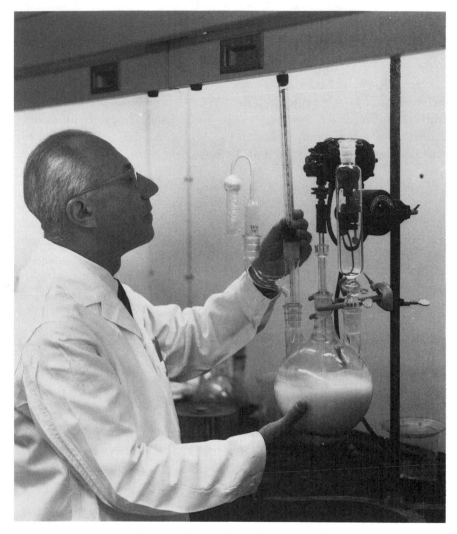

Leo Sternbach, who in the late 1950s synthesized the first of the benzodiazepine tranquilizers ("Librium," "Valium"), here seen in his lab at Roche Laboratories in Nutley, N. J. Valium was introduced in 1963, a year after the photograph was taken (courtesy Hoffmann-La Roche).

had further potential. He was sent back to the lab bench. In 1959, he came up with a related benzo, diazepam, that was considerably more potent and that could be stabilized in pills. Roche marketed diazepam in 1963 as "Valium," which until the introduction of Prozac was the single most successful drug in pharmaceutical history. In 1969, Valium surpassed

Librium as number one on the American drug list.[131] By 1970, one woman in five and one man in thirteen was using "minor tranquilizers and sedatives," meaning mainly the benzos.[132]

The benzodiazepines had a dramatic impact on the practice of psychiatry. For the first time, psychiatrists were able to offer their patients a potent drug, unlike the mild Miltown, that did not sedate them. (The antipsychotics were simply too potent for routine use in psychiatry.) The share of psychiatric patients receiving prescriptions increased from a quarter of all office visits in 1975 to fully one-half by 1990 (from 25.3 percent to 50.2 percent).[133] With the benzodiazepines as the entering wedge, psychiatry became increasingly a specialty oriented to the provision of medication. With the profession's main previous treatment modality, dynamic psychotherapy, now falling into disuse, an alternative lay at hand.

There was, however, one problem: The benzodiazepines turned out to be addictive, in the sense that patients' symptoms after trying to discontinue the drug were often worse than before starting. In recognition of their potential for abuse, in 1975 the Food and Drug Administration put the benzodiazepines and meprobamate on its "schedule IV," controlling refills and imposing on pharmacists special reporting requirements.[134] Sales had already leveled off, and by 1980 Valium (diazepam) stood number 32 on the list of most commonly prescribed drugs, Librium (chlordiazepoxide) number 59.[135] It was the end of "Valiumania." Nonetheless, the drugs had not exactly gone out of style: almost 7 million prescriptions a year continued to be written in the United States for Valium-style products.

Until this point, there had been very little "unscientific" in the narrative. The benzodiazepines were perfectly appropriate for the treatment of anxiety and mild depression, and science-schooled psychiatrists did well to put their patients on them. Yet it had now become apparent that great sums were to be earned in the sale of psychiatry drugs. As Valium soared in popularity, awareness dawned among drugmakers that here lay the markets of the future. As the highly competitive drug companies rushed into psychopharmaceuticals, they began to distort psychiatry's own diagnostic sense. In trying to create for themselves market niches, drug companies would balloon illness categories. A given disorder might have been scarcely noticed until a drug company claimed to have a remedy for it, after which it became epidemic. As historian of psychopharmacology David Healy puts it, "As often happens in medicine, the availability of a treatment leads to an increase in recognition of the disorder that might benefit from that treatment."[136]

Take, for example, panic disorder. The tradition in psychiatry was to see panic as part of anxiety. As *DSM-II* said in 1968 of "anxiety neurosis," "This neurosis is characterized by anxious over-concern extending to panic and frequently associated with somatic symptoms."[137] In 1964, however, Donald Klein, then at Hillside Hospital in Glen Oaks, New York, published an article suggesting that panic was really an illness entity distinct from anxiety. Partially funded by the Geigy and the Smith Kline & French drug companies, the study concluded that one could forestall such attacks by staying on medication.[138] As Klein was a member of the *DSM-III* task force, as well as its subcommittee on "anxiety and dissociative disorders," he was able to persuade other members of the correctness of his views. In 1980, with the publication of *DSM-III*, panic disorder became an illness of its own, characterized, it was said, by "the sudden onset of intense apprehension" and marked by physical sensations such as sweating and faintness.[139] The following year, in 1981, the Upjohn Company of Kalamazoo, Michigan, marketed a new kind of benzodiazepine generically named alprazolam (Xanax). Because the market for benzos was sinking at the time, Upjohn attempted to reposition its benzo as a drug specific for the newly created disease entity "panic disorder." In the 1980s, the company funded extensive field trials—orchestrated by Cornell's Gerald Klerman—to establish that panic was really an independent disease for which alprazolam worked wonders.[140] The results were not entirely convincing.[141] Nonetheless, by the early 1990s Xanax had become one of the hottest drugs in psychiatry, prescribed by many psychiatrists in good faith that they were practicing scientifically and that Xanax offered unique hope in the epidemic of panic disorder sweeping the nation. Among insiders, panic jokingly became known as "the Upjohn illness."

Against this background of psychiatric diagnosis increasingly manipulated by pharmaceutical companies arose the psychiatry drug that was to become the household word of the 1990s: Prozac. When Valium came along, both patients and their doctors were willing to define their problems in terms of anxiety once an effective drug existed for treating it. When Prozac, a drug for depression, arrived on the scene, the accent fell on depression as the hallmark of distress. "Our phone rings off the hook every time someone does a story about Prozac," said one physician at Manhattan's Beth Israel Medical Center. "People want to try it. If you tell them they're not depressed they say, 'Sure I am!' "[142]

Prozac's pathway to fame began in July 1953 when John Gaddum, then at Edinburgh and one of the founders of psychopharmacology in Britain, speculated to a small but influential group of researchers, "It is possible that the 5-HT [serotonin] in our brains plays an essential part in keeping us sane."[143] That utterance became the "signpost in the sky" of a whole generation of young psychopharmacologists.[144] Gaddum himself had done some of the basic scientific work on assessing serotonin, and the early story was one of those triumphs of British pharmacology.[145] But it followed that if serotonin kept us sane, increasing the availability of serotonin in the brain might counter psychiatric illness.

The scene shifted to the National Institutes of Health in Bethesda, where researchers in Bernard Brodie's Laboratory of Chemical Pathology discovered in 1957 that an antipsychotic drug named reserpine could unlock the body's stores of serotonin. The Brodie group correlated behavioral changes with the presence of the various amines, and serotonin became a star. It was the Brodie lab, "LCP," that opened the whole psychiatric side of serotonin research. "LCP," recalled one researcher fondly, "was the Camelot of pharmacology."[146]

But it's often forgotten that there was a British Camelot as well. The young researchers, inspired by Gaddum, were burrowing into brain chemistry at the same time as the Americans. In 1963, Alec Coppen, a biochemist-psychiatrist of the Medical Research Council and staff member at St. Ebba's Hospital, did a crucial experiment showing that serotonin-equivalents could relieve depression.[147] Said Coppen later, "I claim this was the first observation that suggested that 5-HT [serotonin] was important in depression—an idea that is now the centre of a multi-billion pound drug market. But for many years, people said yah-boo sucks—there's nothing in this. Fashions are everything in medicine and 5-HT was not in fashion."[148]

Coppen well knew. In the late 1960s, Arvid Carlsson had reinforced the news that serotonin seemed to control mood and drive.[149] And Carlsson was coaching a Swedish drug company, Astra Pharmaceuticals, in its efforts to bring to market a drug that would inhibit the reuptake of serotonin in fighting depression. In 1981, Astra brought "Zelmid" (zimelidine) onto the market in several European countries.[150] The experience ended in disaster: two years later zimelidine was withdrawn from use as toxic. Nonetheless, Carlsson and Astra count as the initial pioneers of what would later be called SSRIs: selective serotonin reuptake inhibitors.

One might easily bypass these tales of drug companies and their misadventures were they not such a key element in late-twentieth-century psychiatry. For at the Eli Lilly Company in Indianapolis as well, SSRIs were coming into fashion in the 1970s. The firm's senior pharmacologist Ray Fuller had been following international developments in serotonin.

When Fuller came to Lilly in 1971, he tried to interest the firm in the idea that serotonin might have some action against depression in particular. Lilly was resistant. Recalled Alec Coppen of a conference at Lilly's base in Surrey in the early 1970s, "I'll always remember the Vice President of Research saying 'I thank Dr. Coppen for his contribution but I can tell you we won't be developing fluoxetine [Lilly's serotonin drug] as an antidepressant.'"

Yet Fuller, in alliance with Lilly biochemist David Wong, carried the day inside the company. Lilly organized a serotonin-depression team. In the meantime, Lilly had already asked chemist Bryan Molloy to synthesize a series of compounds that might function as antidepressants, minus the side effects of the tricyclics. Wong found that some of these compounds inhibited the reuptake of serotonin at the synapse, thus increasing its availability to the brain. (At present writing, this concept is regarded as simplified: Antidepressants probably do not work by relieving a deficiency of a monoamine such as serotonin.[151]) By 1974, lab tests were in progress on "Lilly 110140,"[152] which shortly received the generic name fluoxetine, later the trade name Prozac. In 1976, Lilly tested a Prozac analogue, nisoxetine, on healthy volunteers, who showed no side effects. The research also established that the drug did not seem to block the reuptake of other neurotransmitters such as noradrenaline,[153] that it too, in other words, seemed to be a SSRI. (The acronym SSRI came into general use only in the early 1990s.[154]) By 1978, Lilly was using the phrase specific serotonin reuptake inhibitor in connection with fluoxetine.[155] Meanwhile, fluoxetine was being put into clinical trials in Indianapolis and Chicago: The results were promising although Lilly—perhaps for competitive reasons—did not publish them.[156]

In 1980, the company decided to go all-out on the drug and sought some big-name biological psychiatrists to help test fluoxetine. John Feighner had left Samuel Guze's department in St. Louis to establish his own private psychiatric clinic in La Mesa, California. Some very good news for the firm flowed from this clinic in 1983: Fluoxetine was just as good as the standard tricyclics in combating depression, and was without huge side effects. There was one more thing: Among the 12 different new antidepressants that Feighner was evaluating, fluoxetine was the only one that had as a "side effect" weight loss.[157] (The first generation antidepressants often caused weight gains.) For millions of individuals, of course, weight loss is not a side effect but an ardently desired goal. A weight-reduction drug requiring no dietary restrictions would have an enormous market. After Lilly mentioned in its 1985 annual report that the company was developing a drug for weight loss, the stock soared.[158]

Yet the more that Lilly tested fluoxetine as an antidepressant, the more the company put weight loss on the back burner, for the findings that came in from a number of field trials between 1984 and 1987 showed that patients would find fluoxetine much superior to the standard tricyclics because it had fewer side effects, making them feel, if anything, euphoric and "wired" rather than leaden and constipated. It also acted earlier and possessed a safer therapeutic window, meaning a wide margin between the therapeutic dose and the toxic dose (hence patients didn't have to be monitored with blood tests).[159] In December 1987, the Food and Drug Administration approved Prozac for use.[160]

In 1990, three years after Prozac was released, two researchers at McLean Hospital published an article suggesting that the drug was effective not merely for depression but for a range of disorders from panic to drop attacks ("cataplexy"). Since all of these conditions responded to Prozac (as well as to other drugs), they must have something in common, perhaps membership in an Affective Spectrum Disorder (ASD). This created an apparent scientific justification for expanding greatly the notion of depression, which now became one of "the most widespread diseases of mankind," as the authors put it.[161] One of the authors, Harrison Pope, was quoted as saying that ASD affected "possibly one third of the population of the world."[162] The prospects for Prozac became incalculable.

And so the word went out. By 1993, almost half of all visits to American psychiatrists were for mood disorders.[163] Just as Valium had assuaged a nation beset by anxiety, the availability of a new drug for depression had produced a pattern of disorder the drug was capable of treating.

What followed was a media psychocircus of suggestion, as Prozac and its competitors were extended to the world public as a panacea for coping with life's problems even in the absence of psychiatric illness (one recalls that the great majority of individuals with a formal psychiatric illness seek no treatment of any kind). Prozac is "much more than a fad," proclaimed *Time* in 1993. "It is a medical breakthrough" that has brought relief to individuals such as "Susan," a self-described workaholic who becomes irritable around the time of her periods and once threw her wedding ring at her husband. Now the edges of her personality had been planed off a bit.[164] It would be ludicrous to argue that such people suffered a formal psychiatric illness in the historic tradition of the agonized and the inconsolable, for real psychiatric disease causes terrible pain and disablement. Yet here lay part of Prozac's core market.

Driven by the promise of problem-free personality and weight loss, Prozac took off more rapidly than any other psychiatric drug in history.

By 1990, less than three years after its appearance, it had become the number one drug prescribed by psychiatrists.[165] "With Millions Taking Prozac, A Legal Drug Culture Arises," headlined the *New York Times*.[166] The black market that was developing for the drug seemed hardly necessary, for physicians were prescribing it for everything imaginable. "Prozac has attained the familiarity of Kleenex and the social status of spring water," said *Newsweek* in 1994. "The drug has shattered old stigmas," as Americans were said to be "swapping stories about it at dinner parties."[167] By 1994, Prozac had become the number two best-selling drug in the world, following, perhaps ironically, an ulcer drug named Zantac.[168]

Inserting Prozac into the history of psychiatry, requires untangling good science from scientism. Good science lay behind the discovery of fluoxetine as a much safer and quicker second-generation antidepressant than imipramine and the other tricyclics, whose discovery Kuhn had launched. Scientism lay behind converting a whole host of human difficulties into the depression scale, and making all treatable with a wonder drug. This conversion was possible only because clinical psychiatry had enmeshed itself so massively in the corporate culture of the drug industry. The result was that a scientific discipline such as psychiatry nurtured a popular culture of pharmacological hedonism, as millions of people who otherwise did not have a psychiatric disorder craved the new compound because it lightened the burden of self-consciousness while making it possible for them to stay slim.

Yet the Prozac episode produced one massive benefit for the public good: It helped psychiatric conditions begin to seem acceptable in the eyes of the public, although we are still far from speaking of a complete destigmatization of mental illness. The "insane," who had transfixed the public view with horror for centuries, had now vanished to be replaced by people suffering from "stress" for whom help was easily available. Said *Newsweek* in 1990, a sure guide to the public pulse, "As Prozac's success stories mount, so does the sense that depression and other mental disorders are just that—treatable illnesses, not failings of character."[169] In the judgment of historian Healy, the pharmacotherapy of mild depression had evidenced itself to be so successful that one might conclude "'biological depression' is a mild illness for the most part and that those who end up being hospitalized for the disorder are an unrepresentative minority."[170]

There were other players in this beginning destigmatization of mental illness. The National Alliance for the Mentally Ill, or NAMI, a Washington-based advocacy group founded in 1979 consisting of parents and friends of those with major mental illnesses, campaigned against such stigmatizing notions as the schizophrenogenic family and insisted that schizophrenia was a biological disease. By 1996, NAMI had 130,000 members and a staff of 38. Were the mentally ill so awful that local communities should ship them away on a bus? In 1985, a National Coalition of Psychiatrists Against Motorcoach Therapy was formed, dedicated to stopping the practice of "procuring one-way bus fares for habitual and undesirable mental health patients" after their release from the hospital.[171] In various ways, therefore, advocacy groups militated to ensure the acceptance of psychiatric illness as just another kind of medical illness and not something outlandish and fearsome.

Nonetheless, if by the end of the twentieth century, "lunacy" ended up seeming less awful, the success was heavily that of psychopharmacology. It was not that people themselves had become more understanding or tolerant, merely that the drug revolution had made it possible to dampen or abolish entirely the symptoms of psychiatric illness, so that individuals with these disorders needed be no more feared than people with a broken arm or a bruise on the head. "After 37 years," said Pierre Deniker, who had helped initiate the pharmacological revolution, "the face of madness has been completely changed, not only by means of psychopharmacology but also by the development of psychotherapy, sociotherapy and the rehabilitation of the patients in the community." For Deniker, "the insane or lunatic" had metamorphosed into "an ordinary patient."[172] Whether one deems drug therapy to be "cosmetic" psychopharmacology or not, this is no small achievement.

Why Psychiatry?

In two hundred years' time, psychiatrists had progressed from being the healers of the therapeutic asylum to serving as gatekeepers for Prozac. Psychiatric illness had passed from a feared sign of bad blood—a genetic curse—to an easily treatable condition not essentially different from any other medical problem, and possessing roughly the same affective valence. Indeed, so much like other medical illnesses had disorders of the mind become that the uncomfortable question arose, who needed psychiatrists?

Physicians themselves began increasingly to avoid the field. The percentage of American medical graduates planning to specialize in psychiatry fell from 3.5 in 1984 to 2.0 in 1994, a decline of almost half. By the mid-1990s fewer than 500 young doctors were entering psychiatry training programs annually.[173]

The crisis of psychiatry at the end of the twentieth century was not dissimilar to that at the beginning, when neurology and internal medicine had threatened to gobble up office-practice psychotherapy and the asylum menaced entombing psychiatry itself in a mausoleum of red brick. The difference was that by the century's end psychiatry possessed a more solid physical basis than the asylum, namely a proprietary knowledge of the use of drugs.

Yet such specialty knowledge could prove a slim reed. Other medical professions with specialized knowledge had gone under as science raced past their wisdom, witness hydrotherapy. Moreover, psychiatry had a long history of losing ground. Every time a psychiatric disorder became medicalized, it disappeared from psychiatry. Thus over the years, psychiatry had lost neurosyphilis to the internists, mental retardation to the pediatricians, and stroke to the neurologists. Now that psychiatry itself had become medicalized, what justification was there for retaining it as a separate specialty? The psychotherapeutic side could easily be hived off to the psychologists and social workers, who were more intensively trained as therapists, and the brain-biological side assigned to the neurologists, who felt more at home looking at CT scans and determining the significance of lesions in the basal ganglia. What was left?[174]

Consider this confrontation. "I'd been feeling tired, rundown, and very weepy," said a patient. "It seemed relentless, and although I rarely go to the doctor, I felt it wise to get a good physical and checkup. He listened for about 2 minutes (not even looking at me), suddenly said, 'You're depressed,' handed me a prescription, and walked out." The patient was so angry that she slammed his office door and rushed home in tears. "I could have been a bit of furniture for all he cared—and I didn't even get a physical!"[175]

Psychiatry is a specialty that specializes in the doctor-patient relationship. Whether one is trained on the psychotherapeutic side or the neuroscientific, one learns as a budding psychiatrist that giving one's patients time is the essence of the art. Whereas the average consultation in internal medicine or obstetrics lasts only around 10 minutes, the average in psychiatry lasts over 40.[176]

Within this 40 minutes, psychiatrists do essentially two things that their competitors on either side—the psychologists on the one side, the neurologists on the other—do not do. Psychiatrists offer psychotherapy, which the neurologists generally speaking do not (the average consultation in neurology lasts only 28 minutes, and goes on that long only because the neurological exam is so time-consuming[177]). And psychiatrists prescribe medications, which the nonmedical competition is not permitted to do.

This combination of psychotherapy plus medication represents the most effective of all approaches in dealing with disorders of the brain and mind. Surveys comparing the effectiveness of psychotherapy alone, medication alone, and the two together, converge on the finding that "neurochem" and "neurochat" augment each other as the optimum form of care. "The advantage for combined treatment is striking," concluded one study. "A combination of treatments may represent more than an additive effect of two treatments." Instead, the one seems to potentiate the other.[178] There may be a synergistic relationship between biological improvement from medication and an opportunity to discuss with a sympathetic physician the kind of cognitive disorientation that occurs in psychiatric illness.

The accent here is on physician. Although the skills of the psychologist and social worker are not to be denigrated, the history of medicine suggests that patients derive some kind of bonus from the knowledge that they are dealing with a physician. It seems to be true that the kind of catharsis achieved from telling one's story to a figure of respect is heightened when that figure is not merely a friend or confidant, but a doctor.[179] "Human suffering responds to the spoken word rendered by compassionate persons cast in the role of healer," said one observer. "Even though men have known this for a long, long time, is it still very good news."[180]

Notes

Abbreviations used in Notes:

AJP   *American Journal of Psychiatry*
BJP   *British Journal of Psychiatry*
BMJ   *British Medical Journal*
BMSJ   *Boston Medical and Surgical Journal*
JAMA   *Journal of the American Medical Association*
JNMD   *Journal of Nervous and Mental Disease*
NEJM   *New England Journal of Medicine*
PNW   *Psychiatrisch-Neurologische Wochenschrift*
Munk's Roll William Munk, *Roll of the Royal College of Physicians of London* (London: RCP, 1861–   )

Chapter 1: The Birth of Psychiatry

1. Cited in William P. Letchworth, *The Insane in Foreign Countries* (New York: Putnam's, 1889), p. 172.

2. *King Lear*, III, iv.

3. Anton Müller, *Die Irren-Anstalt in dem königlichen Julius-Hospitale zu Würzburg* (Würzburg: Stahel, 1824), pp. 44, 46–47, 151, 164–165.

4. K. Ernst, "Geisteskrankheit ohne Institution: eine Feldstudie im Kanton Fribourg aus dem Jahr 1875," *Schweizer Archiv für Neurologie, Neurochirurgie und Psychiatrie*, 133 (1983), pp. 239–262, quotes pp. 250, 251.

5. Louis Caradec, *Topographie médico-hygiènique du département du Finistère* (Brest: Anner, 1860), p. 335.

6. William Perfect, *Select Cases in the Different Species of Insanity* (Rochester: Gillman, 1787), pp. 131–133.

7. Dorothea L. Dix, "Report to the Legislature of Massachusetts of Jan. 1843," *On Behalf of the Insane Poor: Selected Reports* (reprint New York: Arno Press, 1971), quotes pp. 5–7.

8. Michel Foucault writes of the early-modern period, "Madness traces a very familiar silhouette in the social landscape. A new and lively pleasure is taken in the old confraternities of madmen, in their festivals, their gatherings. . . ." "This world of the early seventeenth century is strangely hospitable, in all senses, to madness." *Madness and Civilization: A History of Insanity in the Age of Reason*, Fr. trans. from 1961 ed. (New York: Random House, 1965), pp. 40–41. The historical basis for Foucault's statements is extremely slender. Foucault's work has greatly influenced other historians of psychiatry, for example, Klaus Dörner, *Bürger und Irre: Zur Sozialgeschichte und Wissenschaftssoziologie der Psychiatrie* (Frankfurt/M.: Europäische Verlagsanstalt, 1969), p. 217.

9. See Patricia Allderidge, "Hospitals, Madhouses and Asylums: Cycles in the Care of the Insane," *BJP*, 134 (1979), pp. 321–334, esp. p. 323.

10. See Kathleen Jones, *Asylums and After: A Revised History of the Mental Health Services: From the Early 18th Century to the 1990s* (London: Athlone, 1993), pp. 7–10.

11. Richard Hunter and Ida Macalpine, *Three Hundred Years of Psychiatry 1535–1860* (London: Oxford U. P., 1963), p. 632.

12. Mark Winston, "The Bethel at Norwich: An Eighteenth-Century Hospital for Lunatics," *Medical History*, 38 (1994), pp. 27–51; p. 27 n. 4 lists all eight.

13. See William Ll. Parry-Jones, *The Trade in Lunacy: A Study of Private Madhouses in England in the Eighteenth and Nineteenth Centuries* (London: Routledge, 1972).

14. John Haslam, *Observations on Madness and Melancholy*, 2nd rev. ed. (London: Callow, 1809; first ed. 1798), p. 317.

15. Andrew Halliday, *General View of the Present State of Lunatics and Lunatic Asylums in Great Britain and Ireland* (London: Underwood, 1828), pp. 14–15.

16. Foucault, *Madness and Civilization*; ch. 2 is entitled "The Great Confinement."

17. Cited in Introduction, George Mora, ed. and trans., Vincenzio Chiarugi, *On Insanity and Its Classification* (Canton, MA: Science History Pubs., 1987), p. lxxxiii. Chiarugi's *Della Pazzia* was originally published in Florence in 1793–1794 in three vols.

18. See Jean-Pierre Goubert and Roselyne Rey, eds., *Atlas de la révolution française, vol. 7: Médecine et santé* (Paris: Éditions de l'École des Hautes Études en Sciences Sociales, 1993), pp. 38, 43.

19. See Goubert, *Atlas*, p. 48, for statistics on the *dépôt de mendicité* of Rouen, 1788–1800, where the "fous" were greatly outnumbered by the beggars (both well and unwell), and by patients with infectious illnesses (p. 48).

20. Johann Christian Reil, *Rhapsodieen über die Anwendung der psychischen Curmethode auf Geisteszerüttungen* (Halle, 1803; reprint Amsterdam: Bonset, 1968), pp. 7, 14.

21. For a listing of the principal institutions in Germany together with their founding dates, see Heinrich Laehr, *Ueber Irrsein und Irrenanstalten* (Halle: Pfeffer, 1852), pp. 242–283.

22. Müller, *Julius-Hospitale*, p. 17.

23. Examples from Mary Ann Jimenez, *Changing Faces of Madness: Early American Attitudes and Treatment of the Insane* (Hanover, NH: University Press of New England, 1987), pp. 38–39.

24. For an overview, see Gerald N. Grob, *The Mad among Us: A History of the Care of America's Mentally Ill* (New York: Free Press, 1994), pp. 17–21.

25. On New York Hospital, see Henry M. Hurd, ed., *The Institutional Care of the Insane in the United States and Canada*, 4 vols. (Baltimore: Johns Hopkins Press, 1916–1917), vol. 3, pp. 133–135.

26. Norman Dain, *Disordered Minds: The First Century of Eastern State Hospital in Williamsburg, Virginia, 1766–1866* (Charlottesville: University Press of Virginia, 1971), p. 9.

27. Reil, *Rhapsodieen*, pp. 52–53.

28. Andrew Scull lambasted capitalism strongly in his influential *Museums of Madness: The Social Organization of Insanity in Nineteenth-Century England* (London: Allen Lane, 1979), pp. 30–31 and passim, then returned to gnaw in passing at this bone again in *The Most Solitary of Afflictions: Madness and Society in Britain, 1700–1900* (New Haven: Yale U. P., 1993), a book that is essentially an extensively revised second edition of *Museums*, see pp. 106, 125. For a Foucauldian invocation of the central state as the villain in the piece see, for example, Dirk Blasius, *Der verwaltete Wahnsinn: Eine Sozialgeschichte des Irrenhauses* (Frankfurt/M.:Fischer, 1980, passim). Texts from other such zealot-scholars permeate the literature.

29. Hunter and Macalpine, *Three Hundred Years of Psychiatry*, p. 402.

30. William Battie, *A Treatise on Madness* (London: Whiston, 1758), pp. 68–69.

31. Battie, *Treatise*, p. 93.

32. Henri Ellenberger, *The Discovery of the Unconscious: The History and Evolution of Dynamic Psychiatry* (New York: Basic, 1970) passes over Battie in silence in searching for predecessors of Freud. Psychoanalyst-historian Gregory Zilboorg gives Battie a glancing reference as dealing "primarily with the brain." *A History of Medical Psychology* (New York: Norton, 1941), p. 301.

33. On Chiarugi's life, see P. L. Cabras, *Uno psichiatra prima della psichiatria: Vincenzio Chiarugi* (Florence: Scientific Press, 1993); see also Mora's introduction to Chiarugi's *On Insanity*, esp. pp. lii–liii. On the image of Chiarugi in the historiography of Italian psychiatry, see Patrizia Guarnieri, *La Storia della psichiatria: Un secolo di studi in Italia* (Florence: Olschki, 1991), pp. 17–19.

34. On Pinel's life, see René Semelaigne, *Philippe Pinel et son oeuvre au point de vue de la médecine mentale* (Paris: Imps. Réunies, 1888; reprint Arno Press, 1976), pp. 1–53, p. 20 on Pinel and the Belhomme clinic; Jan Goldstein,

Console and Classify: The French Psychiatric Profession in the Nineteenth Century (New York: Cambridge U. P., 1987), pp. 67–72, 122–123. For a convenient overview, see also Raymond de Saussure, "Philippe Pinel," in Kurt Kolle, ed., *Grosse Nervenärzte*, 2nd ed. vol. 1 (Stuttgart: Thieme, 1970), pp. 216–235. On Pinel as "liberator" of the insane, see also Dieter Jetter, *Zur Typologie des Irrenhauses in Frankreich und Deutschland (1780–1840)* (Wiesbaden: Steiner, 1971), pp. 18–27. On the Belhomme clinic, see René Benard, "Une maison de santé psychiatrique sous la révolution: La maison Belhomme," *Semaine des hôpitaux de Paris*, 32 (Dec. 20, 1956), pp. 3991–4000.

35. Philippe Pinel, *Traité médico-philosophique sur l'aliénation mentale*, 2nd ed. (Paris: Brosson, 1809; first ed. 1801), pp. 252–253.

36. See the testimony of German visitors of the day gathered in Christian Müller, *Vom Tollhaus zum Psychozentrum: Vignetten und Bausteine zur Psychiatriegeschichte in zeitlicher Abfolge* (Hürtgenwald, Switz.: Pressler, 1993), pp. 43–58.

37. Goldstein offers a reliable guide to these events, *Console and Classify*, p. 124 and passim.

38. On Esquirol, see René Semelaigne, *Les pionniers de la psychiatrie française avant et après Pinel*, 2 vols. (Paris: Baillière, 1930), vol. 1, pp. 124–140; Henri Ey, "J. E. D. Esquirol," in Kolle, *Grosse Nervenärzte*, 2nd ed., vol. 2 (1970), pp. 87–97.

39. Mentioned in Pinel, *Traité*, p. 236, n. 1. On this private hospital, see Dora B. Weiner, "Esquirol's Patient Register: The First Private Psychiatric Hospital in Paris, 1802–1808," *Bulletin of the History of Medicine*, 63 (1989), pp. 110–120.

40. See, for example, Esquirol, "De la lypémanie ou mélancolie" (1820), in Esquirol, *Des maladies mentales*, 3 vols. (Paris: Baillière, 1838), vol. 1, p. 470.

41. For an overview of Reil's life and ideas, see Otto M. Marx, "German Romantic Psychiatry," *History of Psychiatry*, 1 (1990), pp. 351–381 esp. pp. 361–368 and 2 (1991), pp. 1–25, esp. p. 1. Despite the title of Marx's article, it is difficult to consider Reil a "Romantic psychiatrist." See also on Reil's life, Adalbert Gregor, "Johann Christian Reil," in Theodor Kirchhoff, ed., *Deutsche Irrenärzte*, 2 vols. (Berlin: Springer, 1921–1924), vol. 1, pp. 28–42. On Reil as the obstacle to the diffusion of Pinel's views in Germany, see Heinrich Neumann, *Die Irrenanstalt zu Pöpelwitz bei Breslau* (Erlangen: Enke, 1862), p. 5. Neumann said that what made Esquirol's views appealing to the Germans was their foundation on experience in a private clinic.

42. Reil, *Rhapsodieen*, pp. 16–17, 19.

43. Reil, *Rhapsodieen*, pp. 185–187, 209–211.

44. Ernst Horn, *Oeffentliche Rechenschaft über meine zwölfjährige Dienstführung* (Berlin: Realschul, 1818), p. 73.

45. Karl Birnbaum, "Ernst Horn," in Kirchhoff, *Deutsche Irrenärzte*, vol. 1, pp. 77–83, quote p. 81. On Horn's reforms, see also George Windholz, "Psychiatric Treatment and the Condition of the Mentally Disturbed at Berlin's

Charité in the Early Decades of the Nineteenth Century," *History of Psychiatry*, 6 (1995), pp. 157–176.

46. For a textbook example of this kind of parochialism, oblivious to international trends, see the American Psychiatric Association's history of itself, Walter E. Barton, *The History and Influence of the American Psychiatric Association* (Washington: APA, 1987).

47. Barton, *History American Psychiatric Association*, p. 302.

48. Benjamin Rush, "An Inquiry into the Influence of Physical Causes upon the Moral Faculty" (1786), in Rush, *Medical Inquiries and Observations*, 4-vols.-in-2 (Philadelphia: Carey, 1815; Arno Press reprint, 1972), vol. 1, pp. 93–124, quote p. 97. As early as 1944 Adolf Meyer called Rush the "Father of American Psychiatry." "Revaluation of Benjamin Rush" (1944), in Eunice E. Winters, ed., *Collected Papers of Adolf Meyer, vol. 3: Medical Teaching* (Baltimore: Johns Hopkins Press, 1951), pp. 503–515, see esp. pp. 503 and 515.

49. Benjamin Rush, *Medical Inquiries and Observations upon the Diseases of the Mind* (1812), 3d ed. (Philadelphia: Grigg, 1827), p. 15.

50. Quoted in Hurd, *Institutional Care of the Insane*, vol. 3, p. 403.

51. Rush, *Medical Inquiries Mind*, pp. 241–242.

52. See Franco Valsecchi, *L'Italia nel Settecento dal 1714 al 1788* (n.p.: Mondadori, 1959), pp. 633 682; Eric Cochrane, *Florence in the Forgotten Centuries 1527–1800* (Chicago: University of Chicago Press, 1973), pp. 449–453.

53. See, for example, Scull, *Most Solitary of Afflictions*, pp. 3–4, 198–199, 233–234. Scull seems to take the viewpoint that there is no such thing as mental illness, which would make psychiatrists' claims to treat such illness superfluous. On the subject of asylum psychiatrists in the nineteenth century, he writes, "By sustaining the illusion that asylums were medical institutions, they placed a humanitarian and scientific gloss on the community's behaviour, legitimizing the removal of difficult and troublesome people whose confinement would have been awkward to justify on other grounds" (p. 246).

54. Reil, *Rhapsodieen*, p. 19.

55. According to Achim Mechler, "Das Wort 'Psychiatrie': Historische Anmerkungen," *Nervenarzt*, 34 (1963), pp. 405–406. Mechler cites Reil's *Beiträge zur Beförderung einer Curmethode auf psychischem Wege* (Halle, 1808), which I have not seen.

56. John Ferriar, *Medical Histories and Reflections*, 4 vols. (London: Cadell, 1810), vol. 2, pp. 109–110. An earlier edition of this work appeared in 1792–1798.

57. See the essay "Begriff der psychischen Medicin als Wissenschaft," apparently written by Adalbert Kayssler, in *Magazin für die psychische Heilkunde*, 1 (i) (1805), pp. 45–77.

58. Battie, *Treatise on Madness*, p. 69.

59. Ferriar, *Medical Histories*, vol. 2, pp. 137–140.

60. Reil, *Rhapsodieen*, pp. 457–462.

61. Horn, *Rechenschaft*, p. 249.

62. Pinel, *Traité*, pp. 237–238.

63. Esquirol, article "De la Folie" (1816), reprinted in *Des maladies mentales*, quotes vol. 1, pp. 126, 128.

64. Pinel, *Traité*; Chapter 8 is entitled, "Préceptes généraux à suivre dans le Traitement moral."

65. Molière, *L'amour médecin* (1665), (Paris: Nouveaux Classiques Larousse, 1975), pp. 50, 53.

66. Reil, *Rhapsodieen*, pp. 28–32.

67. See Jean Camus and Philippe Pagniez, *Isolement et psychothérapie* (Paris: Alcan, 1904), p. 74.

68. Roy Porter, *Mind-Forg'd Manacles: A History of Madness in England from the Restoration to the Regency* (Cambridge: Harvard U. P., 1987), pp. 206–222.

69. Chiarugi, *On Insanity*, pp. 137–138, para. 517. Mora, the translator, suggests that "moral" is best understood as "psychological."

70. Samuel Tuke, *Description of the Retreat, an Institution near York for Insane Persons of the Society of Friends* (York: Alexander, 1813; reprint ed. London: Dawsons, 1964), quote p. 136; see also pp. 139–140. On the Retreat, see Anne Digby, *Madness, Morality and Medicine: A Study of the York Retreat, 1796–1914* (Cambridge: Cambridge U. P., 1985); also Porter's judicious summary in *Mind-Forg'd Manacles*, pp. 222–228.

71. Pinel, *Traité*, p. 219.

72. Pinel, *Traité*, pp. 134, 212.

73. For the general rules of Reil's "psychische Curmethode," see *Rhapsodieen*, pp. 218–253.

74. Haslam, *Observations*, pp. 295–296.

75. Julius Preuss, *Biblisch-talmudische Medizin* (1911) (reprint New York: Ktav, 1971), p. 347.

76. See Stanley W. Jackson, "Unusual Mental States in Medieval Europe I. Medical Syndromes of Mental Disorder: 400–1100 A.D.," *Journal of the History of Medicine*, 27 (1972), pp. 262–297 esp. pp. 284–285 on incubus; on the relative recency of the hysteria diagnosis (NB it does not go back to the Ancients) see Helen King, "Once upon a Text: Hysteria from Hippocrates," in Sander L. Gilman et al., *Hysteria beyond Freud* (Berkeley: University of California Press, 1993), pp. 3–90; on fashionable eighteenth-century diagnoses, see Edward Shorter, *From Paralysis to Fatigue: A History of Psychosomatic Illness in the Modern Era* (New York: Free Press, 1992), pp. 1–25.

77. Jacob Friedrich Isenflamm, *Versuch einiger praktischen Anmerkungen über die Nerven zur Erläuterung . . . hypochondrisch und hysterischer Zufälle* (Erlangen: Walcher, 1774), pp. 248–252.

78. See Alfred Martin, *Deutsches Badewesen in vergangenen Tagen* (Jena: Diederichs, 1906); Roy Porter, ed., *The Medical History of Waters and Spas* (London: Wellcome Institute for the History of Medicine, 1990); Lise Grenier/Institut Français d'Architecture, *Villes d'eaux èn France* (Paris: Hazan, 1985).

79. Phyllis Hembry, *The English Spa, 1560–1815: A Social History* (London: Athlone, 1990), pp. 270–283.

80. Otto Mönkemöller, "Die Neurologie im Beginne des 19. Jahrhunderts," *PNW*, 9 (July 13, 1907), pp. 128–130.

81. [Augustus Bozzi-] Granville, *The Spas of Germany*, 2 vols. (Brussels: Belgian Printing, 1838), vol. 2, p. 386.

82. Granville, *Spas of Germany*, vol. 1 pp. 135–136.

83. Robert Peirce, *The History and Memoirs of the Bath* (London/Bath: Hammond, 1713), pp. 190–191.

84. From an extract of Cheyne's *The Natural Method of Curing the Diseases of the Body* (1742), quoted in Hunter and Macalpine, *300 Years of Psychiatry*, p. 353.

85. George Cheyne, *The English Malady: Or, A Treatise of Nervous Diseases of All Kinds* (London: Powell, 1733; Scholars' Facsimiles reprint ed., 1976), p. 2.

86. [Great Britain], *Dictionary of National Biography*, pp. 217–219; see also Porter, *Mind-Forg'd Manacles*, pp. 83–84; William F. Bynum, "The Nervous Patient in 18th- and 19th-century Britain: The Psychiatric Origins of British Neurology," in R. M. Murray and T. H. Turner, eds., *Lectures on the History of Psychiatry. The Squibb Series* (London: Royal College of Psychiatrists, 1990), pp. 115–127, esp. 117.

87. Charles Perry, *A Mechanical Account and Explication of the Hysteric Passion* (London: Shuckburgh, 1755), pp. 1, 5, 185, 187.

88. Pierre Pomme, *Traité des affections vaporeuses des deux sexes* (1763), 3d ed. (Lyon: Duplain, 1768), quote p. 33.

89. Joseph Daquin [or d'Aquin], *Topographie médicale de la ville de Chambéry* (Chambéry: Gorrin, 1787), pp. 131–133.

90. Daquin, friendly with Pinel, wrote in 1792 an essay on mental illness and the organization of the asylum portion of the Hôtel Dieu, *La philosophie de la folie ou essai philosophique sur les personnes attaquées de folie* (1792), which I have not seen. For a summary, see Marcel Gauchet and Gladys Swain, *La pratique de l'esprit humain: L'institution asilaire et la révolution démocratique* (Paris: Gallimard, 1980), pp. 413–422. The authors, however, end up making the ludicrous claim that it was Daquin who thought up moral therapy: "Le traitement moral, Daquin l'a conçu . . ." (p. 422).

91. Battie, *Treatise*, pp. 35, 36, 57.

92. Battie, *Treatise*, quotes pp. 1, 66.

93. Chiarugi, *On Insanity*, p. 208, para. 813.

94. Chiarugi, *On Insanity*; see the reports of 100 patients at the end of the volume, for example, observation 3, p. 249: "A great deal of lymph was found collected under the pia matter. . . ."

95. Quoted in Eric T. Carlson and Meribeth M. Simpson, "The Definition of Mental Illness: Benjamin Rush (1745–1813)," *AJP*, 121 (1964), pp. 209–214, quote p. 211.

96. Pinel, *Traité*, pp. xix–xx. Pinel praised specifically Johann Greding's postmortem sections on "les maladies les plus ordinaires des aliénés, et sur les lésions de structure ou les vices de conformation qui semblent leur être propres" (p. xx).

97. Reil, *Rhapsodieen*, p. 235. "Indem die zu reizbaren Hirnfasern zur Ruhe gebracht, die trägen erregt werden, kehrt die normale Proportion in der Dynamik des Seelenorgans zurück und der hervorstechende Wahn schwindet."

98. Reil, *Rhapsodieen*, pp. 184, 188–189.

99. Markus Schär, *Seelennöte der Untertanen* (Zurich: Chronos, 1985), pp. 277, 279.

100. Battie, *Treatise*, pp. 59, 60.

101. Haslam, *Observations*, p. 230.

102. Haslam, *Observations*, pp. 231–232.

103. Pinel, *Traité*, p. 13; for his discussion of "Aliénation originaire ou héréditaire," see pp. 13–16.

104. Esquirol, "De la lypémanie ou mélancholie," *Des maladies mentales*, statistics pp. 435–436.

105. Esquirol, "De la Folie" in *Des maladies mentales*, p. 64.

106. Reil, "Medicin und Pädagogik," *Magazin für die psychische Heilkunde*, 1 (1805), 411–446, term on p. 416.

107. Chiarugi, *On Insanity*, p. 285.

108. See Battie, *Treatise*, pp. 5–6, 33–34; Ferriar, *Medical Histories*, vol. 2, pp. 111–114. On the influence of Locke, see Porter, *Mind Forg'd Manacles*, pp. 188–193.

109. Otto Braus, *Akademische Erinnerungen eines alten Arztes an Berlins klinische Grössen* (Leipzig: Vogel, 1901), pp. 155–156.

110. Esquirol, "De la folie," in *Des maladies mentales*, pp. 25–54.

111. On the friendship between the Esquirol and Heinroth, see Ey, "Esquirol," p. 90.

112. Johann Christian August Heinroth, *Lehrbuch der Seelengesundheitskunde*, vol. 1 (Leipzig: Vogel, 1823), pp. 591–592. On Heinroth, see Luc S. Cauwenbergh, "J. Chr. A. Heinroth (1773–1843): A Psychiatrist of the German Romantic Era," *History of Psychiatry*, 2 (1991), pp. 365–383; Emil Kraepelin, "Hundert Jahre Psychiatrie," *Zeitschrift für die gesamte Neurologie und Psychiatrie*, 38 (1917), pp. 161–275, esp. pp. 181–186; and Werner Leibbrand and Annemarie Wettley, *Der Wahnsinn: Geschichte der abendländischen Psychopathologie* (Munich: Alber, 1961), pp. 492–496.

113. Carl Gustav Carus, *Lebenserinnerungen*, 4 vols. (Leipzig, 1865–1866), vol. 1, p. 228.

114. See, for example, Ellenberger, *Discovery of the Unconscious*, p. 212.

Chapter 2: The Asylum Era

1. U.S. Bureau of the Census, *Historical Statistics of the United States, Colonial Times to 1970, Bicentennial Edition*, Part 2 (Washington, DC: GPO,

1975), vol. 1, p. 84, tab. B-427; 183 patients in mental hospitals per 100,000 population.

2. Henry C. Burdett, *Hospitals and Asylums of the World, vol. 1: Asylums* (London: Churchill, 1891), p. 322.

3. *Medical Directory for 1908* (London: Churchill, 1908), p. 389.

4. Heinrich Laehr, *Die Heil- und Pflegeanstalten für Psychisch-Kranke des deutschen Sprachgebietes im J. 1890* (Berlin: Reimer, 1891), pp. vii–xi.

5. Samuel W. Hamilton, "The History of American Mental Hospitals," in American Psychiatric Association, *One Hundred Years of American Psychiatry* (New York: Columbia U. P., 1944), pp. 73–166; see esp. the list of state mental institutions, together with their dates of opening. The Eastern State Hospital in Williamsburg, Virginia (1773), was the first such institution.

6. For an overview, see Kathleen Jones, *Asylums and After: A Revised History of the Mental Health Services: From the Early 18th Century to the 1990s* (London: Athlone, 1993).

7. On Frank and the tradition of medical police, see Erna Lesky, *Die Wiener medizinische Schule im 19. Jahrhundert* (Graz: Böhlau, 1978), garden story p. 175.

8. For a detailed account, see Dieter Jetter, *Zur Typologie des Irrenhauses in Frankreich und Deutschland (1780–1840)* (Wiesbaden: Steiner, 1971), pp. 119–169.

9. Theodor Kirchhoff, ed., *Deutsche Irrenärzte: Einzelbilder ihres Lebens und Wirkens*, 2 vols. (Berlin: Springer, 1921–1924), vol. 1, pp. 94–95. My account of Hayner is based on pp. 94–99; see also Guido Weber, "Sonnenstein: Zur Hundertjahrfeier," *PNW*, 13 (July 1, 1911), pp. 127–133.

10. Heinrich Damerow, psychiatric editor and asylum supervisor at Halle, campaigned against the absolute separation of facilities for acute and chronic care. See his *Über die relative Verbindung der Irren- Heil- und Pflege-Anstalten* (Leipzig: Wigand, 1840).

11. G. A. E. von Nostiz und Jänckendorf's famous *Beschreibung der Königlich-Sächsischen Heil- und Pflegeanstalt Sonnenstein* (1829) was not available to me, and I rely for these details on Otto Bach's manuscript paper, "Soziotherapie in der psychiatrischen Betreuung sächsischer Anstalten des 19. und zu Beginn des 20. Jahrhunderts," p. 5.

12. For some details of Pienitz's administration, see Kirchhoff, *Deutsche Irrenärzte*, vol. 1, pp. 99–103.

13. Emil Kraepelin quotes Damerow on Sonnenstein as "the rising sun of a new day for public psychiatry in and for Germany." Kraepelin, "Hundert Jahre Psychiatrie," *Zeitschrift für die gesamte Neurologie und Psychiatrie*, 38 (1917), pp. 161–275, quote p. 232. In Pienitz's later days and certainly after his death, Sonnenstein lost some of this reformist burnish. See one Dr. Köhler's account of conditions there around 1855, in "Rückblicke auf meine 33jährige Thätigkeit im Bereich des practischen Irrenwesens von Mitte 1855 bis 1888," *Allgemeine Zeitschrift für Psychiatrie*, 46 (1889), pp. 159–167, esp. pp. 141–146.

14. On Langermann, see Kirchhoff, *Deutsche Irrenärzte*, vol. 1, pp. 42–51.

15. These details from Kirchhoff, *Deutsche Irrenärzte*, vol. 1, pp. 83–84.

16. Maximilian Jacobi, *Über die Anlegung und Einrichtung von Irren-Heilanstalten, mit ausführlicher Darstellung der Irren-Heilanstalt zu Siegburg* (Berlin: Reimer, 1834), pp. 16–17 (". . . a hospital organized for the exclusive treatment of mental disturbances associated with organic brain disorders").

17. Maximilian Jacobi, *Die Hauptformen der Seelenstörungen in ihren Beziehungen zur Heilkunde*, vol. 1 (Leipzig: Weidmann, 1844), case pp. 135–143. No further volumes appeared.

18. Carl Pelman, *Erinnerungen eines alten Irrenarztes* (Bonn: Cohen, 1912), p. 47.

19. On provincial French asylums after the Revolution, see Jetter, *Zur Typologie des Irrenhauses*, pp. 44–79. It is evident that departmental administrations soon quenched the reformist zeal of the students of Etienne Esquirol who founded many of these provincial institutions.

20. Jan Goldstein, *Console and Classify: The French Psychiatric Profession in the Nineteenth Century* (Cambridge: Cambridge U. P., 1987), p. 131. Goldstein notes disapprovingly Esquirol's belief in the healing power of the psychiatrist by the force of his personality (pp. 132–133).

21. Etienne [Jean-Etienne-Dominique] Esquirol, "Mémoire historique et statistique sur la maison royale de Charenton" (1835), in Esquirol, ed., *Des maladies mentales*, vol. 2 (Paris: Baillière, 1838), pp. 539–706, quotes pp. 695, 701–702. Among the therapeutic features of Charenton, he cited, "Les avantages de la situation, la régularité et la douceur de l'administration, le zèle des médecins, l'abondance des services domestiques, la tenue générale . . ." (p. 702).

22. On the law of 1838 and its preludes, see Jacques Postel and Claude Quétel, eds., *Nouvelle histoire de la psychiatrie* (Toulouse: Privat, 1983), pp. 171–185. Goldstein's well-researched account becomes diverted into a kind of "doctors' plot" explanation of events. *Console and Classify*, pp. 276–297. For the text of the law of June 30, 1838, see Georges Guillain, "Sémiologie psychiatrique," in Pierre Marie, ed., *Pratique neurologique* (Paris: Masson, 1911), pp. 252–259.

23. See the list of asylums in Burdett, *Hospitals of the World*, vol. 1, pp. 356–397.

24. John Ferriar, *Medical Histories and Reflections* [2nd ed.] (London: Cadell, 1810), vol. 2, pp. 136–137.

25. Quoted in Richard Hunter and Ida Macalpine, *Three Hundred Years of Psychiatry, 1535–1860* (London: Oxford U. P., 1963), p. 690.

26. George Man Burrows, *Commentaries on the Causes, Forms, Symptoms, and Treatment, Moral and Medical, of Insanity* (London: Underwood, 1828), pp. 667, 669. On Burrows, see *Munk's Roll* (*Lives of the Fellows of the Royal College of Physicians of London*), vol. 3, p. 290.

27. *Munk's Roll*, vol. 3, p. 291.

28. William Charles Ellis, *A Treatise on the Nature, Symptoms, Causes, and Treatment of Insanity* (London: Holdsworth, 1838), pp. 6–7.

29. Ellis, *Treatise*, p. 8.

30. Hunter and Macalpine are responsible for the rehabilitation of Ellis's historic reputation (*Three Hundred Years of Psychiatry*, pp. 870–877). To be sure, Ellis was knighted in 1835, "the first psychiatrist to be knighted exclusively for services to the insane." Yet his name does not appear in the standard biographical dictionaries of famous doctors. Andrew Scull, in his scorched-earth assault on psychiatry, taxes Ellis, an otherwise thoroughly progressive figure, with a desire to abandon the cheery physical settings of early moral therapy by making asylums drab. *The Most Solitary of Afflictions: Madness and Society in Britain 1700–1900* (New Haven: Yale U. P., 1993), p. 167.

31. Reprinted by Andrew Scull, along with an extensive introduction as, *The Asylum as Utopia: W. A. F. Browne and the Mid-Nineteenth Century Consolidation of Psychiatry* (London: Tavistock, 1991). Scull flagellates Browne and most of the other alienists of this period for wanting "to make the treatment of madness an exclusively medical prerogative" (p. lxviii, n. 145). But if indeed psychiatrists were not to treat "madness," who else should?

32. Obituary, "W. A. F. Browne," *Lancet*, 1 (Mar. 14, 1885), p. 499.

33. Browne, *What Asylums Were. . . .* (1837), reprinted in Scull, *Asylum as Utopia*, p. 177.

34. "Royal" asylums in Scotland were privately founded but obliged by charter to accept both rich and poor.

35. Quotes in Henry M. Hurd, *The Institutional Care of the Insane in the United States and Canada*, 4 vols. (Baltimore: Johns Hopkins Press, 1916), vol. 3, p. 384. See pp. 439–455 for a detailed narrative of the Frankford Retreat's history.

36. Quote in Hurd, *Institutional Care Insane*, vol. 1, p. 235. For further details on Todd and the Hartford Retreat see ibid., vol. 2, pp. 76–102. See also Gerald N. Grob, *Mental Institutions in America: Social Policy to 1875* (New York: Free Press, 1973), pp. 78–80. On Todd and the Retreat, see Francis J. Braceland, *The Institute of Living: The Hartford Retreat, 1822–1972* (Hartford: Institute of Living, 1972), pp. 28–41.

37. Details on Wyman and the McLean Asylum from Hurd, *Institutional Care of the Insane*, vol. 2, pp. 599–602, vol. 4, pp. 542–543; and from S. B. Sutton, *Crossroads in Psychiatry: A History of the McLean Hospital* (Washington, DC: American Psychiatric Press, 1986), pp. 23–51.

38. Quote from Mary Ann Jimenez, *Changing Faces of Madness: Early American Attitudes and Treatment of the Insane* (Hanover, NH: University Press of New England, 1987), p. 116. For the basic narrative, see Hurd, *Institutional Care of the Insane*, vol. 2, pp. 637–643.

39. On Utica, see Hurd, *Institutional Care of the Insane*, vol. 3, pp. 152–159; Ellen Dwyer has written a study of Utica, *Homes for the Mad: Life Inside Two*

Nineteenth-Century Asylums (New Brunswick: Rutgers U. P., 1987). On Milledgeville, see Peter G. Cranford, *But for the Grace of God: The Inside Story of the World's Largest Insane Asylum, Milledgeville!* (Augusta: Great Pyramid Press, 1981), pp. 24–26 on the origins.

40. Hurd, *Institutional Care of Insane*, vol. 3, pp. 160–164.

41. Grob, *Mental Institutions in America*, pp. 371–372.

42. John Charles Bucknill, "Notes on Asylums for the Insane in America," *Lancet*, 1 (May 13, 1876), pp. 701–703, quote p. 702.

43. David J. Rothman, *The Discovery of the Asylum: Social Order and Disorder in the New Republic*, rev. ed. (Boston: Little Brown, 1990), p. 239. Rothman emphasizes the redistribution of criminals, the poor, and so on, from other institutions to the asylum. In my view, it is likely that a majority of these redistributed individuals had a psychiatric illness as well as being poor, criminal, or unwanted.

44. Adolf Meyer, "Thirty-Five Years of Psychiatry in the United States" (1928), in Eunice E. Winters, ed., *The Collected Papers of Adolf Meyer*, vol. 2 (Baltimore: Johns Hopkins, 1951), pp. 1–23, quote p. 12.

45. Hans Laehr, *Die Anstalten für Psychisch-Kranke in Deutschland, Österreich, der Schweiz und den baltischen Ländern*, 7th ed. (Berlin: Reimer, 1912), p. 245. Data for Prussia.

46. Georg Dobrick, "Videant consules . . . !" *PNW*, 13 (Sept. 30, 1911), pp. 265–269, quote p. 265.

47. Max Schröder, "Heilungsaussichten in den Irrenanstalten," *PNW*, 10 (Sept. 26, 1908), pp. 222–223, quote p. 223.

48. Friedrich Vocke, "Ein Beitrag zur Frage, ob die Zahl der Geisteskranken zunimmt," *PNW*, 8 (Feb. 16, 1907), pp. 427–430, citation p. 428.

49. For these statistics, see Josef Starlinger, "Über die zweckmässige Grösse der Anstalten für Geisteskranke," *PNW*, 15 (June 21, 1913), pp. 143–151, tab. p. 146; and Burnett, *Hospitals of the World*, vol. 1, pp. 383–391.

50. H. A. Wildermuth, "Reiseerinnerungen an Frankreich, England, Schottland und Belgien," *Allgemeine Zeitschrift für Psychiatrie*, 40 (1883–1884), pp. 763–823, quote p. 767.

51. Jones, *Asylums and After*, p. 116.

52. David Budden, *A County Lunatic Asylum: The History of St. Matthew's Hospital* (Burntwood: St. Matthew's Hospital, Pharmacy Department, 1989), pp. 60–62.

53. Montagu Lomax, *The Experiences of an Asylum Doctor* (London: Allen and Unwin, 1921), pp. 14, 41, 206.

54. Thomas Szasz aired a rough version of this thesis in *The Myth of Mental Illness: Foundations of a Theory of Personal Conduct*, rev. ed. (New York: Harper and Row, 1974). For more scholarly renditions, drawing specifically on the work of Michel Foucault, see Dirk Blasius, "Psychiatrische Versorgung in Preussen, 1880–1910," *Sudhoffs Archiv*, 66 (1982), pp. 105–128 ("The insanity boom at the end of the nineteenth and beginning of the twentieth

century [was] less a problem of rising social-pathological metastases than of bureaucratic control of social pathology" p. 111); see also Richard W. Fox, *So Far Disordered in Mind: Insanity in California, 1870–1930* (Berkeley: University of California Press, 1978), who views asylums as "sequester[ing] the nonproductive" (p. 176). Andrew Scull began as a Foucauldian then later distanced himself from the social-constructionists with the argument that psychiatrists were "medicalizing" behavior that was merely "problematic" in order to increase their own power. Scull has never been able to go further than characterizing psychiatric disorder as merely troublesome (for society) and puts the term mental illness in ironical quotation marks. See *Most Solitary of Afflictions*, pp. 378, 381.

55. This view seems to characterize the scholars grouped about the Wellcome Institute for the History of Medicine in London, who, though conceding the existence of "madness," are reluctant to break it into component parts, and feel more comfortable discussing societal "views" than the phenomenon itself. See the introductions to the three-volume work, edited by W. F. Bynum, Roy Porter, and Michael Shepherd, *The Anatomy of Madness: Essays in the History of Psychiatry* (London: Tavistock, 1985–1988).

56. See the pathbreaking articles of Edward Hare, especially "The Changing Content of Psychiatric Illness," *Journal of Psychosomatic Research*, 18 (1974), pp. 283–289; "Was Insanity on the Increase?" *BJP*, 142 (1983), pp. 439–455. Through retrospective diagnosis, going back and reanalyzing the patients' original charts, Trevor H. Turner has demonstrated high levels of psychiatric illness among nineteenth-century patients. See *A Diagnostic Analysis of the Casebooks of Ticehurst House Asylum, 1845–1890* (Cambridge: Cambridge U. P., 1992; Psychological Medicine, monograph supplement 21). Turner dismisses Foucault's ideas: "The florid psychotic material and disturbed patterns of behaviour were striking." As for a supposed medicalization of deviance, Turner concludes, "There is no sense in which a medical model . . . seems to have been imposed on those who were merely deviant from a social point of view or harmlessly eccentric. The picture seen here is one of medical powerlessness." Turner, "Rich and Mad in Victorian England," *Psychological Medicine*, 19 (1989), pp. 29–44, quotes pp. 24–25, 43.

57. Julius Wagner-Jauregg, "Der Rechtsschutz der Geisteskranken," *Wiener Klinische Wochenschrift*, 14 (May 23, 1901), pp. 518–521, quote p. 519.

58. Dwyer, *Homes for the Mad*, p. 87. As for the charge that psychiatrists attempted to medicalize madness, Dwyer concludes that, "asylum doctors most often simply acquiesced in a diagnosis made outside the institution" (p. 117).

59. H. C. Erik Midelfort, *Mad Princes of Renaissance Germany* (Charlottesville: University Press of Virginia, 1994).

60. See Hunter and Macalpine, *Three Hundred Years of Psychiatry*, pp. 13–15.

61. I have given my views of this change in another work and will not repeat the evidence or argument here. See Shorter, *The Making of the Modern Family* (New York: Basic, 1975). On the possible role of closer family sentiments in the

rise of private asylums in England, see Charlotte MacKenzie, *Psychiatry for the Rich: A History of Ticehurst Private Asylum, 1792–1917* (London: Routledge, 1992), pp. 20–21.

62. Bruno Goergen, *Privat-Heilanstalt für Gemüthskranke* (Vienna: Wimmer, 1820), pp. 3–4.

63. Wilhelm Svetlin, *Zweiter Bericht über die Privatheilanstalt für Gemüthskranke auf dem Erdberge zu Wien* (Vienna: Urban & Schwarzenberg, 1891), p. 28, tab. 5.

64. Anon, "Neurological and Psychiatrical Clinics in Germany," BMJ, 1 (June 20, 1908), p. 1534.

65. John Crammer, *Asylum History: Buckinghamshire County Pauper Lunatic Asylum—St. John's* (London: Gaskell, 1990), p. 120.

66. Dwyer, *Homes for the Mad*, p. 101, fig. 4.6.

67. Morton Kramer, et al., *A Historical Study of the Disposition of First Admissions to a State Mental Hospital: Experience of the Warren State Hospital during the Period 1916–50* (Washington, DC: GPO, 1955; Public Health Service Pub. No. 445), p. 9, tab. 6. The initial figure is for 1916–1925.

68. Gerald N. Grob, *From Asylum to Community: Mental Health Policy in Modern America* (Princeton: Princeton U. P., 1991), p. 159.

69. See on this, Burdett, *Hospitals of the World*, vol. 1, pp. 164–165, 151–152, 175.

70. Notably Scull, *Most Solitary of Afflictions*, pp. 361–373.

71. Budden, *History of St. Matthew's Hospital*, pp. 34–35.

72. For a brief overview of the history of neurosyphilis, see Edward Shorter, "What Can Two Historical Examples of Sexually-Transmitted Diseases Teach Us About Aids?" in Tim Dyson, ed., *Sexual Behaviour and Networking: Anthropological and Socio-Cultural Studies on the Transmission of HIV* (Liège: Eds. Derouaux-Ordina, 1992), pp. 49–64.

73. Lewis Thomas, *The Youngest Science: Notes of a Medicine-Watcher* (New York: Viking, 1983), pp. 46–47.

74. Kurt Kolle, *Wanderer zwischen Natur und Geist: Das Leben eines Nervenarztes* (Munich: Lehmann, 1972), p. 28.

75. Maria Rivet, *Les Aliénés dans la famille et dans la maison de santé* (Paris: Masson, 1875), p. 145.

76. For an overview of early writing, see Heinrich Obersteiner, *Die progressive allgemeine Paralyse*, 2nd ed. (Vienna: Hölder, 1908), pp. 3–7. Obersteiner concluded that progressive paralysis was "a modern disease" (p. 7). Scholarly interest in the subject was reawakened with Edward H. Hare's, "The Origin and Spread of Dementia Paralytica," BJP, 105 (1959), pp. 594–626.

77. William Perfect, *Select Cases in the Different Species of Insanity* (Rochester: Gillman, 1787), pp. 68–71. One of Perfect's own patients was a young man who, after experiencing the symptoms of primary and secondary syphilis, also "dwindled into a downright state of idiotism" (pp. 242–246).

78. George Mora, ed. and trans., Vincenzio Chiarugi, *On Insanity and Its Classification* (1793) (Canton, MA: Science History Pubs., 1987), obs. 3, pp. 248–249; obs. 83, p. 302.

79. John Haslam, *Observations on Madness and Melancholy*, 2nd rev. ed. (London: Callow, 1809), pp. 208–209n., 259.

80. Etienne Esquirol, "Démence," in *Dictionnaire des sciences médicales*, vol. "Dac-des" (Paris: Panckoucke, 1814), pp. 280–293, tables and quotes pp. 285–293; only female patients were at the Salpêtrière; the private patients were of both sexes.

81. Etienne Esquirol, "De la démence" (1814 [*sic*]), published in Esquirol, *Des maladies mentales*, vol. 2 (Paris: Baillière, 1838), pp. 219–282, quotes pp. 271–272; Bayle's dissertation, *Traité des maladies du cerveau et de ses membranes* (1826), is the most recent reference cited by Esquirol in this essay, p. 275.

82. Christian Friedrich Harless, "Noch einige praktische Bemerkungen über die Myelitis," in Harless and Valerian Aloys Brera, eds., *Über die Entzündung des Rückenmarks* (Nürnberg: Schrag, 1814), pp. 36–73, quote p. 54.

83. Moritz Heinrich Romberg, *Lehrbuch der Nervenkrankheiten des Menschen*, vol. 1, pt. 2 (Berlin: Duncker, 1846), section on "Tabes dorsualis" [*sic*], pp. 794–801, quote p. 801.

84. Stephanie Austin, "The History of Malariotherapy for Neurosyphilis," *JAMA*, 268 (July 22, 1992), pp. 516–519.

85. On 6 percent, see E. Gurney Clark and Niels Danbolt, "The Oslo Study of the Natural Course of Untreated Syphilis," *Medical Clinics of North America*, 48 (1964), pp. 613–623. H. J. Källmark put the percentage ultimately dying of neurosyphilis at only 2–4 percent, *Eine statistische Untersuchung über Syphilis* (Uppsala: med. diss., 1931), pp. 196, 226.

86. Heinrich Neumann, *Die Irrenanstalt zu Pöpelwitz bei Breslau* (Erlangen: Enke, 1862), p. 41.

87. John Punton, "The Results of Six Years' Work in a Sanitarium for Nervous and Mental Diseases," *The Kansas City Medical Index-Lancet*, 28 (1907), pp. 177–186, tab. opp. p. 178.

88. Max Sichel, "Die progressive Paralyse bei den Juden," *Archiv für Psychiatrie und Nervenkrankheiten*, 52 (1913), pp. 1030–42, esp. p. 1034.

89. Joseph Workman, "On Paresis," *Canada Lancet*, 10 (1878), pp. 357–359, quotes pp. 358, 359.

90. Lomax, *Experiences of an Asylum Doctor*, p. 93.

91. Caesar Heimann, *Bericht über Sanitätsrath Dr. Karl Edel's Asyl für Gemüthskranke* (Berlin: Hirschwald, 1895), pp. 75–78. Data are for the period 1869–1893.

92. On alcohol and the central nervous system, see William A. Lishman, *Organic Psychiatry: The Psychological Consequences of Cerebral Disorder* (Oxford: Blackwell, 1978), pp. 699–715.

93. William L. Langer, *The Rise of Modern Europe: Political and Social Upheaval, 1832–1852* (New York: Harper & Row, 1969), p. 14.

94. B. R. Mitchell, *Abstract of British Historical Statistics* (Cambridge: Cambridge U. P., 1971), pp. 260–261.

95. W. J. Rorabaugh, "Estimated U.S. Alcoholic Beverage Consumption, 1790–1860," *Journal of Studies on Alcohol*, 37 (1976), pp. 357–364, p. 361, tab. 2. American alcohol consumption had been very high in the eighteenth century and fell off sharply in the early nineteenth.

96. T. J. Markovitch, *L'industrie française de 1789 à 1964* (Paris: Institut de science économique appliquée, 1966; cahier no. 173), p. 213. See also Michael R. Marrus, "Social Drinking in the Belle Époque," *Journal of Social History*, 7 (1974), pp. 115–141, p. 123, fig. 1.

97. Alexander von Oettingen, *Die Moralstatistik in ihrer Bedeutung für eine Socialethik*, 3d ed. (Erlangen: Deichert, 1882), pp. 688n2, 691.

98. Hermann Grunau, *Über Frequenz, Heilerfolge und Sterblichkeit in den öffentlichen preussischen Irrenanstalten von 1875 bis 1900* (Halle a. S.: Marhold, 1905), p. 45; "Delirium potatorum."

99. Karl Bonhoeffer, *Nervenärztliche Erfahrungen und Eindrücke* (Berlin: Springer, 1941), p. 48. "Today" meant Hitler's Germany, where Bonhoeffer's sons were martyred under the Nazi regime.

100. Grunau, *Über Frequenz*, p. 41, tab. B.

101. Paul Garnier, *La Folie à Paris* (Paris: Baillière, 1890), p. 24.

102. K. Pandy, *Die Irrenfürsorge in Europa* (Berlin, Reimer, 1908), pp. 305–306.

103. Margaret S. Thompson, "The Wages of Sin: The Problem of Alcoholism and General Paralysis in Nineteenth-Century Edinburgh," in Bynum, *Anatomy of Madness*, vol. 3, pp. 316–340, see figure 12:1, p. 319.

104. *Medical Directory*, 1908, pp. 1958–66.

105. Grunau, *Über Frequenz*, p. 41, tab. B.

106. John Haslam, *Observations on Madness and Melancholy*, 2nd ed. (London: Callow, 1809), pp. 49–51, 64–67. Haslam attributed the problems of the young man to drink, yet the case likely constitutes a very early description of schizophrenia.

107. Philippe Pinel, *Traité médico-philosophique sur l'aliénation mentale*, 2nd ed. (Paris: Brosson, 1809), p. 182.

108. Edward Hare, "Schizophrenia as a Recent Disease," *BJP*, 153 (1988), pp. 521–531; see also his "Commentary One," remarks offered on another paper, in the *Australian and New Zealand Journal of Psychiatry*, 21 (1987), pp. 315–316. Hare's notion that schizophrenia might be caused by a virus, and that the dissemination of this hypothesized virus was the cause of the nineteenth-century increase, has not won general acceptance. Hare, "Epidemiological Evidence for a Viral Factor in the Aetiology of the Functional Psychoses," P. V. Morozov, ed., *Research on the Viral Hypothesis of Mental Disorders* (Basel: Karger, 1983), pp. 52–75.

109. Hare, "Insanity on Increase," p. 449.

110. See, for example, Andrew Scull, "Was Insanity Increasing? A Response to Edward Hare," *BJP*, 144 (1984), pp. 432–436. Scull's answer to Hare was that, rather than schizophrenia rising, "the boundaries of what constituted committable madness expanded over the course of the nineteenth century" (p. 434). In other words, as time went on, patients became less and less sick (rather than more and more, as Hare and others would argue).

111. Dilip V. Jeste et al., "Did Schizophrenia Exist before the Eighteenth Century?" *Comprehensive Psychiatry*, 26 (1985), pp. 493–503; Nigel M. Bark, "On the History of Schizophrenia: Evidence of Its Existence before 1800," *New York State Journal of Medicine*, 88 (1988), pp. 374–383.

112. Rajendra Persaud, "The Reporting of Psychiatric Symptoms in History: The Memorandum Book of Samuel Coates, 1785–1825," *History of Psychiatry*, 4 (1993), pp. 499–510, quote p. 510.

113. Robert Wilkins, "Hallucinations in Children and Teenagers Admitted to Bethlem Royal Hospital in the Nineteenth Century and Their Possible Relevance to the Incidence of Schizophrenia," *Journal of Child Psychology and Psychiatry*, 28 (1987), pp. 569–580; Wilkins, "Delusions in Children and Teenagers Admitted to Bethlem Royal Hospital in the 19th Century," *BJP*, 162 (1993), pp. 487–492.

114. Edward B. Renvoize and Allan W. Beveridge, "Mental Illness and the Late Victorians: A Study of Patients Admitted to Three Asylums in York, 1880–1884," *Psychological Medicine*, 19 (1989), pp. 19–28, quotes pp. 25, 27.

115. Hermann Lenz, *Vergleichende Psychiatrie: eine Studie über die Beziehung von Kultur, Soziologie und Psychopathologie* (Vienna: Maudrich, 1964), based on the records of the Niedernhart asylum in Austria, see esp. tab. p. 41. Turner, *Ticehurst Casebooks*, p. 19; R. R. Parker et al., "County of Lancaster Asylum, Rainhill: 100 Years Ago and Now," *History of Psychiatry*, 4 (1993), pp. 95–105.

116. Karl Kahlbaum, "Über jugendliche Nerven- und Gemüthskranke und ihre pädagogische Behandlung in der Heilanstalt," *Allgemeine Zeitschrift für Psychiatrie*, 40 (1883–84), pp. 863–873, quote p. 863. "Hebephrenie." p. 865.

117. Rivet, *Les Aliénés*, pp. 188–190.

118. William A. White, *Forty Years of Psychiatry* (New York: Nervous and Mental Disease Publishing Company, 1933), pp. 12–13.

119. Crammer, *Asylum History: Buckinghamshire*, p. 181.

120. Eliot Slater, "Psychiatry in the Thirties," *Contemporary Review*, 226 (1975), pp. 70–75, quotes pp. 71–72.

121. Lomax, *Experiences of an Asylum Doctor*, p. 94.

122. Emil Kraepelin, *Lebenserinnerungen* (Berlin: Springer, 1983), pp. 11–12.

123. Werner Heinz (pseud.), *Tagebuch eines alten Irrenarztes* (Lindenthal: Wellersberg, 1928), pp. 1–2.

124. Birgit Schoop-Russbült, ed., *Psychiatrischer Alltag in der Autobiographie von Karl Gehry (1881–1962)* (Zurich: Juris, 1989), pp. 50–51.

125. Grob, *Mental Institutions in America*, p. 149.

126. Silas Weir Mitchell, "Address before the Fiftieth Annual Meeting of the American Medico-Psychological Association, Held in Philadelphia, May 16th, 1894," *JNMD*, 21 (1894), pp. 413–437, quotes pp. 415, 422, 427.

127. William N. Bullard, "The New Era in Neurology," *JNMD*, 39 (1912), pp. 433–439, quote p. 438.

128. White, *Forty Years of Psychiatry*, p. 18.

129. John Romano, "On Becoming a Psychiatrist," *JAMA*, 261 (Apr. 21, 1989), pp. 2240–43, quote p. 2241.

Chapter 3: The First Biological Psychiatry

1. Ernest Billod, *Les Aliénés en Italie* (Paris: Masson, 1884), quote p. 6; "le stygmate" p. 5. Here he was speaking of France.

2. Richard Hunter and Ida Macalpine, *Three Hundred Years of Psychiatry, 1535–1860* (London: Oxford U. P., 1963), p. 404.

3. Mentioned in Richard von Krafft-Ebing, *Der klinische Unterricht in der Psychiatrie* (Stuttgart: Enke, 1890), p. 15.

4. *Dorland's Illustrated Medical Dictionary*, 26th ed. (Philadelphia: Saunders, 1981), pp. 1200–1206.

5. On developments at the Charité, see Paul Sérieux, *L'assistance des aliénés en France, en Allemagne, en Italie et en Suisse* (Paris: Imprimerie municipale, 1903), p. 292.

6. Basic information on the history of psychiatric teaching in German universities may be gleaned from Hans-Heinz Eulner, *Die Entwicklung der medizinischen Specialfächer an den Universitäten des deutschen Sprachgebietes* (Stuttgart: Enke, 1970), pp. 670–680.

7. See Franz Kohl, "Das erste Projekt einer 'akademischen Irrenklinik' in Heidelberg (1826 bis 1842)," *Historia Hospitalium*, no. 18 (1989–1992), pp. 181–184. Ioannis Pilavas, *Psychiatrie im Widerstreit der Konzepte: Zur Entstehungsgeschichte der Tübinger Nervenklinik* (Sigmaringen: Thorbecke, 1994), p. 14.

8. See Krafft-Ebing, *Psychiatrischer Unterricht*, pp. 16–17.

9. Alfred E. Hoche, *Jahresringe: Innenansicht eines Menschenlebens* (Munich: Lehmann, 1934), p. 120. "Sonderbare Eigenbrötler."

10. Wilhelm Griesinger, *Die Pathologie und Therapie der psychischen Krankheiten für Aerzte und Studirende* (Stuttgart: Krabbe, 1845).

11. Griesinger, *Die Pathologies und Therapie der psychischen Krankheiten*, 2nd revised and very enlarged ed. (Stuttgart, 1861, reprinted unchanged 1867; the E. J. Bonset firm of Amsterdam published a reprint of this 1867 edition in 1964).

12. Wernicke was quoted in Karl Bonhoeffer, "Lebenserinnerungen," in J. Zutt et al., eds., *Karl Bonhoeffer zum Hundertsten Geburtstag* (Berlin: Springer, 1969), p. 45.

13. On pedagogic aspects, see "Nachrichten von der psychiatrischen Clinik zu Berlin," *Archiv für Psychiatrie und Nervenkrankheiten*, 1 (1868), pp. 232–234.

14. Robert Wollenberg, *Erinnerungen eines alten Psychiaters* (Stuttgart: Enke, 1931), pp. 64–65.

15. Wilhelm Griesinger, "Über Irrenanstalten und deren Weiter-Entwickelung in Deutschland," *Archiv für Psychiatrie und Nervenkrankheiten*, 1 (1868), pp. 8–43, esp. 11–12.

16. Griesinger, "Vorwort," *Archiv für Psychiatrie und Nervenkrankheiten*, 1 (1868), p. III.

17. For basic accounts of Griesinger's life and work, see Theodor Kirchhoff, ed., *Deutsche Irrenärzte*, 2 vols. (Berlin: Springer, 1921–1924), vol. 2, pp. 1–14; Rudolf Thiele, "Wilhelm Griesinger," in Kurt Kolle, ed., *Grosse Nervenärzte*, 2nd ed., vol. 1 (Stuttgart: Thieme, 1970), pp. 115–127; see also Werner Janzarik, "Die klinische Psychopathologie zwischen Griesinger und Kraepelin im Querschnitt des Jahres 1878," in Janzarik, ed., *Psychopathologie als Grundlagenwissenschaft* (Stuttgart: Enke, 1979), pp. 51–61. At the hands of such students of "professionalization" as Paul Weindling, Griesinger has been reduced to a simplistic caricature, to wit: "Griesinger discovered 'neuroses' which were prevalent among the bourgeoisie and particularly among young female governesses and teachers. Such stigmatizing of an emancipating group warned that hereditary predisposition to mental disease could undermine the self-confident success of the bourgeoisie." Weindling, *Health, Race and German Politics between National Unification and Nazism, 1870–1945* (Cambridge: Cambridge U. P., 1989), pp. 83–84.

18. Kirchhoff, *Deutsche Irrenärzte*, vol. 2, pp. 75–82.

19. On Gudden, see Franz Kohl, "Bernhard von Gudden (1824–1886): Anstaltspsychiater, Hirnanatom und einflussreicher Universitätslehrer," *Psychiatrische Praxis*, 21 (1994), pp. 162–166.

20. On Meynert's life and work, see Erna Lesky, *Die Wiener medizinische Schule im 19. Jahrhundert* (Graz: Böhlau, 1978), pp. 373–382; see also Franz Günther von Stockert, "Theodor Meynert," in Kolle, *Grosse Nervenärzte*, vol. 2, pp. 98–105.

21. Meynert's first psychiatric textbook was mainly a manual of neuroanatomy, punctuated with hypothetical observations about the frontal lobes as the inhibitory centers and the subcortical regions as the stimulative ones. *Psychiatrie: Klinik der Erkrankungen des Vorderhirns* (Vienna: Braumüller, 1884), see, for example, p. 268 on the relationship between cortex and subcortex.

22. Theodor Meynert, *Klinische Vorlesungen über Psychiatrie* (Vienna: Braumüller, 1890), p. v.

23. Arthur Schnitzler, *Jugend in Wien: Eine Autobiographie* (1918) (Frankfurt/M.: Fischer Taschenbuch, 1981), p. 260.

24. Adolf Strümpell, *Aus dem Leben eines deutschen Klinikers* (Leipzig: Vogel, 1925), p. 108. For a recent treatment of Meynert, unsympathetic and

highly favorable to psychoanalysis, see Albrecht Hirschmüller, *Freuds Begegnung mit der Psychiatrie: von der Hirnmythologie zur Neurosenlehre* (Tübingen: Diskord, 1991), pp. 93–104, 109–117.

25. Theodor Meynert, "Über die Nothwendigkeit und Tragweite einer anatomischen Richtung in der Psychiatrie," *Wiener Medizinische Wochenschrift*, 18 (May 3, 1868), pp. 573–576.

26. For an introduction, see Mary A. B. Brazier, *A History of Neurophysiology in the 19th Century* (New York: Raven, 1988).

27. Emil Kraepelin, *Lebenserinnerungen* (Berlin: Springer, 1983), pp. 20–21. Flechsig had appeared at Gudden's clinic in Munich to learn something of practical psychiatry but failed to turn up at rounds.

28. Daniel Paul Schreber, *Denkwürdigkeiten eines Nervenkranken* (Leipzig: Mutze, 1903), see, for example, p. 23, "Flechsig als Urheber des Seelenmords."

29. Sigmund Freud, "Psychoanalytische Bemerkungen über einen autobiographischen beschriebenen Fall von Paranaoia (Dementia Paranoides)" (1911), in Freud, *Gesammelte Werke*, vol. 8 (Frankfurt/M.: Fischer, 1945), pp. 239–320.

30. This was Julius Wagner-Jauregg's cutting opinion of Hitzig, expressed in his MS memoirs (1939), "Nachgelassene Lebenserinnerungen...," p. 58, at Institut für Geschichte der Medizin, Vienna, shelf no. HS 3290. See also Alfred W. Grubser and Erwin H. Ackerknecht, eds., *Constantin von Monakow, Vita Mea. Mein Leben* (c. 1927) (Berne: Hans Huber, 1970), p. 125.

31. Carl Wernicke, *Lehrbuch der Gehirnkrankheiten für Aerzte und Studirende*, 3 vols. (Kassel: Fischer, 1881–1883).

32. Carl Wernicke, *Grundriss der Psychiatrie* (Leipzig: Thieme, 1900).

33. Karl Kleist, "Carl Wernicke," in Kolle, *Grosse Nervenärzte*, vol. 2, pp. 106–128, quote p. 114. See also Mario Lanczik, *Der Breslauer Psychiater Carl Wernicke* (Sigmaringen: Thorbecke, 1988), and Lanczik and G. Keil, "Carl Wernicke's Localization Theory and Its Significance for the Development of Scientific Psychiatry," *History of Psychiatry*, 2 (1991), pp. 171–180.

34. Karl Jaspers, *Allgemeine Psychopathologie für Studierende, Ärzte und Psychologen* (1913), 3d ed. (Berlin: Springer, 1923), p. 13. "Solche anatomischen Konstruktionen sind durchaus plastisch ausgefallen (Meynert, Wernicke) und werden mit Recht 'Hirnmythologien' genannt." Oswald Bumke, however, claimed that Franz Nissl was first to use the phrase. Bumke, "Fünfzig Jahre Psychiatrie," *Münchener Medizinische Wochenschrift*, 72 (July 10, 1925), pp. 1141–43; see p. 1141.

35. Emil Kraepelin, "Hundert Jahre Psychiatrie," *Zeitschrift für die gesamte Neurologie und Psychiatrie*, 38 (1917), pp. 161–275; see p. 234.

36. Jan Goldstein, *Console and Classify: The French Psychiatric Profession in the Nineteenth Century* (Cambridge: Cambridge U. P., 1987), pp. 135–136.

37. Sérieux catalogues the deficiencies in French psychiatric training, making unfavorable comparisons with Germany, *L'Assistance des aliénés*, pp. 397–417.

38. See Stefan Müller, *Antoine-Laurent Bayle: Sein grundlegender Beitrag zur Erforschung der progressiven Paralyse* (Zurich: Juris, 1965), esp. p. 16.

39. See René Semelaigne, *Les pionniers de la psychiatrie française*, 2 vols. (Paris: Baillière, 1930–1932), vol. 1, pp. 244–249.

40. Vincente J. Iragui, "The Charcot-Bouchard Controversy," *Archives of Neurology*, 43 (1986), pp. 290–295, esp. pp. 292–293.

41. Bénédict-Auguste Morel, *Traité des dégénérescences physiques, intellectuelles et morales de l'espèce humaine* (Paris: Baillière, 1857), p. 46.

42. This account is based on Semelaigne, *Pionniers psychiatrie française*, vol. 1, pp. 342–351.

43. Semelaigne, *Pionniers psychiatrie française*, vol. 2, pp. 40–49. For Lasègue's description of anorexia nervosa, see "De l'anorexie hystérique," *Archives générales de médecine*, 21 (1873), pp. 385–403. On the creation of Lasègue's half-chair in the 1860s, see Goldstein, *Console and Classify*, pp. 347–348.

44. On Ball's appointment, see Pierre Pichot, *A Century of Psychiatry* (Paris: Dacosta, 1983), pp. 25–27. The bitter negotiations, touching particularly on how many clinical beds Ball was to have, may be followed in the *Progrès médical* throughout October and November, 1877, November and December 1878, and May 24 and Nov. 22, 1879. On Ball's life, see Semelaigne, *Pionniers psychiatrie française*, vol. 2, pp. 201–209.

45. The story of Charcot's "hysteria" is told in detail in Edward Shorter, *From Paralysis to Fatigue: A History of Psychosomatic Illness in the Modern Era* (New York: Free Press, 1992), pp. 166–200.

46. "Centenaire de Charcot," *Revue neurologique*, 32 (1925), pp. 746–1168.

47. On Magnan's life see Paul Sérieux, "V. Magnan: sa vie et son oeuvre," *Annales médico-psychologiques*, 10 ser., 8 (1917), pp. 273–329, 449–507; 9 (1918), pp. 5–59; basic biographical data on pp. 274–300. This was reprinted as Paul Sérieux, *V. Magnan: Sa vie et son oeuvre (1835–1916)* (Paris: Masson, 1921).

48. Sérieux, *Magnan*, p. 291. Sérieux claimed in his intensely nationalistic account, "In the history of psychiatry this period is still with us, marked by the unique combination of eminent teachers and distinguished students, an elite cohort of scientific pioneers who have transformed contemporary psychiatry."

49. Sérieux, *Ann. méd.-psych.*, 9 (1918), p. 46.

50. See Pichot, *Century of Psychiatry*, pp. 75–76. See also Pichot, "The Diagnosis and Classification of Mental Disorders in French-Speaking Countries: Background, Current Views and Comparison with Other Nomenclatures," *Psychological Medicine*, 12 (1982), pp. 475–492.

51. Clarence B. Farrar, MS diary of his trip to Europe c. 1902–04, in possession of Queen Street Mental Health Centre, Greenland-Griffin Archive, Toronto, Canada. On Stoddart, see the biographical note in *Munk's Roll*, vol. 4, p. 495.

52. Walter Rivington, *The Medical Profession* (Dublin: Fannin, 1879), pp. 315–316.

53. John Haslam, *Observations on Madness and Melancholy*, 2nd rev. ed. (London: Callow, 1809), p. 238.

54. William Charles Ellis, *A Treatise on the Nature, Symptoms, Causes, and Treatment of Insanity* (London: Holdsworth, 1838), p. 22.

55. David Skae, "A Rational and Practical Classification of Insanity," *Journal of Mental Science*, 9 (1863), pp. 309–319, quote p. 318.

56. See, for example, W. H. W. Sankey, "On Melancholia," *Journal of Mental Science*, 9 (1863–1864), pp. 176–196, esp. p. 195.

57. On Sankey's life see *Munk's Roll*, vol. 4, pp. 147–148, which dates the beginning of his lectureship to 1864. See also the obituary in *BMJ*, 1 (March 23, 1889), pp. 689–690.

58. Michael Collie, *Henry Maudsley: Victorian Psychiatrist* (London: St. Paul's Bibliographies, 1988), p. 20.

59. John Conolly, *The Treatment of the Insane without Mechanical Restraint* (1850). I consulted the later edition: London: Smith, 1856. On Conolly, see Richard Hunter and Ida Macalpine, *Three Hundred Years of Psychiatry* (London: Oxford U. P., 1963), pp. 805–806, 1030–34. James Crichton-Browne leaves a sympathetic portrait of him in *Victorian Jottings from an Old Commonplace Book* (London: Etchells, 1926), pp. 326–329.

60. Collie, *Maudsley*, p. 23. For some details on Lawn House, see William Ll. Parry-Jones, *The Trade in Lunacy: A Study of Private Madhouses in England in the Eighteenth and Nineteenth Centuries* (London: Routledge, 1972), pp. 80, 231.

61. Henry Maudsley, *Body and Mind* (London: Macmillan, 1870), p. 41. Maudsley attributed the "fingers' ends" observation to his colleague John Charles Bucknill.

62. See Aubrey Lewis, "Henry Maudsley," in Kolle, *Grosse Nervenärzte*, vol. 3, pp. 101–108, quote p. 106; on founding the Maudsley Hospital, see also Aubrey Lewis, "Henry Maudsley: His Work and Influence" (1950), reprinted in Lewis, *The State of Psychiatry: Essays and Addresses* (London: Routledge, 1967), pp. 29–48, esp. p. 45.

63. Eunice E. Winters, ed., *The Collected Papers of Adolf Meyer*, vol. 2 (Baltimore: Johns Hopkins, 1951), pp. 237–255, quote p. 250; from his essay "Medicinische Studien in Paris, Edinburgh und London" (1891).

64. Rosemary Stevens, *American Medicine and the Public Interest* (New Haven: Yale U. P., 1971), p. 60 n. 13.

65. Edward R. Hun, "Haematoma Auris," *American Journal of Insanity*, 27 (1870), pp. 13–28. "Preceding the appearance of the tumor we find that one, or in rare cases both, of the ears become red and swollen, while at the same time the face and eyes give evidence of a strong determination of blood toward the head [!]" (p. 14). On Hun, see Henry M. Hurd, *The Institutional Care of the Insane in the United States and Canada*, vol. 1 (Baltimore: Johns Hopkins, 1916), p. 282.

66. John Charles Bucknill, "Notes on Asylums for the Insane in America," *Lancet*, 1 (June 3, 1876), pp. 810–812, quote p. 811. See also D. Hack Tuke's

favorable assessment of Deecke, in *The Insane in the United States and Canada* (London: Lewis, 1885), p. 116. Although Deecke was said to have studied in Berlin, it is unclear what he might have studied. See his obituary notice in *JAMA*, 45 (Dec. 23, 1905), p. 1973.

67. Hurd, *Institutional Care Insane*, vol. 1, pp. 282–283.

68. See William A. White, "Presidential Address," *AJP*, 5 (1925), pp. 1–20, phrase pp. 4–5.

69. Meyer, *Collected Papers*, vol. 2, pp. 220–221.

70. Meyer, *Collected Papers*, vol. 1, pp. 239–240.

71. See Hans H. Walser, ed., *August Forel: Briefe/Correspondance, 1864–1927* (Berne: Huber, 1968), for example, Meyer's letter to August Forel, Jan. 3, 1893, p. 285.

72. On Kankakee, see Hurd, *Institutional Care Insane*, vol. 2, pp. 222–259; on Meyer's recruitment, p. 239.

73. Meyer, *Collected Papers*, vol. 2, p. 93.

74. Meyer, *Collected Papers*, vol. 2, p. 59.

75. Meyer, *Collected Papers*, vol. 2, p. 274.

76. On these events, see Gerald N. Grob, *Mental Illness and American Society, 1875–1940* (Princeton: Princeton U. P., 1983), pp. 127 131.

77. For some recollections of the Manhattan State Hospital during Meyer's tenure, see David Kennedy Henderson, *The Evolution of Psychiatry in Scotland* (Edinburgh: Livingstone, 1964), pp. 156–167.

78. Meyer, *Collected Papers*, vol. 2, p. 115.

79. See Meyer's tour of the horizon, *Collected Papers*, vol. 2, p. 70.

80. Strictly speaking, the psychopathic hospitals, first established in Ann Arbor, Michigan, in 1906, combined teaching and research even before Meyer opened the Henry Phipps Psychiatric Clinic as part of the Johns Hopkins Hospital in 1913. See Hurd, *Institutional Care Insane*, vol. 2, pp. 815–824. The Psychopathic Department of the Boston State Hospital, which opened in 1912, had a connection to Harvard where its director Elmer Southard was professor of neuropathology (ibid., p. 653). Yet the impact of the Phipps was much greater.

81. S. L. Sherman et al., "Further Segregation Analysis of the Fragile X Syndrome with Special Reference to Transmitting Males," *Human Genetics*, 69 (1985), pp. 289–299, discovered the phenomenon of genetic anticipation in fragile X syndrome, meaning that the "penetrance" of a disorder increases over successive generations; Ying-Hui Fu et al., "Variation of the CGG Repeat at the Fragile X Site Results in Genetic Instability: Resolution of the Sherman Paradox," *Cell*, 67 (1991), pp. 1047–58, which found, "The risk of mental impairment in fragile X pedigrees is contingent upon position of individuals in pedigrees; brothers of NTMs [normal transmitting males] are at low (~9%) risk, while grandsons and great grandsons have much higher risks (40% and 50%)." (p. 1047); Robert I. Richards and Grant R. Sutherland, "Dynamic Mutations: A New Class of Mutations Causing Human Disease," *Cell*, 70 (1992), pp. 709–712, called attention to dynamic mutation as the

process behind several important human genetic diseases including fragile X; for the isolation of the gene in fragile X, see Gregory J. Tsongalis and Lawrence M. Silverman, "Molecular Pathology of the Fragile X Syndrome," *Archives of Pathology and Laboratory Medicine*, 117 (1993), pp. 1121–25; Stephen T. Warren and David L. Nelson, "Advances in Molecular Analysis of Fragile X Syndrome," *JAMA*, 271 (Feb. 16, 1994), pp. 536–553, observed that as the gene (a succession of trinucleotide repeats, namely CGG) is handed on, the number of repeats increases dramatically, from 6 to 52 repeats in a nonsymptomatic individual, from 230 to 1,000 repeats in an affected individual. The authors concluded, "As the premutation is transmitted vertically through a family it tends to increase in size, and therefore greater numbers of affected children are observed in later generations . . ." (pp. 538–539). On Huntington's disease, one source points out that, "the repeat sequence may decrease in size as well as expand." Editorial, *Journal of Medical Genetics*, 30 (1993), pp. 975–977, quote p. 975.

82. Morel, *Traité dégénérescences*, pp. iii–ix, 5–6, 62, 72, 346.

83. Morel, *Traité dégénérescences*, on alcoholism, his main bugbear, see pp. 79–140; on slums, pp. 635–644; on sequestration, p. 691. For a brief overview of Morel's theories, see Rafael Huertas, "Madness and Degeneration, I: From 'Fallen Angel' to Mentally Ill," *History of Psychiatry*, 3 (1992), pp. 391–411; Huertas gives the large secondary literature on the history of degeneration in "Disease and Crime in Spanish Positivist Psychiatry," ibid., 4 (1993), pp. 459–481, see pp. 459–460, n. 2.

84. Richard von Krafft-Ebing, "Die Erblichkeit der Seelenstörungen und ihre Bedeutung für die forensische Praxis," *Friedreich's Blätter für gerichtliche Medicin*, 19 (1868), pp. 188–211.

85. Richard von Krafft-Ebing, "Über die prognostische Bedeutung der erblichen Anlage im Irresein," *Allgemeine Zeitschrift für Psychiatrie*, 26 (1869), pp. 438–456, quote p. 439; he mentioned some of the stigmata of Morelian degeneration, p. 443.

86. Richard von Krafft-Ebing, *Lehrbuch der Psychiatrie* (1879), 3d ed. (Stuttgart: Enke, 1888), p. 424.

87. Richard von Krafft-Ebing, *Psychopathia Sexualis: Eine klinisch-forensische Studie* (Stuttgart: Enke, 1886).

88. Moritz Benedikt, *Aus meinem Leben: Erinnerungen und Eröterungen* (Vienna: Konegen, 1906), p. 392.

89. Valentin Magnan and Maurice Paul Legrain, *Les Dégénérés (État mental et syndromes épisodiques)* (Paris: Rueff, 1895), p. 79. On the course of the concept of degeneration in France, see Ian R. Dowbiggin, *Inheriting Madness: Professionalization and Psychiatric Knowledge in Nineteenth-Century France* (Berkeley: University of California Press, 1991).

90. Magnan, *Les Dégénérés*, p. 235.

91. Anon. [W. H. O. Sankey], "On the Degeneracy of the Human Race," *Journal of Psychological Medicine*, 10 (1857), pp. 159–208.

92. Maudsley, *Body and Mind*, pp. 61, 63.

93. On degeneration doctrines in England, see Janet Oppenheim, *"Shattered Nerves": Doctors, Patients, and Depression in Victorian England* (New York: Oxford U. P., 1991), pp. 265–292.

94. Samuel Alexander Kenny Strahan, "Propagation of Insanity and Allied Neuroses," *Journal of Mental Science*, 36 (1890), pp. 325–338, quotes pp. 329–330. Strahan left medicine to become a lawyer, going on to write *Marriage and Disease: A Study of Heredity and the More Important Family Degenerations* (New York: Appleton, 1892).

95. Laurence J. Ray, "Models of Madness in Victorian Asylum Practice," *Archives européenes de sociologie*, 22 (1981), pp. 229–264, data p. 252.

96. François Ritti's obituary of Magnan made only a glancing reference to his doctrines of "la folie des dégénérés" and "le délire chronique" as controversial. François Ritti, "Mort de M. Magnan," *Annales médico-psychologiques*, 10 ser., 8 (1917), pp. 74–79, esp. p. 76.

97. [Wilhelm Stekel] Med. Dr. Serenus (pseud.), *Äskulap als Harlekin: Humor, Satire und Phantasie aus der Praxis* (Wiesbaden: Bergmann, 1911), p. 3.

98. Oswald Bumke, *Landläufige Irrtümer in der Beurteilung von Geisteskranken* (Wiesbaden: Bergmann, 1908), pp. 13–14.

99. See Jaspers, *Allgemeine Psychopathologie*, pp. 13–37.

100. Émile Zola, *Germinal*, trans. Stanley and Eleanor Hochman (New York: NAL, 1970), pp. 38, 106.

101. Alfred Hoche and Karl Binding, *Die Freigabe der Vernichtung lebensunwerten Lebens* (Leipzig: Meiner, 1920). Although the authors argued mainly for the euthanasia of terminal medically ill individuals who themselves desired death, Hoche did suggest that institutionalized people with severe mental retardation might also be subject to euthanasia. The book found a mixed reception in the medical press; compare the negative review in the *Berliner Klinische Wochenschrift*, 57 (July 19, 1920), pp. 695–696, and the brief positive notice in the *Münchener Medizinische Wochenschrift*, 67 (Sept. 3, 1920), p. 1048. The racist *Archiv für Rassen- und Gesellschaftsbiologie* found the work "devoid of eugenic viewpoints" (vol. 13, 1921, p. 211). On the generally negative response to these proposals during the Weimar Republic, see Hans-Walter Schmuhl, *Rassenhygiene, Nationalsozialismus, Euthanasie: Von der Verhütung zur Vernichtung "lebensunwerten Lebens," 1890–1945* (Göttingen: Vandenhoeck, 1987), pp. 115–125. By conflating degeneration, eugenics, and genetics, Weindling manages, in my view incorrectly, to suggest that psychiatrists were among the worst of those propagating doctrines that led to Nazism. See, for example, his *Health, Race and German Politics*, pp. 336–338. For an especially tendentious example of academic efforts to blame psychiatrists, a style of historical writing in which every biological thought leads inevitably to Hitler, see Hans-Georg Güse and Norbert Schmacke, *Psychiatrie zwischen bürgerlicher Revolution und Faschismus*, 2 vols. (Kronberg: Athenäum, 1976), esp. vol. 2, pp. 387f. Gustav W.

Schimmelpennig attempts to rehabilitate Hoche's reputation on the grounds that he was philo-Semitic and did not pave the way for Hitler's practice of euthanasia. *Alfred Erich Hoche. Das wissenschaftliche Werk: "Mittelmässigkeit?"* (Göttingen: Vandenhoeck, 1990), pp. 5–11, on Jews p. 9 n. 25.

102. On medicine before and during the Nazi period, see Robert N. Proctor, *Racial Hygiene: Medicine under the Nazis* (Cambridge: Harvard U. P., 1988); and Michael Kator, *Doctors under Hitler* (Chapel Hill: University of North Carolina Press, 1989). Kator points out that one of the major Nazi specialists in racial genetics, Otmar von Verschuer, had been trained as an internist (p. 232).

103. In addition to the standard accounts of Kraepelin's life in such sources as Kolle, *Grosse Nervenärzte*, vol. 1, pp. 175–186, see: R. Avenarius, "Emil Kraepelin, seine Persönlichkeit und seine Konzeption," in Janzarik, *Psychopathologie als Grundlagenwissenschaft*, pp. 62–73; Hans W. Gruhle, "Emil Kraepelin 100. Geburtstag," *Nervenarzt*, 27 (1956), pp. 241–244; P. Hoff, "Nosologische Grundpostulate bei Kraepelin: Versuch einer kritischen Würdigung des Kraepelinischen Spätwerkes," *Zeitschrift für klinische Psychologie*, 36 (1988), pp. 328–336; on Kraepelin's personality and clinical manner, see Shorter, *From Paralysis to Fatigue*, pp. 241–244.

104. Emil Kraepelin, *Compendium der Psychiatrie* (Leipzig: Abel, 1883). Weindling is determined to see villainy everywhere and in reference to Kraepelin's move to Munich in 1904 makes him one of the "leading racial hygienists in Munich." Weindling, *Health, Race and German Politics*, p. 307.

105. On Kraepelin's early years, see his, *Lebenserinnerungen*, pp. 1–24; Wilhelm Wirth, "Emil Kraepelin zum Gedächtnis!" *Archiv für die gesamte Psychologie*, 58 (1927), pp. 1–32.

106. Franz Nissl, *Die Neuronenlehre und ihre Anhänger* (Jena: Fischer, 1903). Unfortunately, Nissl set out to refute the neuron theory, which is why he is mainly known for his stains and not for his discoveries in the neurosciences.

107. See, for example, Ugo Cerletti, "Erinnerungen an Franz Nissl," *Münchener Medizinische Wochenschrift*, 101 (1959), pp. 2368–71.

108. Aloys Alzheimer, "Über eine eigenartige Erkrankung der Hirnrinde," in resumé of the 37th "Versammlung Südwestdeutscher Irrenärzte in Tübingen . . . 1906," *Allgemeine Zeitschrift für Psychiatrie*, 64 (1907), pp. 146–147.

109. On Hellpach's misadventures with Kraepelin, see Willy Hellpach, *Wirken in Wirren: Lebenserinnerungen*, vol. 1: *1877–1914* (Hamburg: Wegner, 1948), pp. 277–278, 354–355.

110. See, for example, Anton Delbrück's review of the 5th ed. *Zeitschrift für Hypnotismus*, 5 (1897), pp. 362–365, esp. p. 362.

111. On Neumann (and on previous representatives of the *Einheitspsychose* view), see M. Lanczik, "Heinrich Neumann und seine Lehre von der Einheitspsychose," *Fundamenta Psychiatrica*, 3 (1989), pp. 49–54. On Neumann's life, see Arthur Leppmann, "Heinrich Neumann. Nekrolog," *Allgemeine Zeitschrift*

für Psychiatrie, 42 (1885), pp. 180–186. Neumann, virtually the only Jew in the German psychiatric establishment at the time, had switched in the 1850s from medicine to psychiatry at Breslau, directing a university psychiatric clinic situated in the city hospital from 1874 until 1884, when Wernicke succeeded him.

112. Karl Kahlbaum, *Die Gruppirung der psychischen Krankheiten und die Eintheilung der Seelenstörungen* (Danzig: Kafemann, 1863), p. 129.

113. Ewald Hecker, "Die Hebephrenie: ein Beitrag zur klinischen Psychiatrie," *Archiv für pathologische Anatomie und Physiologie und für klinische Medicin*, 52 (1871), pp. 394–429. On Hecker, See Mark J. Sedler, "The Legacy of Ewald Hecker: A New Translation of 'Die Hebephrenie,'" *AJP*, 142 (1985), pp. 1265–71.

114. See Mark J. Sedler, "Falret's Discovery: The Origin of the Concept of Bipolar Affective Illness," *AJP*, 140 (1983), pp. 1127–33.

115. Kraepelin, *Erinnerungen*, pp. 68–69.

116. Emil Kraepelin, *Psychiatrie. Ein kurzes Lehrbuch für Studirende und Aerzte*, 4th ed. (Leipzig: Abel, 1893); I have translated "die Erreichung möglichster Naturwahrheit" (p. v) as cutting nature at the joints.

117. Bénédict-Auguste Morel, *Études cliniques, traité théorique et pratique des maladies mentales. . . .* 2 vols. (Paris: Baillière, 1852–1853), I have not seen this; *Traité des maladies mentales* (Paris: Masson, 1860), p. 566. The term was scarcely a central category for Morel in 1860, and he used it *en passant*.

118. Thomas S. Clouston, "The Morisonian Lectures on Insanity for 1873," *Journal of Mental Science*, 19 (1874), pp. 491–507, see pp. 496–498 on the "insanity of pubescence." In this same lecture series, Clouston later spoke of "the hereditary insanity of adolescence," ibid., 21 (1875), pp. 205–206. Clouston later adopted the phrase "neuroses of development"; see his "Some of the Physician's Developmental Problems—Bodily and Mental," [London] *Medical Magazine*, 1 (1892), pp. 425–440, see p. 431.

119. Thomas S. Clouston, "The Neuroses of Development: Adolescent Insanity and its Secondary Dementia," *Edinburgh Medical Journal*, 36 (1891), pp. 104–124.

120. For a summary of Charpentier's paper, see *Revue de l'hypnotisme*, 5 (1891), pp. 90–91. Among other writers on adolescent insanity, see, for example, Heinrich Schüle, a physician at the Illenau asylum in Baden, *Handbuch der Geisteskrankheiten* (Leipzig: Vogel, 1878), "das pubische Irresein" [pubic insanity], p. 232.

121. Kraepelin, *Psychiatrie*. 4th ed. (1893), pp. 434–442. On the psychiatric context of Kraepelin's ideas, see G. E. Berrios and R. Hauser, "The Early Development of Kraepelin's Ideas on Classification: A Conceptual History," *Psychological Medicine*, 18 (1988), pp. 813–821.

122. Emil Kraepelin, *Psychiatrie: Ein Lehrbuch für Studirende und Aerzte*, 5th ed. (Leipzig: Barth, 1896), p. v. "In dem Entwicklungsgange des vorliegenden

Buches bedeutet die jetztige Bearbeitung den letzen, entscheidenden Schritt von der symptomatischen zur klinischen Betrachtungsweise des Irreseins. Diese Wandlung des Standpunktes. . . . zeigt sich vor allem in der Abgrenzung und Gruppirung der Krankheitsbilder. Ueberall hat hier die Bedeutung der äusseren Krankheitszeichen hinter den Gesichtspunkten zurücktreten müssen, die sich aus den Entstehungsbedingungen, aus Verlauf und Ausgang der einzelnen Störungen ergeben haben. Alle reinen 'Zustandsbilder' sind damit aus der Formenlehre verschwunden."

123. Kraepelin, *Psychiatrie*, 5th ed. (1896), pp. 14–15.

124. Emil Kraepelin, *Psychiatrie: ein Lehrbuch für Studirende und Aerzte*, 6th ed., vol. 2: *Klinische Psychiatrie* (Leipzig: Barth, 1899), p. 5.

125. Kraepelin, *Psychiatrie*, 6th ed. (1899), p. 359; for the classification, see the table of contents, pp. v–x. Kraepelin split some melancholia off from manic-depressive illness and adjoined it to "involutional psychosis" *(das Irresein des Rückbildungsalters)*, supposedly attributed to ageing. Some cases of depression were still assigned to "psychopathic conditions (degenerative psychosis)." Yet in the eighth edition of this text, the clinical volume which was published in 1913, he abandoned these categories. Kraepelin, *Psychiatrie: ein Lehrbuch*, 8th ed., 4 vols. 1909–1915, vol. 3: *Klinische Psychiatrie*, part 2 (Leipzig: Barth, 1913), pp. 1353–58. Kraepelin acknowledged the influence of the work of his student, Georges L. Dreyfus, *Die Melancholie: ein Zustandsbild des manisch-depressiven Irreseins* (Jena: Fischer, 1907), for which he wrote the preface. In 1920 Kraepelin softened slightly the watertight division between affective and nonaffective psychoses by admitting that the prognosis could not always be made on the basis of the presenting symptoms. Kraepelin, "Die Erscheinungsformen des Irreseins," *Zeitschrift für die gesamte Neurologie und Psychiatrie*, 62 (1920), pp. 1–29, see p. 27.

126. Summary of paper by Bleuler, "Die Prognose der Dementia praecox (Schizophreniegruppe)," *Allgemeine Zeitschrift für Psychiatrie*, 65 (1908), pp. 436–437 (". . . Erlaube ich mir, hier das Wort Schizophrenie zur Bezeichnung des Kraepelinschen Begriffes zu benützen").

127. Eugen Bleuler, *Dementia Praecox oder Gruppe der Schizophrenien* (1911) (reprint Tübingen: Diskord, 1988). See Manfred Bleuler's preface on his father's self-image as a true pupil of Kraepelin.

128. Meyer, *Collected Papers*, vol. 2, p. 393.

129. Oswald Bumke, "Alfred Erich Hoche," *Archiv für Psychiatrie und Nervenkrankheiten*, 116 (1943), pp. 339–346, quote p. 342. On Hoche, see Schimmelpennig, *Alfred Erich Hoche*.

130. Quoted in Erwin Stransky, MS "Autobiographie," in Vienna, Institut für Geschichte der Medizin, shelf no. HS 2065, p. 272. "Ein norddeutscher Dorfschulmeister in Riesenformat."

131. Reported by Bonhoeffer, "Lebenserinnerungen," p. 46.

132. Clarence B. Farrar, "I Remember Nissl," *AJP*, 110 (1954), pp. 621–624, story pp. 623–624.

133. Franz Nissl, "Über die Entwicklung der Psychiatrie in den letzten 50 Jahren," *Verhandlungen des Naturhistorisch-Medizinischen Vereins*, N.F., 8 (1908), pp. 510–525, quote p. 520.

134. S. B. Sutton, *Crossroads in Psychiatry: A History of the McLean Hospital* (Washington: American Psychiatric Press, 1986), pp. 149–150.

135. Meyer, *Collected Papers*, vol. 3, p. 523.

136. Meyer, *Collected Papers*, vol. 2, p. 280.

137. Henderson, *Evolution Psychiatry Scotland*, p. 183.

138. Meyer, *Collected Papers*, vol. 2, p. 199. For a brief account, see Hurd, *Institutional Care Insane*, vol. 2, pp. 571–573; see also A. McGhee Harvey et al., *A Model of Its Kind, vol. 1: A Centennial History of Medicine at Johns Hopkins* (Baltimore: Johns Hopkins, 1989), pp. 62–63 and passim.

139. According to Theodore Lidz, ". . . When [Meyer] took a firm stand against Kraepelin's 1896 nosology which considered mental disorders as specific disease entities it was a decisive step for American psychiatry." Lidz, "Adolf Meyer and the Development of American Psychiatry," *AJP*, 123 (1966), pp. 320–332, quote pp. 326–327. For a précis of Meyer's multifaceted views, see U. H. Peters, "Adolf Meyer und die Beziehungen zwischen deutscher und amerikanischer Psychiatrie," *Fortschritte der Neurologie und Psychiatrie*, 58 (1990), pp. 332–338.

140. Meyer, *Collected Papers*, vol. 2, p. 266. The claim appeared in Meyer's article, "A Review of the Signs of Degeneration and of Methods of Registration," *American Journal of Insanity*, 52 (1895), pp. 344–363.

141. Apropos Meyer's comments on the fifth edition of Kraepelin's text in 1896. See Meyer, *Collected Papers*, vol. 3, p. 523.

142. Meyer, *Collected Papers*, vol. 3, pp. 536–539. Cotton's work "now will have to be carried on without the leading and active spirit of the sincere and convinced protagonist" (p. 537). On Cotton, see Andrew Scull, "Desperate Remedies: a Gothic Tale of Madness and Modern Medicine," in R. M. Murray and T. H. Turner, eds., *Lectures on the History of Psychiatry* (London: Gaskell, 1990), pp. 144–169.

143. See Meyer, *Collected Papers*, vol. 3, pp. 102, 285–314, 309–310.

144. For an appreciation of this style, see C. Macfie Campbell, "Adolf Meyer," *Archives of Neurology and Psychiatry*, 37 (1937), pp. 715–724, esp. p. 723.

145. See Lidz, *AJP*, p. 327.

Chapter 4: Nerves

1. *The Works of Edgar Allan Poe, vol. 2: Tales* (London: Oxford U. P., 1927), pp. 376–381, quotes pp. 376, 378. For an overview of the disparate literature on what, if anything, was wrong with Poe, see Alexander Hammond, "On Poe Biography: A Review Essay," *ESQ*, 28 (1982), pp. 197–208. See also Robert Patterson, "Once upon a Midnight Dreary: The Life and Addictions of

Edgar Allan Poe," *Canadian Medical Association Journal*, 147 (1992), pp. 1246–48.

2. See Richard Hunter and Ida Macalpine, *Three Hundred Years of Psychiatry, 1535–1860* (London: Oxford U. P., 1963), p. 695 on Norris; pp. 696–703 for excerpts from the report of the select parliamentary committee whose investigations in 1814 and 1815 created such a stir.

3. Bruno Goergen, *Privat-Heilanstalt für Gemüthskranke* (Vienna: Wimmer, 1820), p. 10.

4. Charles Reade, *Hard Cash: A Matter-of-Fact Romance* (c. 1863); I consulted the 2nd ed. (London, Sampson Low, 1864), vol. 2, p. 290. The first editions were undated. So popular was this work that the last of its many editions appeared in 1927.

5. Adolf Grohmann, *Technisches und Psychologisches in der Beschäftigung von Nervenkranken* (Stuttgart: Enke, 1899), pp. 64, 68–69, 70. The first-quoted set of parents actually wanted their son to volunteer quietly for asylum care rather than making a messy committal necessary.

6. Hugo Gugl and Anton Stichl, *Neuropathologische Studien* (Stuttgart: Enke, 1892), p. 18.

7. David Drummond, "The Mental Origin of Neurasthenia and its Bearing on Treatment," *BMJ*, vol. 2 (Dec. 28, 1907), pp. 1813–16, quote p. 1814.

8. Georg Dobrick, "Odium psychiatricum," *PNW*, 13 (Dec. 16, 1911), pp. 381–383.

9. Short notice, *PNW*, 27 (Nov. 28, 1925), p. 496.

10. Georg Lomer, "Ein antipsychiatrisches Zentralorgan," *PNW*, 11 (Oct. 23, 1909), pp. 273–278.

11. Alfred E. Hoche, *Jahresringe: Innenansicht eines Menschenlebens* (Munich: Lehmann, 1934), p. 121.

12. Zbigniew J. Lipowski observes that patients like the term "stress" much better than any specific psychiatric diagnosis. He therefore sends somatizing patients for "stress management" and the like. "Somatization and Depression," *Psychosomatics*, 31 (1990), pp. 13–21, see p. 19.

13. [George] Bernard Shaw, "Preface" (1911) to *The Doctor's Dilemma: A Tragedy* (Harmondsworth: Penguin, 1946), p. 76. The play was first performed in 1906.

14. Gregory Bateson, ed., *Perceval's Narrative: A Patient's Account of His Psychosis, 1830–1832* (Stanford: Stanford U. P., 1961), p. 178.

15. J. Evans Riadore, *Introductory Lectures to a Course on Nervous Irritation, Spinal Affections . . .* (London: Churchill, 1835), p. 59.

16. See for example Jean-Amédée Dupau, *De l'éréthisme nerveux ou analyse des affections nerveuses* (Montpellier: Martel, 1819), pp. 6–7.

17. Heinrich Laehr, *Über Irrsein und Irrenanstalten* (Halle: Pfeffer, 1852), p. 244; "Zusammenstellung der Irren-Anstalten Deutschlands," *Allgemeine Zeitschrift für Psychiatrie*, 15 (1858), "Anhang" [appendix], p. 2.

18. "Anhang," *Allg. Z. Psych.* 1858, p. 7; the *Index-Catalogue of the Library of the Surgeon-General's Office, United States Army,* series 1, vol. 9, p. 780 refers to a prospectus for the "Heil- und Pflegeanstalt für Nervenkranke zu Eitorf," published by August Meyer (Eitorf, 1876).

19. Ewald Hecker, *Über das Verhältniss zwischen Nerven- und Geisteskrankheiten* (Kassel: Fischer, 1881), p. 13; Hecker's asylum, founded in 1881, was called a "Kuranstalt für Nervenleidende" (Hospital for Nervous Sufferers).

20. Robert Sommer, "Kliniken für psychische und nervöse Krankheiten," *Medicinische Woche,* 7 (1906), pp. 4–6, quotes p. 4. Name changed from *Irrenklinik* (Clinic for the Insane) to *Klinik für psychische und nervöse Krankheiten* (Clinic for Psychic and Nervous Diseases). He chose the new term also to spare the sensibilities of the department of medicine, which had control over neurology and did not wish Sommer to arrogate to himself "Nervenpathologie."

21. Ferdinand Adalbert Kehrer, "Erinnerungen eines Neuro- und Psychopathologen," *Hippokrates,* 35 (1964), pp. 22–29, quote p. 27. This brief memoir stands as a monument to the ability of the generation of psychiatrists contaminated by Nazism to pass in silence over the years from 1933 to 1945.

22. John R. Lord, "The Evolution of the 'Nerve' Hospital as a Factor in the Progress of Psychiatry," *Journal of Mental Science,* 75 (1929), pp. 307–315, esp. p. 313.

23. Johannes Bresler, "Eine Oberschlesische Nervenklinik," *PNW,* 26 (Aug. 9, 1924), pp. 104–106, quote p. 105. The institution in question was the provincial psychiatric hospital in Kreuzburg, Oberschlesien (Upper Silesia).

24. Paul Näcke, "Die Trennung der Neurologie von der Psychiatrie und die Schaffung eigener neurologischer Kliniken," *Neurologisches Zentralblatt,* 31 (1912), pp. 82–89, quotes p. 88. Näcke was then director of the Hubertusburg asylum.

25. On this early history, see Richard Metcalfe, *The Rise and Progress of Hydrotherapy in England and Scotland* (London: Simpkin, 1906), pp. 58–76; see also Phyllis Hembry, *The English Spa, 1560–1815: A Social History* (London: Athlone, 1990).

26. Janet Browne makes this point in "Spas and Sensibilities: Darwin at Malvern," *Medical History,* Supplement no. 10 (1990), pp. 102–113; see p. 106.

27. Edward Bulwer Lytton, *Confessions of a Water-Patient* (London: Colburn, 1845), pp. 13–15.

28. Edward Sparks, who had TB and lived permanently in Mentone on the French Riviera, advised against the Riviera for nervous disorders, calling patients with them "rather injured than improved by the climate of the Western Riviera." *The Riviera: Sketches of the Health Resorts* (London: Churchill, 1879), p. 140.

29. Hermann Weber, "Klimatotherapie," in Hugo von Ziemssen, ed., *Handbuch der allgemeinen Therapie* (Leipzig: Vogel, 1880), vol. 2, pt. 1, pp. 1–212. I was able to consult only the French translation of this guide, *Climatothérapie*

(Paris: Alcan, 1886), see pp. 276–278; on Hermann Weber, see *Munk's Roll*, vol. 4, pp. 121–122.

30. Hermann Weber and Frederick Parkes Weber, *The Mineral Waters and Health Resorts of Europe* (London: Smith, 1898), p. 334.

31. Frederick Parkes Weber, Casebooks, vol. for 1907–1909, p. 200. Contemporary Medical Archives Centre, Wellcome Institute for the History of Medicine, London.

32. Notice, *BMJ*, vol. 1 (Apr. 1, 1922), p. 533.

33. Neville Wood, "British Spas and Their Waters," *The Prescriber*, 15 (1921), pp. 113–119, quote p. 119.

34. Paul Gerbod, "Les 'fièvres thermales' en France au XIXe siècle," *Revue historique*, 277 (1987), pp. 309–334. esp, p. 312.

35. A. Bellanger, *Le Magnétisme: verités et chimères de cette science occulte* (Paris: Guilhermet, 1854), p. 219; "une sorte de république champêtre de buveurs d'eau."

36. Octave Mirbeau, *Les vingt et un jours d'un neurasthénique* (Paris: Charpentier, 1901), p. 337.

37. Fernand Levillain, *Les maladies nerveuses et arthritiques à Royat* (Clermont-Ferrand: Malleval, 1894), p. 60.

38. Edouard Egasse and Joseph-Frédéric Guyenot, *Eaux minérales naturelles autorisés de France* (Paris: Éditions scientifiques, 1891), pp. 130–148.

39. On these themes in the history of the spa Pougues-les-Eaux, see Jean Certhoux, "De la neurasthénie aux névroses: le traitement des névroses dans le passé," *Annales médico-psychologiques*, 119 (1961), pp. 913–932.

40. Dr. Sauvage, "Les maladies nerveuses sur le littoral méditerranéen," *Poitou médical*, 22 (1907), pp. 206–212; Albert Rosenau, "Monte Carlo als Winterstation," *Zeitschrift für Balneologie, Klimatologie und Kurort-Hygiene*, 1 (1908–09), pp. 594–596.

41. Dr. Vogelsang, "Montreux," *Zeitschrift für Balneologie . . . .*, 2 (1909–1910), pp. 442–446, statistics p. 445, quote p. 446.

42. Alfred Béni-Barde, *La Neurasthénie* (Paris: Masson, 1908), pp. 367–369.

43. Béni-Barde, *Neurasthénie*, p. 52.

44. See Gerbod, *Revue historique*, pp. 316–317, on the tendency of the French to favor Baden-Baden, Wiesbaden, Bad Homburg, and the Bohemian spas.

45. J. Charvát, "Eine analytische Betrachtung der Karlsbader Kurfrequenz 1756–1960," *Balneologia e Balneotherapia*, 21 (1961), pp. 407–420, statistics pp. 417–419.

46. Dr. Rompel, "Der Fremdenverkehr der bedeutenderen deutschen Badeorte," *Zeitschrift für Balneologie, Klimatologie und Kurort-Hygiene*, 6 (1913), pp. 391–399, statistics p. 399.

47. David Hess, *Die Badenfahrt* (Zurich: Füssli, 1818), p. 85, notation of an anonymous physician.

48. See *Jahrbücher für Deutschlands Heilquellen und Seebäder* (1837), pp. 104–105, 141–146, 154 et seq., 191.

49. Louis Lehmann, *Die chronischen Neurosen als klinische Objekte in Oeynhausen (Rehme)* (Bonn: Cohen, 1880), data pp. 7–9, comment on "manustupration" p. 58. The author's largest category was "scrofula and oligemia," a mixed group of orthopedic, gynecologic, and other disorders.

50. Alfred Martin, "Die Reilsche Badeanstalt in Halle mit ihrem Kur und Badebetrieb," *Zeitschrift für physikalische und diätetische Therapie*, 26 (1922), pp. 131–138.

51. See "Philo vom Walde" [pseud. for Johannes Reinelt], *Vincenz Priessnitz: Sein Leben und sein Wirken* (Berlin: Möller, 1898).

52. For an overview, see Edward Shorter, "Private Clinics in Central Europe, 1850–1933," *Social History of Medicine*, 3 (1990), pp. 159–195, esp. pp. 168–175.

53. He did not advertise his psychiatric past, and this information was gleaned from his personnel file at the Vienna Universitätsarchiv.

54. Landes-Irren-Anstalt Kierling-Gugging (today Niederösterreichisches Landeskrankenhaus für Psychiatrie und Neurologie Klosterneuburg), house archive, discharge number 1903/171.

55. Dr. Walther, "Die offenen Anstalten für Nervenkranke und Leicht Verstimmte," *Correspondenz-Blatt der deutschen Gesellschaft für Psychiatrie*, 20 (1874), pp. 81–91, quotes p. 86, p. 87n.

56. Caspar M. Brosius, *Aus meiner psychiatrischen Wirksamkeit: Eine zweite Adresse* (Wiesbaden: Bergmann, 1881), p. 19.

57. Karl E. Hoestermann, *Zur Erinnerung an die Feier des fünfzigjährigen Bestehens der Wasserheilanstalt Marienberg zu Boppard am Rhein* (Boppard: Richter, 1889), pp. 29–30.

58. Paul Wiedeburg, "Über die psychischen Einflüsse auf Patienten in offenen Heilanstalten mit Ausschluss der direkten ärztlichen Behandlung," *Zeitschrift für diätetische und physikalische Therapie*, 4 (1900–1901), pp. 409–415, quote p. 412. "eine angebliche Vorstufe zu Irrenanstalten."

59. Salomon Federn (also known as S. Bunzel-Federn), *Blutdruck und Darmatonie* (Leipzig: Deuticke, 1894), p. 25.

60. George Beard, "Neurasthenia, or Nervous Exhaustion," *BMSJ*, 80 (Apr. 29, 1869), pp. 217–221, quotes pp. 217, 218. On Beard's life, see Charles M. Rosenberg, "The Place of George M. Beard in American Psychiatry," *Bulletin of the History of Medicine*, 36 (1962), pp. 245–259. Quite independently of Beard, in April 1869, Edwin Van Deusen, an asylum superintendent, also used the term neurasthenia. "Observations on a Form of Nervous Prostration (Neurasthenia) Culminating in Insanity," *American Journal of Insanity*, 25 (1869), pp. 445–461. Yet Beard's contribution was far more influential.

61. George Beard, *A Practical Treatise on Nervous Exhaustion (Neurasthenia): Its Symptoms, Nature . . .* (New York: Wood, 1880), p. vi.

62. Federn, *Blutdruck*, p. 24.

63. William Perfect, *Select Cases in the Different Species of Insanity* (Rochester: Gillman, 1787), pp. 3–7.

64. Caspar M. Brosius, *Aus meiner psychiatrischen Wirksamkeit* (Berlin: Hirschwald, 1878), p. 35.

65. See, for example, Goergen, *Privatheilanstalt*, p. 28.

66. S. Weir Mitchell, "The Evolution of the Rest Treatment," *JNMD*, 31 (1904), pp. 368–373, case pp. 370–372.

67. S. Weir Mitchell, "Rest in Nervous Disease," in Edouard C. Seguin, *A Series of American Clinical Lectures*, vol. 1: Jan.–Dec., 1875 (New York: Putnam, 1876), pp. 83–102, quote p. 84.

68. Theodore H. Weisenburg, "The Weir Mitchell Rest Cure Forty Years Ago and Today," *Archives of Neurology and Psychiatry*, 14 (1925), pp. 384–389, quote p. 385.

69. Weber, *Mineral Waters*, pp. 439–440.

70. William S. Playfair, "Notes on the Systematic Treatment of Nerve Prostration and Hysteria Connected with Uterine Disease," *Lancet*, 2 (May 28, 1881), pp. 857–859, quote p. 857.

71. See the memorable account of how to conduct a rest cure, even on patients suspicious of it, in Alfred T. Schofield, *The Management of a Nerve Patient* (London: Churchill, 1906), pp. 190–229.

72. [Jean-Martin Charcot], "De l'isolement dans le traitement de l'hystérie," *Progrès médical*, 13 (Feb. 28, 1885), pp. 161–164; Georges Gilles de la Tourette took responsibility for writing up Charcot's lecture for publication, a task too menial for the master himself.

73. See, for example, Rudolph Burkart, "Zur Behandlung schwerer Formen von Hysterie und Neurasthenie," *[Volkmann] Sammlung klinischer Vorträge*, no. 245 (1884), pp. 1771–1818.

74. See *American Medical Directory*, 1906, advertisement pages lvi, lxv.

75. *Bäder-Almanach*, 1910, pp. 484, 661–662.

76. Schofield, *Management Nerve Patient*, p. 225.

77. Elizabeth Robins, *A Dark Lantern: A Story with a Prologue* (New York: Macmillan, 1905), quotes pp. 134–135, 146–149, 153–156, 169, 209, 220. On Robins's life, see Joanne E. Gates, *Elizabeth Robins, 1862–1952: Actress, Novelist, Feminist* (Tuscaloosa: University of Alabama Press, 1994), see pp. 136–143 for her rest cure, which was, according to Gates, an almost complete failure.

78. Fernand Levillain, *La Neurasthénie: Maladie de Beard (Méthodes de Weir-Mitchell et Playfair. Traitement de Vigouroux, avec une préface du Professeur Charcot)* (Paris: Maloine, 1891), pp. 238, 243. Romain Vigouroux, an electrotherapist at the Salpêtrière, added a "therapeutic postscript" to the book.

79. In the discussion of a paper by Edward W. Taylor, "The Attitude of the Medical Profession toward the Psychotherapeutic Movement," *JNMD*, 35 (1908), pp. 401–403 paper summarized; Dercum in discussion p. 406.

80. George A. Waterman, "The Treatment of Fatigue States," *Journal of Abnormal Psychology*, 4 (1909), pp. 128–139, quote p. 134.

81. Edwin Bramwell, "A Lecture on Psychotherapy in General Practice," *Edinburgh Medical Journal*, NS, 30 (1923), pp. 37–59, quote p. 46.

82. Gabriel Gustav Valentin, *Traité de névrologie* (Paris: Baillière, 1843), the French translation of Valentin's work on neuroanatomy.

83. "Report of the Council to the American Medico-Psychological Association," *American Journal of Insanity*, 67 (1910), pp. 400–411, list of those attending pp. 405–410.

84. See Bonnie Ellen Blustein, "'A Hollow Square of Psychological Science': American Neurologists and Psychiatrists in Conflict," in Andrew Scull, ed., *Madhouses, Mad-Doctors, and Madmen: The Social History of Psychiatry in the Victorian Era* (Philadelphia: University of Pennsylvania Press, 1981), pp. 241–270. J. Pantel, "Streitfall Nervenheilkunde—eine Studie zur disziplinären Genese der klinischen Neurologie in Deutschland," *Fortschritte der Neurologie und Psychiatrie*, 61 (1993), pp. 144–156.

85. *Bäder Almanach*, 1910, p. 655; "Psychische Beeinflussung." Friedländer, who had worked in several "open" nervous sanatoriums, had never to my knowledge been employed in an asylum.

86. Details on the rise and fall of hypnotism may be found in Edward Shorter, *From Paralysis to Fatigue: A History of Psychosomatic Illness in the Modern Era* (New York: Free Press, 1992), pp. 129–165, 246–247. Among the many histories of hypnotism, see Adam Crabtree, *From Mesmer to Freud: Magnetic Sleep and the Roots of Psychological Healing* (New Haven: Yale U. P., 1993).

87. Hippolyte Bernheim, "De la Suggestion dans l'état hypnotique et dans l'état de veille," *Revue médicale de l'Est*, 15 (1883), pp. 610–619; this was pt. 4 of a multipart series. See also the continuation, pt. 8, 16 (1884), pp. 7–20. Bernheim published these articles in expanded form as *De la suggestion dans l'état hypnotique et dans l'état de veille* (Paris: Doin, 1884). On Bernheim's influence, see Jean Camus and Philippe Pagniez, *Isolement et psychothérapie* (Paris: Alcan, 1904). "Il faut, en réalité, arriver à l'école de Nancy pour qu'avec la théorie de la suggestion solidement assise s'établisse une thérapeutique réglée" (p. 54).

88. Frederik van Eeden, *Happy Humanity* (Garden City: Doubleday, 1912), p. 35. On van Eeden, see R. Th. R. Wentges, "De psychiater Frederik van Eeden," *Nederland. Tijdschrift voor Geneeskunde*, 120 (1976), pp. 927–934.

89. See Liébeault to August Forel, May 18, 1887, "Nous avons eu la visite. . . ." in Hans H. Walser, ed., *August Forel Briefe/Correspondance, 1864–1927* (Berne: Huber, 1968), p. 196.

90. Albert Willem van Renterghem and Frederik Willem van Eeden, *Clinique de psycho-thérapie suggestive* (Brussels: Manceaux, 1889).

91. This account has been compiled from van Eeden, *Happy Humanity*, pp. 33–40; van Eeden, "Les Principes de la psychothérapie," *Revue de l'hypnotisme*, 7 (1893), pp. 97–120; see also the discussion on p. 119; van Renterghem,

"Liébeault et son École," *Zeitschrift für Hypnotismus*, 4 (1896), pp. 333–375; continued vol. 5 (1897), pp. 46–55, 95–127, vol. 6 (1897). pp. 11–44; see vol. 4, pp. 333–334, and vol. 6, pp. 11–15, for details of van Renterghem's life. The claim that Daniel Hack Tuke, youngest son of Samuel Tuke, has priority in 1872 with his use of the term "psycho-therapeutics" is not credible because Tuke did not go beyond vague generalities about the influence of mind over body to spell out a therapeutic technique. Daniel Hack Tuke, *Illustrations of the Influence of the Mind upon the Body in Health and Disease* (1872) (Philadelphia: Lea, 1873): "The influence of the Will upon disease, apart from voluntary Attention, is a very important agent in Psycho-therapeutics" (p. 393).

92. The asylum tradition of moral therapy, also a form of psychotherapy, had never died out. Nonasylum voices in medicine also called attention to psychological approaches even before the advent of Bernheim-style suggestion. See, for example, Paul Julius Möbius, "Über den Begriff der Hysterie," *Zentralblatt für Nervenheilkunde*, 11 (1888), pp. 66–71, who said "There is no other treatment for hysteria than the psychic [*die psychische*]" p. 69.

93. Forel believed that hypnotism effected objective brain changes. *Der Hypnotismus: seine psycho-physiologische, medicinische, strafrechtliche Bedeutung und seine Handhabung* (1889), 2nd ed. (Stuttgart: Enke, 1891), see, for example, pp. 13–19.

94. See Dumeng Bezzola to Forel, Apr. 9, 1908, in Christian Müller, "August Forel und Dumeng Bezzola: ein Briefwechsel," *Gesnerus*, 46 (1989), pp. 55–79, letter p. 68.

95. August Forel, "Bemerkungen zu der Behandlung der Nervenkranken durch Arbeit und zur allgemeinen Psychotherapie," *Zeitschrift für Hypnotismus*, 10 (1902), pp. 1–5, esp. p. 3.

96. Heinrich Obersteiner, *Der Hypnotismus mit besonderer Berücksichtigung seiner klinischen und forensischen Bedeutung* (Vienna: Breitenstein, 1887), p. 67.

97. Heinrich Obersteiner, *Die Privatheilanstalt zu Ober-Döbling* (Vienna: Deuticke, 1891), pp. 144–147.

98. Hugo Gugl and Anton Stichl, *Neuropathologische Studien* (Stuttgart: Enke, 1892), pp. 20–21, 34–35, 108, 137–138. They do not explicitly mention hypnotism, but that does not necessarily mean they did not perform it. See also Richard von Krafft-Ebing, "Zur Verwerthung der Suggestionstherapie (Hypnose) bei Psychosen und Neurosen," *Wiener Klinische Wochenschrift*, 4 (Oct. 22, 1891), pp. 795–799.

99. This is mentioned in Albert von Schrenck-Notzing's doctoral dissertation, *Ein Beitrag zur therapeutischen Verwerthung des Hypnotismus* (Leipzig: Vogel, 1888), p. 76. Schrenck-Notzing was able to interview patients whom Hösslin had hypnotized.

100. See Karl Gerster, "Beiträge zur suggestiven Psychotherapie," *Zeitschrift für Hypnotismus*, 1 (1892–1893), pp. 319–335. Hypnosis was meant. A later advertisement for the sanatorium mentions "Psychotherapie." *Zeitschrift für physikalische Therapie*, 3 (1899–1900), advertisement p. 5.

101. Caesar Heimann, *Bericht über Sanitätsrath Dr. Karl Edel's Asyl für Gemüthskranke zu Charlottenburg, 1869–1894* (Berlin: Hirschwald, 1895), pp. 103–104.

102. Benedict-Augustin Morel, *Traité des dégénérescences* (Paris: Baillière, 1857), p. 685.

103. V. -A. Amédée Dumontpallier, "Séance d'ouverture," *Revue de l'hypnotisme*, 4 (1890), pp. 79–85, see p. 79.

104. Van Renterghem, *Zeitschrift für Hypnotismus*, 5 (1897), pp. 115–119. Dumontpallier et al. also practiced hypnotism.

105. Pierre Janet, *L'État mental des hystériques: Les Stigmates mentaux . . . . le traitement psychologique de l'hystérie* (1893). I consulted the 2nd ed. (Paris: Alcan, 1911); see pp. 645 657 on hypnotism, pp. 657–660 on "suggestion," by which is meant non-hypnotic psychotherapy. For a highly sympathetic account of Janet and his life, see Henri F. Ellenberger, *The Discovery of the Unconscious: The History and Evolution of Dynamic Psychiatry* (New York: Basic, 1970), pp. 331–417. The present author finds the oblivion into which Janet's work had previously fallen largely justified.

106. Smith Ely Jelliffe, "Glimpses of a Freudian Odyssey," *Psychoanalytic Quarterly*, 2 (1933), pp. 318–329, quote p. 323.

107. Smith Ely Jelliffe, "Deaths of M. Allen Starr and Joseph Francis Babinski," JAMA, 100 (Jan. 14, 1933), p. 134.

108. See Camus and Pagniez, *Isolement et psychothérapie*, pp. 1–3; see pp. 99–107 for a description of the service; see also Dejerine's preface to this volume. Dejerine coauthored his big book on psychoneurosis with Ernest Gauckler, *Les manifestations fonctionnelles des psychonévroses* (Paris: Masson, 1911), pp. v–viii. On Dejerine's life, see Gauckler, *Le Professeur J. Dejerine* (Paris: Masson, 1922).

109. Jules-Joseph Dejerine, "Le Traitement des psycho-névroses à l'hôpital par la méthode de l'isolement," *Revue neurologique*, 10 (1902), pp. 1145–48.

110. Jelliffe, *Psychoanalytic Quarterly*, 1933, p. 324.

111. Jelliffe, *Psychoanalytic Quarterly*, 1933, p. 324. C. B. Farrar records that people were asking whether Dejerine has neurasthenia or general paralysis. "Diary 1902–04," undated entry.

112. Catherine Ducommun, "Paul Dubois (1848–1918)," *Gesnerus*, 41 (1984), pp. 61–99, career details p. 64.

113. Paul Dubois, *Les psychonévroses et leur traitement moral* (1904), 3d ed. (Paris: Masson, 1909), p. xxiii.

114. Dejerine, *Psychonévroses*, p. viii.

115. Jules-Joseph Dejerine, "Clinique des maladies du systéme nerveux: Leçon inaugurale," *Presse médicale*, Apr. 1, 1911, pp. 253–259.

116. Gilbert Ballet, "Le domaine de la psychiatrie," *Presse médicale*, May 10, 1911, pp. 377–380.

117. Jules-Joseph Dejerine, "Le domaine de la psychiatrie, réponse à M. le Professeur Gilbert Ballet," *Presse médicale*, May 24, 1911, pp. 425–426.

118. Byrom Bramwell, "Functional Paraplegia," *Clinical Studies*, NS, 1 (1903), pp. 332–344, esp. pp. 340, 343.

119. On the relationship between psychiatry and neurology in Britain, see William F. Bynum, "The Nervous Patient in 18th- and 19th-Century Britain: the Psychiatric Origins of British Neurology," in R. M. Murray and T. H. Turner, eds., *Lectures on the History of Psychiatry* (London: Gaskell, 1990), pp. 115–127.

120. Ernest Jones, *Free Associations: Memories of a Psycho-analyst* (New York: Basic, 1959), p. 123.

121. Quentin Bell, *Virginia Woolf: A Biography*, 2 vols. (New York: Harvest, 1972), vol. 1, pp. 90, 94, 166.

122. William A. Hammond, "The Non-Asylum Treatment of the Insane," *Medical Society of the State of New York, Transactions*, 1879, pp. 280–297. See also Gerald N. Grob, *Mental Illness and American Society, 1875–1940* (Princeton: Princeton U. P., 1983), pp. 49–55.

123. Lewellys F. Barker, *Time and the Physician* (New York: Putnam, 1942), pp. 168–170. Barker had wanted to establish a "psychopathological" division at Hopkins but lacked the funds (p. 175).

124. See, for example, Joseph Collins, "The General Practitioner and the Functional Nervous Diseases," *JAMA*, 52 (Jan. 9, 1909), pp. 87–92, esp. p. 91, who was mildly miffed at the puffing up as "psychotherapy" of techniques, that he claimed neurologists had always known.

125. Charles L. Dana, "The Future of Neurology," *JNMD*, 40 (1913), pp. 753–757, quotes pp. 754, 755, 756.

Chapter 5: The Psychoanalytic Hiatus

1. Gary B. Cohen, "Die Studenten der Wiener Universität von 1860 bis 1900," in Richard Georg Plaschka and Karlheinz Mack, *Wegenetz europäischen Geistes II: Universitäten und Studenten* (Munich: Oldenbourg, 1987), pp. 290–316, tab. 4, p. 297.

2. Steven Beller, *Vienna and the Jews, 1867–1938: A Cultural History* (Cambridge: Cambridge U.P., 1989), p. 36.

3. Beller, *Vienna and the Jews*, p. 37.

4. The basic dates of Freud's life are conveniently available in Peter Gay, ed., *The Freud Reader* (New York: Norton, 1989), pp. xxxi–xlvii.

5. Robert A. Kann, ed., *Theodor Gomperz: ein Gelehrtenleben im Bürgertum der Franz-Josefs-Zeit* (Vienna: Akademie der Wissenschaften, 1974), pp. 236–237.

6. Erwin Stransky, MS "Autobiographie," undated, Vienna, Institut für Geschichte der Medizin, HS. 2.065, p. 117.

7. Jeffrey M. Masson, ed., *The Complete Letters of Sigmund Freud to Wilhelm Fliess, 1887–1904* (Cambridge: Harvard U.P., 1985), p. 378.

8. MS "Nachgelassene Lebenserinnerungen von Julius Wagner-Jauregg," Vienna, Institut für Geschichte der Medizin, HS. 3290, p. 95a.

9. Josef Breuer and Sigmund Freud, *Studies on Hysteria* (1895), James and Alix Strachey, Eng. trans. (London: Hogarth Press, 1955); Albrecht Hirschmüller, *Physiologie und Psychoanalyse in Leben und Werk Josef Breuers* (Berne: Huber, 1978), see pp. 348–364 for Breuer's actual case history of Pappenheim, as opposed to the account in *Studies on Hysteria*, which is partly fanciful; on Anna von Lieben and other patients, see Peter J. Swales, "Freud, His Teacher, and the Birth of Psychoanalysis," in Paul E. Stepansky, ed., *Freud: Appraisals and Reappraisals* (Hillsdale, NJ: Analytic Press, 1986), pp. 3–82.

10. Freud, *Studies on Hysteria* (Harmondsworth: Pelican, 1974), pp. 225–226.

11. See, for example, Freud's letter to his friend Wilhelm Fliess on Dec. 12, 1897, "Can you imagine what 'endopsychic myths' are? The latest product of my mental labor." Masson, *Freud/Fliess*, p. 286.

12. Masson, *Freud/Fliess*, p. 57.

13. Masson, *Freud/Fliess*, pp. 155–158.

14. Eva Brabant et al., eds., *Sigmund Freud/Sandor Ferenczi: Briefwechsel*, vol. 1, pt. 1 (Vienna: Böhlau, 1993), p. 221.

15. Emil Raimann, *Die hysterischen Geistesstörungen* (Vienna: Deuricke, 1901), p. 217.

16. Emil Raimann, *Zur Psychoanalyse* (Vienna: Urban, 1924), pp. 32–33.

17. Sigmund Freud, "L'Hérédité et l'étiologie des névroses" (1896), in Freud, *Gesammelte Werke*, vol. 1 (Frankfurt/M.: Fischer, 1952), pp. 407–422, esp. p. 416.

18. These three elements were firmly established by 1899. See, for example, Freud's "Über Deckerinnerungen" (1899), *Gesammelte Werke*, vol. 1, pp. 531–554.

19. Franz Alexander, "A Review of Two Decades," in Alexander and Helen Ross, eds., *Twenty Years of Psychoanalysis* (New York: Norton, 1953), pp. 13–27, quote p. 16.

20. Masson, *Freud/Fliess*, p. 398.

21. Wilhelm Stekel, "Zur Geschichte der analytischen Bewegung," *Fortschritte der Sexual-Wissenschaft*, 2 (1926), pp. 539–575, esp. p. 551.

22. Paul Roazen, *Freud and His Followers* (1971) (reprint ed. New York: New York U. P., 1984), p. 302n.

23. Sigmund Freud, *Das Unbehagen in der Kultur* (1930), in *Gesammelte Werke*, vol. 14, pp. 421–506.

24. Anecdote reported in Hermann Keyserling, *Reise durch die Zeit*, vol. 2: *Abenteuer der Seele* (Darmstadt: Holle, 1958), p. 281. The colleague was unnamed.

25. Gerhard Fichtner, ed., *Sigmund Freud/Ludwig Binswanger: Briefwechsel, 1908–1938* (Frankfurt/M.: Fischer, 1992), p. 81.

26. Grete Meisel-Hess, *Die Intellektuellen* (Berlin: Oesterheld, 1911), pp. 341–346.

27. See Max Eitingon, *Bericht über die Berliner psychoanalytische Poliklinik (März 1920 bis Juni 1922)* (Vienna: Internationaler Psychoanalytischer Verlag, 1923).

28. Martin Gumpert, *Hölle im Paradies: Selbstdarstellung eines Arztes* (Stockholm: Bermann-Fischer, 1939), p. 185.

29. Elias Canetti, *Das Augenspiel: Lebensgeschichte, 1931–1937* (1985) (Frankfurt/M.: Fischer Taschenbuch, 1988), pp. 142–143. ". . . zu jener Zeit in Gesprächen nichts gesagt werden konnte, ohne dass es durch die Motive, die dafür sofort bei der Hand waren, entkräftet wurde. . . ." Canetti used the phrase, "die psychoanalytische Verseuchung."

30. Elias Canetti, *Die Fackel im Ohr, Lebensgeschichte, 1921–1931* (1982) (Frankfurt/M.: Fischer Taschenbuch, 1988), pp. 134–135.

31. Andreas Kluge, "Über Psychoanalyse," *PNW,* 25 (Aug. 25, 1923), pp. 131–134, quotes pp. 132, 133.

32. See Abram de Swaan, "On the Sociogenesis of the Psychoanalytic Setting," in *Human Figurations: Essays for Norbert Elias* (Amsterdam: Sociologisch Tijdschrift, 1977), pp. 381–413, esp. pp. 385–386.

33. Gustav Aschaffenburg, "Die Beziehungen des sexuellen Lebens zur Entstehung von Nerven-und Geisteskrankheiten," *Münchener Medizinische Wochenschrift,* 53 (Sept. 11, 1906), pp. 1793–1798.

34. Adolf Albrecht Friedländer, "Hysterie und moderne Psychoanalyse," *PNW,* 11 (Jan. 29, 1910), pp. 393–396, esp. p. 395.

35. Friedländer, "Hysterie und moderne Psychoanalyse" (concl.), *PNW,* 11 (Mar. 5, 1910), pp. 442–445, quote p. 444.

36. Johannes Heinrich Schultz, *Lebensbilderbuch eines Nervenarztes* (Stuttgart: Thieme, 1964), p. 71. On links between Bonhoeffer's psychiatric clinic and the psychoanalytic clinic in Berlin, see Uwe Henrik Peters, *Psychiatrie im Exil: Die Emigration der dynamischen Psychiatrie aus Deutschland, 1933–1939* (Düsseldorf: Kupka, 1992), pp. 99–100.

37. Adolf Strümpell, *Aus dem Leben eines deutschen Klinikers: Erinnerungen und Beobachtungen* (Leipzig: Vogel, 1925), pp. 278–279.

38. Christian Müller, "August Forel und Dumeng Bezzola: ein Briefwechsel," *Gesnerus,* 46 (1989), pp. 55–79, quote p. 64; see also pp. 69–70.

39. Hannah Decker's otherwise differentiated analysis of Freud's reception in Germany does not bring out this point. *Freud in Germany: Revolution and Reaction in Science, 1893–1907* (New York: International U.P., 1977), pp. 179–188.

40. Konrad Rieger, "Über die Behandlung 'Nervenkranker,'" *Schmidt's Jahrbücher der in- und ausländischen Gesammten Medicin,* 251 (1896), pp. 193–198, quote p. 196.

41. Viktor von Weizsäcker, *Natur und Geist: Erinnerungen eines Arztes* (Göttingen: Vandenhoeck, 1955), p. 190.

42. See, for example, Ernst Romberg, "Über Wesen und Behandlung der Hysterie," *Deutsche Medizinische Wochenschrift*, 36 (Apr. 21, 1910), pp. 737–742, who believed the cathartic effect of the patient telling the doctor the story to be curative.

43. For some background on the world of private clinics, see Edward Shorter, "Private Clinics in Central Europe, 1850–1933," *Social History of Medicine*, 3 (1990), pp. 159–195.

44. Wolfgang Warda, "Ein Fall von Hysterie, dargestellt nach der kathartischen Methode von Breuer und Freud," *Monatsschrift für Psychiatrie und Neurologie*, 7 (1900), pp. 471–489.

45. [Ludwig Binswanger], *Zur Geschichte der Heilanstalt Bellevue in Kreuzlingen, 1857–1932* (N.p. [Zurich], n.d.), p. 29.

46. Fichtner, *Freud/Binswanger*, pp. 53–54.

47. See Juliusburger's exchange with the anti-Semitic psychiatrist Johannes Bresler over whether asylum directors should be Christians. Juliusburger, "Psychiater und Religion," *PNW*, 31 (June 1, 1929), pp. 270–272.

48. Fritz Eichelberg, *Jahrbuch der ärztlich geleiteten Heilanstalten und Privatkliniken Deutschlands* (Berlin: Pulvermacher, 1927), p. 31.

49. Landes-Irren-Anstalt Kierling-Gugging (today Niederösterreichisches Landeskrankenhaus für Psychiatrie und Neurologie Klosterneuburg), house archive, discharge number 1903/73.

50. Heinrich Meng, *Leben als Begegnung* (Stuttgart: Hippokrates, 1971), p. 65.

51. Alfred Döblin, *Berlin Alexanderplatz* (1929), Eng. trans. (Penguin: Harmondsworth, 1978), pp. 448–450. Döblin had gone to the Buch asylum in 1906; in the 1920s he and Heinrich Meng, then in his 30s, did in fact attempt together to analyze a patient.

52. Menachem Amitai and Johannes Cremerius, "Dr. med. Arthur Muthmann: Ein Beitrag zur Frühgeschichte der Psychoanalyse," *Psyche*, 38 (1984), pp. 738–753, story pp. 743–744.

53. Birgit Schoop-Russbült, ed., *Psychiatrischer Alltag in der Autobiographie von Karl Gehry (1881–1962)* (Zurich: Juris, 1989), pp. 52–53, 63, 135.

54. Of the 496 physicians from Germany, Austria, and Switzerland present, 70.4 percent gave street addresses, and 25.0 percent institutional addresses of some kind (usually public asylums and private clinics but occasionally general hospitals and other medical institutions). It was impossible to identify further 4.6 percent. See Wladimir Eliasberg, ed., *Psychotherapie: Bericht über den I. Allgemeinen ärztlichen Kongress für Psychotherapie in Baden-Baden, 17.–19. April 1926* (Halle/S.: Marhold, 1927), "Teilnehmerverzeichnis," pp. 319–327. Physicians with an interest in psychiatric and neurological illness often did not identify themselves as such in the *Ärztliches Handbuch nebst Verzeichnis der Ärzte im Deutschen Reich*, 10th ed., for 1924–1925 (Leipzig: Verlagsbuchhandlung des Verbandes der Ärzte Deutschlands, 1925) and so exact figures on the proportion of "psychiatrists" are impossible to obtain. It must be kept in mind that many

asylum psychiatrists in particular would not have attended a congress on psychotherapy. Thus it would be incorrect to maintain that 70 percent of all psychiatrists showed a strong interest in psychoanalysis.

55. At the international level, this development may be rapidly limned from the content of medical articles of a psychological nature. Although in the last two decades of the nineteenth century hypnosis had been the rage, by 1910–1919 the number of articles on hypnosis had declined by almost 90 percent. Conversely, between the 1880s and 1910–1919, the number of articles on "psychotherapy" rose from 4 to 76. In 1910–1919 there were 148 additional articles on "psychoanalysis." Clearly, the analytic dog was wagging the therapeutic tail. By the end of the 1920s, the international psychotherapeutic literature was dominated completely by psychoanalysis. In the decade 1920–1929, 302 articles on psychoanalysis appeared, compared with 136 on hypnosis, 84 on psychotherapy, and 31 on suggestion. These statistics are based on an analysis of articles under the rubrics of "hypnosis-hypnotism," "psychotherapy," "suggestion," and "psychoanalysis" appearing between 1880 and 1929 in the three successive series of the *Index-Catalogue of the Library of the Surgeon-General's Office, United States Army* (Washington, DC: GPO, 1880–).

56. E. Stanley Abbot, "Out-Patient or Dispensary Clinics for Mental Cases," *American Journal of Insanity*, 77 (1920), pp. 218–225, esp. p. 218.

57. Walter Channing, "Dispensary Treatment of Mental Diseases," *American Journal of Insanity*, 58 (1901), pp. 109–119, quote p. 119.

58. Abbot, *American Journal of Insanity*, pp. 220–221.

59. See Gerald N. Grob, *Mental Illness and American Society, 1875–1940* (Princeton: Princeton U.P., 1985), pp. 144–166.

60. George M. Kline, "Presidential Address," *AJP*, 7 (1927), pp. 1–22, quote p. 4.

61. On the figure for 1910, see "Report of the Council to the American Medico-Psychological Association," *American Journal of Insanity*, 67 (1910), pp. 400–411; list of members attending pp. 405–411; "Proceedings of the Seventy-Seventh Annual Meeting," *AJP*, 1 (1921), pp. 216–240; list of members attending pp. 225–235. I took a street address rather than an institutional address as evidence of private practice.

62. James Jackson Putnam, "Recent Experiences in the Study and Treatment of Hysteria at the Massachusetts General Hospital; with Remarks on Freud's Method of Treatment by 'Psycho-analysis,'" *Journal of Abnormal Psychology*, 1 (1906), pp. 26–41. On these events, see Isador H. Coriat, "Some Personal Reminiscences of Psychoanalysis in Boston," *Psychoanalytic Review*, 32 (1945), pp. 1–8; Eugene Taylor, "On The First Use of 'Psychoanalysis' at the Massachusetts General Hospital, 1903 to 1905," *Journal of the History of Medicine*, 43 (1988), pp. 447–471.

63. On Brill, see May E. Romm, "Abraham Arden Brill," in Franz Alexander et al., eds., *Psychoanalytic Pioneers* (New York: Basic, 1966), pp. 210–223.

64. Peters, *Psychiatrie im Exil*, p. 123.

65. Of the many articles praising Freud, typical was that of George M. Parker, a neurologist at Roosevelt Hospital, "Hysteria under Psychoanalysis," *Medical Record* 78 (Aug. 6, 1910), pp. 219–226: "Psychoanalysis, as a procedure, is showing a strong growth curve in this country . . ." (p. 219). For "arrogant ass," see Freud to Jung, March 3, 1911, in William McGuire, ed., *The Freud/Jung Letters* (Princeton: Princeton U.P., 1974), p. 399.

66. Although several local societies and institutes had long previously limited themselves to accepting physicians, this became formal policy of the national association only in 1938. Robert P. Knight, "The Present Status of Organized Psychoanalysis in the United States," *Amer. Pa. Assn. J.*, 1 (1953), pp. 197–221, esp. p. 214. European physicians, who stood less in awe of themselves generally, were more tolerant of lay analysis. Whereas in Central Europe a whole host of titles, such as Herr Hofrat, Herr Geheimrat, Herr Professor, and Herr General came before "Herr Doktor," in the United States MDs were at the top of the pecking order.

67. Nathan G. Hale, Jr., *Freud and the Americans: The Beginnings of Psychoanalysis in the United States, 1876–1917* (New York: Oxford U. P., 1971), p. 317, and pp. 527–528 n. 12.

68. Henry M. Hurd, *Institutional Care of the Insane in the United States and Canada* (Baltimore: Hopkins, 1916), vol. 3, p. 272.

69. David Kennedy Henderson, *The Evolution of Psychiatry in Scotland* (Edinburgh: Livingstone, 1964), p. 165.

70. "Foreword and Corrections," *Amer. Pa. Assn. Bull.*, 2 (1938), p. 8.

71. See Arcangelo R. T. D'Amore, "Historical Reflections on the Organizational History of Psychoanalysis in America," in Jacques M. Quen and Eric T. Carlson, eds., *American Psychoanalysis: Origins and Development* (New York: Brunner, 1978), pp. 127–140, esp. p. 131.

72. For information on the founding of the local societies, see their reports to the council at the 1938 meeting of the American Psychoanalytic Association. *Amer. Pa. Assn. Bull.*, 1 (1938), pp. 79f.

73. "Proceedings" of annual meeting, AJP, 8 (1928), pp. 355–359.

74. Knight, *Amer. Pa. Assn. J.*, 1953, p. 216. This three-year policy was reaffirmed in 1954. See *Amer. Pa. Assn. Bull.*, 10 (1954), p. 358.

75. "Proceedings of Societies," AJP, 90 (1933), pp. 381–382; A. A. Brill was elected chairman of the section, therewith becoming a vice-president of the APA, and Leo Bartemeier was elected section secretary.

76. Kubie in discussion, "Round Table on Problems of Training," *Amer. Pa. Assn. Bull.*, 3 (1940), p. 27.

77. *Amer. Pa. Assn. Bull.*, 1940, pp. 33–34.

78. Franklin G. Ebaugh and Charles A. Rymer, *Psychiatry in Medical Education* (New York: Commonwealth Fund, 1942), pp. 193–194.

79. Sally Willard and Jefferson Trask Pierce, *The Layman Looks at Doctors* (New York: Harcourt, 1929), quote p. 200; on Sally Willard's encounter with psychoanalysis, see pp. 199–226.

80. "The 'Nervous Breakdown,'" *Fortune*, April 1935, pp. 84–88 et seq., quote p. 182.

81. Knight characterized the American analysts of the 1920s and 1930s as "primarily introspective individuals, inclined to be studious and thoughtful, [who] tended to be highly individualistic and to limit their social life to clinical and theoretical discussions with colleagues." *Amer. Pa. Assn. J.*, 1953, p. 218.

82. On the figure of 4,000 medical emigrés, see Kathleen M. Pearle, *Preventive Medicine: The Refugee Physician and the New York Medical Community, 1933–1945* (Bremen: University of Bremen, Research Center on Social Conditions, 1981), p. 14. The other statistics are from Peters, *Psychiatrie im Exil*, p. 16.

83. Otto Fenichel, *Outline of Clinical Psychoanalysis* (New York: Norton, 1934).

84. "List of Colleagues from Abroad . . . ," *Amer. Pa. Assn. Bull.*, 3 (1940), pp. 59–61; the eight who had joined the Berlin Psychoanalytic Society were Otto Fenichel (who actually was Viennese), Paul Friedmann, Joachim and Irene Haenel, Bernard Kamm, Ernst Simmel, Edith Weigert-Vowinckel, and Siegfried Bernfeld (the only nonmedical analyst from Berlin).

85. The story is told by Russell Jacoby, *The Repression of Psychoanalysis: Otto Fenichel and the Political Freudians* (New York: Basic, 1983), p. 119.

86. Heinrich Meng, "Paul Federn: Teacher and Reformer," in Ernst Federn, *Thirty-Five Years with Freud in Honour of the Hundredth Anniversary of Paul Federn, M.D.* (Brandon, VT: Clinical Psychology Pub., 1972; *Journal of Clinical Psychology*, suppl. no. 32), pp. 34–40, quote p. 38.

87. For a list of emigré analysts from Vienna, see Johannes Reichmayr, *Spurensuche in der Geschichte der Psychoanalyse* (Frankfurt: Nexus, 1990), pp. 154–157.

88. Franz Werfel, "Der Arzt von Wien" (1938), in Werfel's *Erzählungen aus zwei Welten*, vol. 3 (Frankfurt/M.: Fischer, 1954), pp. 40–45, quotes pp. 42–43. Werfel ends his drama, however, with the protagonist's suicide, a not uncommon outcome for such Viennese psychoanalysts as Paul Federn and Wilhelm Stekel, who however suicided abroad.

89. On Schilder's life in America, see the sketch in Walter Bromberg, *Psychiatry between the Wars, 1918–1945: A Recollection* (Westport: Greenwood, 1982), pp. 83–90.

90. On these events, see Dieter Langer, *Paul Ferdinand Schilder: Leben und Werk* (Erlangen: med. diss., 1979), pp. 86–88.

91. Else Pappenheim, "Zeitzeugin," in Friedrich Stadler, *Vertriebene Vernunft, vol. 2: Emigration und Exil österreichischer Wissenschaft* (Munich: Jugend und Volk, 1988), pp. 221–229, quote p. 226.

92. Pappenheim, *Emigration*, p. 225.

93. Roazen, *Freud and His Followers*, p. 520.

94. On this alliance, see Lewis A. Coser, *Refugee Scholars in America: Their Impact and Their Experiences* (New Haven: Yale U.P., 1984), pp. 49–50. See

also Nathan G. Hale, Jr., "From Berggasse XIX [*sic*] to Central Park West: The Americanization of Psychoanalysis, 1919–1940," *Journal of the History of the Behavioral Sciences*, 14 (1978), pp. 299–315.

95. Arnold A. Rogow, *The Psychiatrists* (New York: Putnam, 1970), p. 109.

96. Lewis A. Coser, *Refugee Scholars*, p. 53. The top seven were Heinz Hartmann, Ernst Kris, Erik Erikson, Margaret Mahler, Phyllis Greenacre, Ruth Jacobson, and Rudolph Loewenstein. Numbers eight and nine—Otto Fenichel and Helene Deutsch—were also refugees.

97. Martin Grotjahn, *My Favorite Patient: The Memoirs of a Psychoanalyst* (Frankfurt/M.: Lang, 1987), pp. 76–77.

98. Seymour B. Sarason, *The Making of an American Psychologist: An Autobiography* (San Francisco: Jossey-Bass, 1988), p. 214.

99. Arnold A. Rogow, *Psychiatrists*, p. 37.

100. Coser, *Refugee Scholars*, p. 47.

101. One group of psychoanalysts opposed an analytic takeover of psychiatry, fearing that the real takeover would be psychiatry imposing itself on psychoanalysis. On such figures as Otto Fenichel, who generally favored lay analysis as well, see Jacoby, *Repression of Psychoanalysis*, p. 130.

102. "Alphabetical List of All Members," *Amer. Pa. Assn. Bull.*, 3 (1939–1940), pp. 145–152.

103. Report on American Institute for Psychoanalysis, *American Journal of Psychoanalysis*, 2 (1942), p. 28.

104. On these schisms in New York, see John Frosch, "The New York Psychoanalytic Civil War," *Amer. Pa. Assn. J.*, 39 (1991), pp. 1037–64.

105. On Yale, see Sarason, *Making of a Psychologist*, pp. 215–216; Eugene B. Brody, "The New Biological Determinism in Socio-Cultural Context," *Australian and New Zealand Journal of Psychiatry*, 24 (1990), pp. 464–469, esp. p. 466.

106. "Bulletin," *Amer. Pa. Assn. J.*, 4 (1956), p. 374.

107. Edith Weigert, "Die Entwicklung der psychoanalytischen Ausbildung in USA," *Psyche*, 6 (1953), pp. 632–640, quotes p. 633.

108. Henri Ellenberger, "A Comparison of European and American Psychiatry," *Bulletin of the Menninger Clinic*, 19 (1955), pp. 43–52, quote p. 46. See Ellenberger, *The Discovery of the Unconscious: The History and Evolution of Dynamic Psychiatry* (New York: Basic, 1970).

109. See the list in Walter E. Barton, *The History and Influence of the American Psychiatric Association* (Washington, DC: APA Press, 1987), pp. 336–339. Between the presidencies of Hardin Branch in 1962–1963 and Raymond Waggoner in 1969–1970, every president was either an analyst, or a member of GAP or of the American Academy of Psychoanalysis.

110. Committee on Social Issues of the Group for the Advancement of Psychiatry, *The Social Responsibility of Psychiatry, A Statement of Orientation*, Report No. 13 (New York: GAP, July, 1950), quote p. 3.

111. Grob, *Asylum to Community*, p. 32.

112. Weigert, *Psyche*, p. 633.

113. *The Psychiatrist, His Training and Development. Report of the 1952 Conference on Psychiatric Education . . . Organized and Conducted by the American Psychiatric Association and the Association of American Medical Colleges* (Washington, DC: APA, 1953), p. 99.

114. Karl Menninger, "The Contribution of Psychoanalysis to American Psychiatry" (1953), in Barnard H. Hall, ed., *A Psychiatrist's World: The Selected Papers of Karl Menninger* (New York: Viking, 1959), quote p. 837.

115. Howard W. Potter and Henriette R. Klein, "Toward Unification of Training in Psychiatry and Psychoanalysis," *AJP*, 108 (1951), pp. 193–197, quote p. 193.

116. *New York Times*, Oct. 9, 1994, p. 1.

117. Committee on Medical Education of the Group for the Advancement of Psychiatry, *Trends and Issues in Psychiatric Residency Programs*, report no. 31 (New York: GAP, March 1955), pp. 13, 15.

118. Potter, *AJP*, p. 194.

119. GAP, *Trends and Issues*, 1955, p. 13.

120. Joan B. Woods et al., "Basic Psychiatric Literature as Determined from the Recommended Reading Lists of Residency Training Programs," *AJP*, 124 (1967), pp. 217–224, see tab. 1, p. 223.

121. Rogow, *Psychiatrists*, pp. 62, 64.

122. *Freud/Ferenczi Briefwechsel*, pp. 52–53.

123. See Federn's early articles, "The Analysis of Psychotics," *International Journal of Psychoanalysis*, 15 (1934), pp. 209–214; "Psychoanalysis of Psychoses," *Psychiatric Quarterly*, 17 (1943), pp. 3–19. Meng says that early in his work Federn incriminated the mother in the genesis of psychotic illness. Meng, in Federn, *Thirty-Five Years of Freud*, p. 38.

124. Meyer to Abraham Myerson, Nov. 26, 1937, quoted in Gerald N. Grob, *The Inner World of American Psychiatry, 1890–1940: Selected Correspondence* (New Brunswick: Rutgers U.P., 1985), p. 132.

125. Donald L. Burnham, "Orthodoxy and Eclecticism in Psychoanalysis: The Washington-Baltimore Experience," in Quen, ed., *American Psychoanalysis*, pp. 88–91. St. Elizabeths Hospital is customarily written without the apostrophe.

126. On Sullivan at the Sheppard, see Bliss Forbush, *The Sheppard & Enoch Pratt Hospital, 1853–1970: A History* (Philadelphia: Lippincott, 1971), pp. 80–81, 106–109. For an early statement of his views, see Harry Stack Sullivan, "The Modified Psychoanalytic Treatment of Schizophrenia," *AJP*, 11 (1931), pp. 519–540.

127. *Amer. Pa. Soc. Bull.*, 1 (1938), pp. 122–123.

128. On Fromm-Reichmann's life, see Peters, *Psychiatrie im Exil*, pp. 173–188.

129. Frieda Fromm-Reichmann, "Notes on the Development of Treatment of Schizophrenics by Psychoanalytic Psychotherapy," *Psychiatry*, 11 (1948), pp. 263–273, quote p. 265.

130. John Neill, "Whatever Became of the Schizophrenogenic Mother?" *American Journal of Psychotherapy*, 44 (1990), pp. 499–505, quote p. 502.

131. Bertram Lewin, *The Psychoanalysis of Elation* (London: Hogarth, 1951), p. 137.

132. Sandor Rado, "The Problem of Melancholia," *International Journal of Psychoanalysis*, 9 (1928), pp. 420–438, esp. p. 423. Rado initially used the phrase in "An Anxious Mother: A Contribution to the Analysis of the Ego," ibid., 9 (1928), pp. 219–226; see p. 225.

133. Melanie Klein, "A Contribution to the Psychogenesis of Manic-Depressive States" (1934), in Klein, *Contributions to Psycho-Analysis, 1921–1945* (London: Hogarth, 1948; reprint New York: McGraw-Hill, 1964), pp. 282–310, esp. p. 284.

134. "Bulletin," *Amer. Pa. Assn. J.*, 6 (1958), p. 692; 600 members and candidates indicated an interest in teaching in the program.

135. F. A. Freyhan, "Vier Jahrzehnte klinische Psychiatrie—aus persönlicher Sicht," *Fortschritte der Neurologie und Psychiatrie*, 47 (1979), pp. 436–441, quote p. 437. After his return to Germany, "Fritz" Freyhan became one of the founders of psychopharmacology there.

136. Karl Menninger, *Selected Papers*, p. 851.

137. Karl Menninger, *The Vital Balance: The Life Process in Mental Health and Illness* (New York: Viking, 1963), p. 33.

138. Lothar B. Kalinowsky, [Memoir], in Ludwig J. Pongratz, ed., *Psychiatrie in Selbstdarstellungen* (Berne: Huber, 1977), pp. 147–164, quote p. 158.

139. Frieda Fromm-Reichmann believed, in the words of one of her students, "that there were no qualitative differences between people, psychotic or otherwise, only quantitative ones." Ralph M. Crowley, "Frieda Fromm-Reichmann: Recollections of a Student," *Psychiatry*, 45 (1982), pp. 105–107, quote p. 106. See also Mitchell Wilson, "*DSM-III* and the Transformation of American Psychiatry: A History," *AJP*, 150 (1993), pp. 399–410, quote p. 400.

140. Ellenberger, *Bull. Menninger Clinic*, p. 43.

141. Ellenberger, *Bull. Menninger Clinic*, p. 49.

142. Kalinowsky, *Selbstdarstellungen*, p. 161. It is not apparent from the project's report which patients these might have been, as only patients from the mental hospital were candidates for "topectomy." Yet the Neurological Institute of Presbyterian Hospital performed other lobotomies, and the patients of these analysts may have been among them. See Fred A. Mettler and Columbia-Greystone Associates, eds., *Selective Partial Ablation of the Frontal Cortex* (New York: Hoeber, 1949); the 49 patients are listed by number on pp. 16–17. The report of Lawrence Pool and Robert G. Heart gives 58 as the number of patients. "Topectomy," *Psychosurgery, 1st International Conference* (Aug. 4th–7th, 1948) (Lisbon: no publ., 1949), pp. 328–329.

143. Israel Zwerling et al., "Personality Disorder and the Relationships of Emotion to Surgical Illness in 200 Surgical Patients," *AJP*, 112 (1955), pp. 270–277, quote p. 273.

144. See Judd Marmor, *Psychiatrists and Their Patients: A National Study of Private Office Practice* (Washington: American Psychiatric Association, 1975), pp. 34f.

145. Herman M. van Praag, *"Make-Believes" in Psychiatry or The Perils of Progress* (New York: Brunner/Mazel, 1993), pp. 10–11.

146. According to an APA survey, in 1970 10 percent of all American psychiatrists were psychoanalysts. Franklyn N. Arnhoff and A. H. Kumbar, *The Nation's Psychiatrists–1970 Survey* (Washington, DC: APA, 1973), tab. 7, p. 6.

147. Hale, *Journal of the History of the Behavioral Sciences* 1978, see p. 313 n. 15.

148. This statistic is based on a sample of 97 psychiatrists in six states practicing in 1941 who were still in practice in 1962, taken from the *Biographical Directory of the Fellows and Members of the American Psychiatric Association as of May 8, 1962* (New York: Bowker, 1963). Since the sample is weighted toward those who were young in 1941, it is all the more surprising that almost two-thirds of young psychiatrists then were doing solely institutional work.

149. Arnhoff and Kumbar, *The Nation's Psychiatrists*, p. 16.

150. Robert A. Dorwart et al., "A National Study of Psychiatrists' Professional Activities," *AJP*, 149 (1992), pp. 1499–1505, see p. 1502. Up from 3.7 percent of the total in 1982.

151. Leon Eisenberg, "Mindlessness and Brainlessness in Psychiatry," *BJP*, 148 (1986), pp. 497–508, quote p. 498.

152. For the story, see Grob, *Asylum to Community*, p. 278. Jeremy Lazarus, "The Goldwater Rule Revisited," *Psychiatric News*, Aug. 5, 1994, p. 14.

153. See, for example, Hale, *J. Hist. Behav. Sci.*, p. 300.

154. John Demos, "Oedipus and America: Historical Perspectives on the Reception of Psychoanalysis in the United States," *Annals of Psychoanalysis*, 6 (1978), pp. 23–39.

155. On the role of these "two great stresses" in the genesis of psychosomatic illness in Jews, see Edward Shorter, *From the Mind into the Body: The Cultural Origins of Psychosomatic Symptoms* (New York: Free Press, 1994), pp. 92–94.

156. John Murray Cuddihy, *The Ordeal of Civility: Freud, Marx, Lévi-Strauss, and the Jewish Struggle with Modernity* (New York: Basic, 1974), p. 46.

157. Robert Musil, *Der Mann ohne Eigenschaften*, vol. 1 (1930) (Reinbek: Rowoholt, 1987), p. 388. "Dieser so durchseelte Mittelstand." The reference was to Jews and non-Jews alike, though the former were arguably more "durchseelt."

158. Beller, *Vienna and the Jews*, p. 208.

159. Paul Harmat, "Die zwanziger Jahre—die Blütezeit der Budapester psychoanalytischen Schule," *Medizinhistorisches Journal*, 23 (1988), pp. 359–366,

quote p. 360. He cites the writer István Vas on psychoanalysis as a secret ceremony.

160. Hilda C. Abraham and Ernst L. Freud, eds., *Sigmund Freud/Karl Abraham: Briefe, 1907–1926*, 2nd ed. (Frankfurt/M.: Fischer, 1980), pp. 47, 57.

161. Vincent Brome, *Ernest Jones: Freud's Alter Ego* (New York: Norton, 1983), p. 109.

162. Salomo Friedländer's 1922 story "Der operierte Goj" is reprinted as a note in Oskar Panizza, *Der Korsettenfritz: Gesammelte Erzählungen* (Munich: Matthes, 1981), pp. 279–292, quote p. 287. For background on Friedländer, see Sander L. Gilman, *The Case of Sigmund Freud: Medicine and Identity at the Fin de Siècle* (Baltimore: Hopkins, 1993), pp. 39–41.

163. Max Müller, *Erinnerungen: Erlebte Psychiatriegeschichte, 1920–1960* (Berlin: Springer, 1982), p. 23.

164. Stransky, "Autobiographie," p. 557. Stransky himself was somewhat anti-Semitic and felt complimented at the remark. Regarding Jung's anti-Semitism, there is debate only about its degree. See Andrew Samuels, "Psychologie nationale, national-socialisme et psychologie analytique: réflexions sur Jung et l'antisémitisme," *Revue internationale d'histoire de la psychanalyse*, 5 (1992), pp. 183–219.

165. Ernest Jones, *Free Associations: Memories of a Psycho-analyst* (New York: Basic, 1959), p. 209.

166. Stransky, "Auto-Biographie," pp. 142–143.

167. Grotjahn, *My Favorite Patient*, p. 76.

168. Alexander, *Twenty Years of Psychoanalysis*, p. 16.

169. Sarason, *Making of an American Psychologist*, p. 215.

170. John MacIver and Frederick C. Redlich, "Patterns of Psychiatric Practice," *AJP*, 115 (1959), pp. 692–697, esp. pp. 693–694. Based on a survey of 40 physicians.

171. Rogow, *Psychiatrists*, pp. 58–59.

172. Rogow, *Psychiatrists*, p. 78.

173. Victor D. Sanua, "Mental Illness and Other Forms of Psychiatric Deviance among Contemporary Jewry," *Transcultural Psychiatric Research Review*, 29 (1992), pp. 197–233, esp. pp. 198–199. Walter Weintraub and H. Aronson, "Patients in Psychoanalysis: Some Findings Related to Sex and Religion," *American Journal of Orthopsychiatry*, 44 (1974), pp. 102–108; Leo Srole et al., *Mental Health in the Metropolis: The Midtown Manhattan Study* (New York: McGraw-Hill, 1962), pp. 300–324, who concluded, "It is our opinion that the acceptance of psychiatry probably accounts for the inordinately high rate of psychoneurosis among Jews" (p. 317).

174. Joseph Veroff, Richard A. Kulka, and Elizabeth Douvan, *Mental Health in America: Patterns of Help-Seeking from 1957 to 1976* (New York: Basic, 1981), tab. 5.30, p. 172. Respondents were asked if they had ever sought help from a psychiatrist or a psychologist, a question I interpret to

mean, received psychotherapy. The percentage for non-Jews represents an average among the six Protestant denominations plus the Catholics.

175. On the actual facts of Joanne Greenberg's case, see Laurice L. McAfee, "Interview with Joanne Greenberg," in Ann-Louise S. Silver, ed., *Psychoanalysis and Psychosis* (Madison: International U.P., 1989), pp. 519–531.

176. Joanne Greenberg [pseud. "Hannah Green"], *I Never Promised You a Rose Garden* (1964) (New York: Signet, 1965), pp. 34, 61, 96, 98, 203. On details of the supposed trauma, see "Frieda Fromm-Reichmann Discusses the 'Rose Garden' Case," *Psychiatry*, 45 (1982), pp. 128–136, esp. p. 129.

177. Greenberg, *Rose Garden*, p. 42

178. *American Jewish Year Book*, 64 (1963), pp. 16–17; *American Jewish Year Book*, 92 (1992), see p. 66 on Jewish education of children by marriage type; pp. 43–46 on various risk factors in intermarriage.

179. "A Gift to Help . . . ," *New York Times*, Oct. 13, 1994, p. A18.

180. Leslie Y. Rabkin, "Mental Health . . . ," in Jack Fischel and Sanford Pinsker, eds., *Jewish-American History and Culture: An Encyclopedia* (New York: Garland, 1992), pp. 387–392, quote p. 387.

Chapter 6: Alternatives

1. [American Psychiatric Association], *One Hundred Years of American Psychiatry* (New York: Columbia U.P., 1944), pp. 150–151.

2. John R. Lord, "The Evolution of the 'Nerve' Hospital as a Factor in the Progress of Psychiatry," *Journal of Mental Science*, 75 (1929), pp. 307–315, statistics and quote p. 309. The author was a psychiatrist at Horton, one of the vast London county mental hospitals.

3. Lothar B. Kalinowsky, "The Discoveries of Somatic Treatments in Psychiatry: Facts and Myths," *Comprehensive Psychiatry*, 21 (1980), pp. 428–435, quote, p. 428.

4. Henry Rollin, "The Dark before the Dawn," *Journal of Psychopharmacology*, 4 (1990), pp. 109–114, quotes pp. 109, 110.

5. On the relatively high discharge rates, see Morton Kramer et al., *A Historical Study of the Disposition of First Admissions to a State Mental Hospital: Experience of the Warren State Hospital during the Period 1916–1950* (Washington: GPO, 1955, PHS pub. no. 445), who found for the period 1916–1935 that more than half of all patients admitted under 65 (who did not die in hospital) were released within two years. tab. 8, p. 12. On the low status of psychiatry, see Max Müller, *Erinnerungen: Erlebte Psychiatriegeschichte, 1920–1960* (Berlin: Springer, 1982,), p. 5.

6. On Wagner-Jauregg's anti-Semitism and his choice of psychiatry as a field, see his manuscript autobiography, entitled, "Medicinische Laufbahn," in the Vienna Institut für Geschichte der Medizin, shelf no. HS 3290, pp. 27–28a, as well as Erwin Stransky's manuscript autobiography, "Autobiographie," shelf no. HS 2065, pp. 172, 227–230.

7. Julius Wagner-Jauregg, "Über die Einwirkung fieberhafter Erkrankungen auf Psychosen," *Jahrbücher für Psychiatrie und Neurologie*, 7 (1887), pp. 94–131, esp. pp. 115, 130.

8. For a detailed account of this research, see Magda Whitrow, *Julius Wagner-Jauregg (1857–1940)* (London: Smith-Gordon, 1993), pp. 155–159.

9. The last part of a multipart series describing this research appeared in the first week of January 1919. This part contained the actual case histories. Julius Wagner-Jauregg, "Über die Einwirkung der Malaria auf die progressive Paralyse," *PNW*, 20 (Jan. 4, 1919), pp. 251–255.

10. By 1930, the Sanatorium Rockwinkel bei Bremen was offering "fever cures" for schizophrenia in addition to malaria cures for neurosyphilis. See note "Referate," *PNW*, 32 (Nov. 29, 1930), pp. 583–584.

11. Abram E. Bennett, "Evaluation of Artificial Fever Therapy for Neuropsychiatric Disorders," [*American Medical Association*] *Archives of Neurology and Psychiatry*, 40 (1938), pp. 1141–1158. In view of the substantial proof of the effectiveness of malarial therapy in prolonging life, halting the progression of the illness and giving relief of symptoms in patients with neurosyphilis, it is almost mischievous to comment, as Gerald Grob does, that "evidence to support the efficacy of fever therapy was extraordinarily weak." Grob, *The Mad among Us: A History of the Care of America's Mentally Ill* (New York: Free Press, 1994), p. 180. On the issue of effectiveness, see John H. Stokes et al., *Modern Clinical Syphilology* (Philadelphia: Saunders, 1944), pp. 181, 333. One authority suggests that the success of fever therapy on nonparalytic psychoses may be owing to the placebo effect. Otfried K. Linde, *Pharmakopsychiatrie im Wandel der Zeit* (Klingenmünster: Tilia-Verlag, 1988), p. 94.

12. On the pros and cons of malarial therapy, see Stokes, *Modern Clinical Syphilology*, pp. 333–347.

13. For some details, see Edward Shorter, *The Health Century* (New York: Doubleday, 1987), pp. 40–44.

14. John Mahoney et al., "Penicillin Treatment of Early Syphilis," *American Journal of Public Health*, 33 (Dec. 1943), pp. 1387–91.

15. See Stokes, *Modern Clinical Syphilology*, passim. The book apparently went to press in August 1944. The first published report of penicillin's efficacy in neurosyphilis was John H. Stokes, et al., "The Action of Penicillin in Late Syphilis Including Neurosyphilis . . . ," *JAMA*, 126 (Sept. 9, 1944), pp. 74–79. Penicillin does not normally cross the blood-brain barrier unless the meninges are inflamed, as they usually are in neurosyphilis. See Alfred Goodman Gilman, ed., *Goodman and Gilman's The Pharmacological Basis of Therapeutics*, 8th ed. (New York: McGraw-Hill, 1990), p. 1070.

16. Stokes, *Modern Clinical Syphilology*, p. 1265.

17. Stokes, *JAMA*, 1944, p. 76.

18. John Haslam, *Observations on Madness and Melancholy*, 2nd ed. (London: Callow, 1809), quotes pp. 324, 328.

19. Montagu Lomax, *The Experiences of an Asylum Doctor* (London: Allen & Unwin, 1921), quote p. 99. It was also administered as a punishment. See p. 100.

20. Eugène Asse, ed., *Lettres de Mlle. de Lespinasse* (Paris: Charpentier, 1876), p. 14. On opium generally, see Matthias M. Weber, "Die 'Opiumkur' in der Psychiatrie: Ein Beitrag zur Geschichte der Psychopharmakotherapie," *Sudhoffs Archiv*, 71 (1987), pp. 31–61, esp. pp. 44–45 on the work of the Engelken family, owners of several private clinics near Bremen.

21. See Nancy Tomes, *A Generous Confidence: Thomas Story Kirkbride and the Art of Asylum-Keeping, 1840–1883* (Cambridge: Cambridge U.P., 1984), pp. 194–195.

22. Alexander Wood, "A New Method of Treating Neuralgia by the Direct Application of Opiates to the Painful Points," *Edinburgh Medical and Surgical Journal*, 82 (1855), pp. 265–281, quote p. 267.

23. See Hermann Grunau, *Über Frequenz, Heilerfolge und Sterblichkeit in den öffentlichen preussischen Irrenanstalten von 1875 bis 1900* (Halle/S: Marhold, 1905), p. 34, who dates 1863 for the introduction of subcutaneous morphine injections into German asylums.

24. Robert Lawson, "On the Physiological Actions of Hyoscyamine," *West Riding Pauper Lunatic Asylum Medical Reports*, 5 (1875), pp. 40–84; "A Contribution to the Investigation of the Therapeutic Actions of Hyoscyamine," *Practitioner*, 17 (1876), pp. 7–19.

25. See Béla Issekutz, *Die Geschichte der Arzneimittelforschung* (Budapest: Kiadó, 1971), p. 132.

26. Alan Norton, "Depression," *BMJ*, 2 (Aug. 18, 1979), pp. 429–430, quote p. 429.

27. On the history of chloral hydrate, see Linde, *Pharmakopsychiatrie*, pp. 60–65.

28. *Aerztlicher Bericht der Private-Heilanstalt des Dr. Albin Eder von dem Jahre 1888* (Vienna: Ueberreuter, 1889), case 11, p. 267.

29. Virginia Woolf to Vita Sackville-West, Mar. 6, 1928, in *A Change of Perspective, The Letters of Virginia Woolf, vol. III: 1923–1928*, ed. Nigel Nicolson (London: Chatto-Windus, 1977), p. 469.

30. Heinz E. Lehmann, "Before They Called It Psychopharmacology," *Neuropsychopharmacology*, 8 (1993), pp. 291–303, esp. p. 294.

31. Mental Health Institute, Independence, Iowa, MS "Days of Yore," 1993, p. 6.

32. Evelyn Waugh, *The Ordeal of Gilbert Pinfold* (London: Chapman and Hall, 1957). The protagonist had been taking a mixture of bromine and chloral hydrate.

33. Comment in discussion of Edward H. Sieveking, "Analysis of Fifty-Two Cases of Epilepsy," *Lancet*, 2 (1857), pp. 136–138, comment p. 138. For details of Locock's work and the application of the bromides, see Robert J. Joynt, "The Use of Bromides for Epilepsy," *American Journal of Diseases of Children*, 128

(1974), pp. 362–363; R. H. Balme, "Early Medicinal Use of Bromides," *Journal of the Royal College of Physicians*, 10 (1976), pp. 205–208.

34. W. Petit, "Du bromure de potassium dans les maladies nerveuses," *Progrès médical*, 19 (Feb. 28, 1891), pp. 177–178, quote, p. 177.

35. Charles A. Roberts, "Myths and Truths in Psychiatry," an address to the Canadian Psychiatric Association, Oct. 1991, copy in Queen Street Mental Health Centre, Archives, Toronto, quote p. 15.

36. For the few facts of Macleod's life that are available, I am grateful to Mrs. Jo Currie of the Edinburgh University Library. Born in 1847 at Woolwich, Macleod became MB in 1875 and MD (Commended) in 1880, with a thesis on hepatic abscess. See *Medical Directory*, 1906, p. 1570, for his various appointments in Shanghai. He remained in the city until 1919 at least.

37. Neil Macleod, "Morphine Habit of Long Standing Cured by Bromide Poisoning," BMJ, 2 (July 10, 1897), pp. 76–77.

38. This account of her illness has been put together from information in Neil Macleod, "Cure of Morphine, Chloral, and Cocaine Habits by Sodium Bromide," BMJ, 1 (April 15, 1899), pp. 896–898, details of "lady 48 years old" from p. 898; and from Macleod, "The Bromide Sleep: A New Departure in the Treatment of Acute Mania," BMJ, 1 (Jan. 20, 1900), pp. 134–136, "case 8," p. 135.

39. Macleod, BMJ 1900, pp. 134–136.

40. Wilhelm Griesinger, for example, was able to procure a temporary remission of depression and mania through the application of chloroform narcosis. *Die Pathologie und Therapie der psychischen Krankheiten* (1861/1867) (reprint Amsterdam: Bonset, 1964), p. 489.

41. See Philip M. Ragg, "The Bromide Sleep in a Case of Mania," BMJ, 2 (Nov. 3, 1900), pp. 1309–10. Ragg noted that his good therapeutic results contradicted Thomas Clouston's notion that bromine was ineffective in the treatment of acute mania. See also Wolff, "Trionalcur," *Zentralblatt für Nervenkrankheiten und Psychiatrie*, 24 (1901), pp. 281–283, who used a sulfone-derivative rather than bromide at an asylum near Beirut.

42. Emil Fischer and Joseph von Mering, "Über eine neue Klasse von Schlafmitteln," *Therapie der Gegenwart*, 44 (1903), pp. 97–101.

43. Linde, *Pharmakopsychiatrie*, pp. 71–72; Kristina Goder, *Zur Einführung synthetischer Schlafmittel in die Medizin im 19. Jahrhundert* (Frankfurt/M.: Lang, 1985), pp. 44–53. In the United States, the Winthrop Chemical Company had the Veronal license.

44. W. Fischer, "Über die Wirkung des Veronal," *Therapeutische Monatshefte*, 17 (1903), pp. 393–395.

45. Hermann von Husen, "Über Veronal," *PNW*, 6 (May 7, 1904), pp. 57–61, quote p. 59.

46. Jane Hillyer, *Reluctantly Told* (New York: Macmillan, 1935), p. 8.

47. Roberts, "Myths and Truths," pp. 15–16.

48. William Sargant and Eliot Slater, *An Introduction to Physical Methods of Treatment in Psychiatry* (Edinburgh: Livingstone, 1944), p. 112.

49. Epifanio administered the first dose of Luminal to a 19-year-old manic patient, "F. L.," on March 25, 1913. The injections were continued for four days, until she was in a "profound slumber." She slept until April 9, experienced a slow recovery from what had started to seem like depression, and was discharged well toward the end of June. Two years later, she was still in remission from an apparent manic-depressive illness. See Giuseppe Epifanio, "L'ipnosi farmacologica prolungata e sua applicazione per la cura di alcune psicopatie," *Rivista di patologia nervosa e mentale*, 20 (1915), pp. 273–308, case 1, pp. 280–282.

50. On Klaesi's personality and on Cloetta's role, see Müller, *Erinnerungen*, pp. 16, 405–407.

51. For details of "Karoline S's" case, see Jakob Klaesi, "Über die therapeutische Anwendung der 'Dauernarkose' mittels Somnifens bei Schizophrenen," *Zeitschrift für die gesamte Neurologie und Psychiatrie*, 74 (1922), pp. 557–592, where it is presented as case 3, p. 573. Klaesi gave a fuller summary in his memoirs: "Jakob Klaesi," in Ludwig J. Pongratz, ed., *Psychiatrie in Selbstdarstellungen* (Berne: Huber, 1977), pp. 165–193, case pp. 183–185, referring to her as the "Versuchsfall" or experimental patient.

52. G. de M. Rudolf later pointed out that 20 percent of schizophrenia patients improve spontaneously and that Klaesi's Somnifen therapy scarcely did better than chance. "Experimental Treatments of Schizophrenia," *Journal of Mental Science*, 77 (1931), pp. 767–791, esp. p. 769.

53. Two of Müller's 24 patients treated with Somnifen died; of the 33 he treated with another barbiturate (Dial), three developed life-threatening complications, though none died. Max Müller, "Die Dauernarkose mit flüssigem Dial bei Psychosen, speziell bei manisch-depressivem Irresein;" *Zeitschrift für die gesamte Neurologie und Psychiatrie*, 107 (1927), pp. 522–543; see p. 528 for mortality and morbidity. On 5 percent and "therapeutic resignation," see Müller, *Erinnerungen*, p. 17.

54. Of the 22 other kinds of treatments for schizophrenia that Rudolf discussed, virtually all fell by the wayside on grounds of toxicity or ineffectiveness. *Journal of Mental Science 1931*.

55. See, for example, Harold D. Palmer and Alfred L. Paine, "Prolonged Narcosis as Therapy in the Psychoses," *AJP*, 12 (1932), pp. 143–164: "Verbatim records of the productions of patients who have been subjected to this form of treatment have been of great value in understanding the dynamics of their psychoses" (p. 153).

56. Eliot Slater, "Psychiatry in the 'Thirties," *Contemporary Review*, 226 (1975), pp. 70–75, quote p. 74.

57. "Referate: das Sanatorium Rockwinkel," *PNW*, 32 (Nov. 29, 1930), pp. 583–584.

58. Harry Stack Sullivan, "The Modified Psychoanalytic Treatment of Schizophrenia," *AJP*, 11 (1931), pp. 519–540, quote p. 533.

59. Kalinowsky, *Comprehensive Psychiatry* 1980, quote p. 429. For an evaluation of the cure, see G. Windholz and L. H. Witherspoon, "Sleep as a Cure for Schizophrenia: A Historical Episode," *History of Psychiatry*, 4 (1993), pp. 83–93. In fact, the sleep cure had little success with schizophrenic patients, but it did offer promise in the affective disorders.

60. Efforts at sleep therapy continued after World War II. Reserpine, an antipsychotic drug introduced into psychiatry by Nathan Kline in 1954, was initially used at the Burghölzli in Zurich as a drug for curative sleep. The mortality from thrombosis was evidently quite high. See David Healy's interview of Jules Angst, pp. 3–4. I am grateful to Dr. Healy for making a copy of this interview available to me.

61. D. Ewen Cameron, "Psychic Driving," *AJP*, 112 (1956), pp. 502–509.

62. Anne Collins, *In the Sleep Room: The Story of the CIA Brainwashing Experiments in Canada* (Toronto: Lester & Orpen Dennys, 1988), pp. 126–127. In my opinion, the CIA angle is irrelevant, in that Cameron would have done exactly the same experiments without any CIA money.

63. D. Ewen Cameron et al., "The Depatterning Treatment of Schizophrenia," *Comprehensive Psychiatry*, 3 (1962), pp. 65–76.

64. Obituary notice for Cameron, *New York Times*, Sept. 9, 1967, p. 31.

65. One is mindful of the dramatic preface to Max Müller's *Die körperlichen Behandlungsverfahren in der Psychiatrie*, vol. I: *Die Insulinbehandlung* (Stuttgart: Thieme, 1952): "Born of the striving even within psychiatry for medical activity, carried along by the resolve to relieve suffering and to heal, [the shock and coma therapies] are to be understood only in the framework of the total development of psychiatry since the turn of the century. In place of the dogma of incurability of mental illness, in place of resigned custodial care, comes belief in the possibility of therapy, comes the burning dedication to bring state-of-the-art medicine even to this previously fallow field" (p. iii).

66. Manfred Sakel, "Neue Behandlung der Morphinsucht," *Deutsche Medizinische Wochenschrift*, 56 (Oct. 17, 1930), pp. 1777–78.

67. David M. Cowie et al., "Insulin and the Mental State of Depression—A Preliminary Report," *Journal of the Michigan State Medical Society*, 22 (Sept. 1923), p. 383. Yet the observation was a flash in the pan. Their further studies at the Psychopathic Hospital in Ann Arbor showed that insulin did not bring patients out of depression. David M. Cowie et al., "Insulin and Mental Depression," [*American Medical Association*] *Archives of Neurology and Psychiatry*, 12 (1924), pp. 522–533.

68. See Annibale Puca, "La insulino-terapia nei malati di mente," *Rassegna di studi psichiatrici*, 16 (1927), pp. 461–468; Paul Schmidt, "Über Organtherapie und Insulinbehandlung bei endogenen Geistesstörungen," *Klinische Wochenschrift*, 7 (Apr. 29, 1928), pp. 839–842. For an overview of insulin's preshock history in psychiatry, see Müller, *Körperliche Behandlungsverfahren*, pp. 1–3; Müller was determined to detract as much credit from Sakel as possible.

69. Manfred Sakel, "Neue Behandlung der Morphinsucht," *Zeitschrift für die gesamte Neurologie und Psychiatrie,* 143 (1933), pp. 506–534, esp. p. 530. "I do not, however, want to draw from these few observations any overly sweeping conclusions."

70. Karl Theo Dussik, comment (pp. 1252–53) following D. Ewen Cameron and R. G. Hoskins, "Experiences in the Insulin-Hypoglycemia Treatment of Schizophrenia," *JAMA,* 109 (Oct. 16, 1937), pp. 1246–49.

71. See Sakel's 13-part series, "Schizophreniebehandlung mittels Insulin-Hypoglykämie sowie hypoglykämischer Schocks," *Wiener Medizinische Wochenschrift,* beginning vol. 84 (Nov. 3, 1934), pp. 1211–13, and ending vol. 85 (Feb. 9, 1935), pp. 179–180. There is no evidence that Sakel was initially aware of previous efforts to treat psychosis with insulin. On such efforts, see F. E. James, "Insulin Treatment in Psychiatry," *History of Psychiatry,* 3 (1992), pp. 221–235, esp. p. 221.

72. Manfred Sakel, *Neue Behandlungsmethode der Schizophrenie* (Vienna: Perles, 1935), p. 111. The 13-part series on which this book was based did not include this statistic.

73. This page is reproduced in Linde, *Pharmakopsychiatrie,* p. 99.

74. Müller, *Erinnerungen,* p. 136. Vienna's politics of ethnicity may have played a role in all this cattiness. Josef Berze, the previous director of the Steinhof Mental Hospital in Vienna, and a Catholic, was a well-known leader of the anti-Sakel coterie. See his "Die Insulin-Chok-Behandlung der Schizophrenie," *Wiener Medizinische Wochenschrift,* 83 (Dec. 2, 1933), pp. 1365–69. Stransky, a pro-insulin psychiatrist (and Jewish), recalled Berze as a difficult individual. "Autobiographie," p. 292.

75. Peters believes that Sakel's tawdry treatment of other émigré psychiatrists may have been responsible for his initial rejection. Peters, "Die Einführung der Schockbehandlungen und die psychiatrische Emigration," *Fortschritte der Neurologie und Psychiatrie,* 60 (1992), pp. 356–365, see p. 358.

76. On Sakel's life and the history of insulin-shock therapy, see Walter Freeman, *The Psychiatrist* (New York: Grune and Stratton, 1968), pp. 31–39; Linde, *Pharmakopsychiatrie,* pp. 96–103.

77. Müller, *Erinnerungen,* p. 152. Although an engaging man in many respects, Müller was as anti-Semitic as any of the Swiss of his day, and referred to Sakel as "a typical East European Jew" (*ein richtiger Ostjude*), his "boundless ambition" being a result of the "his race's resentment" (pp. 153–154).

78. See his report at the 1937 world meeting on physical therapies on schizophrenia in Münsingen, "Erfahrungen mit der Insulinbehandlung in England," *Schweizer Archiv für Neurologie und Psychiatrie,* 39, supp. (1937), pp. 178–179.

79. Isabel G. H. Wilson, *Study of Hypoglycaemic Shock Treatment in Schizophrenia* (London: HMSO; Board of Control, England and Wales, 1937), quote p. 60. The report was dated July 1936.

80. Interview with Eliot Slater (1981), in Greg Wilkinson, ed., *Talking about Psychiatry* (London: Gaskell, 1993), pp. 1–12, quote p. 4.

81. Farrar private archive, letter of J. Allan Walters to C. B. Farrar, July 11, 1937. David Neil Parfitt had written on barbiturate narcosis, "Treatment of Psychosis by Prolonged Narcosis," *Lancet*, 1 (Feb. 22, 1936), pp. 424–426. On the introduction of insulin-coma therapy in England, see James, *History of Psychiatry* 1992, pp. 221–235.

82. Norton, *BMJ* 1979, p. 429.

83. Sargant and Slater, *Physical Methods*, pp. 16–38. In a study of 160 schizophrenic patients who had received the new physical therapies, and a control group of 80 who received routine hospital care, Linford Rees at Whitchurch Hospital in Cardiff found that insulin-coma therapy was clearly superior to other physical therapies, as well as to letting nature take its course. Rees, " A Comparative Study of the Value of Insulin Coma, Electronarcosis, Electro-Shock and Leucotomy in the Treatment of Schizophrenia," *Premier Congrès Mondial de Psychiatrie, Paris, 1950, vol. 4: Thérapeutique Biologique* (Paris: Hermann, 1952), pp. 303–308.

84. Joseph Wortis, *Fragments of an Analysis with Freud* (New York: McGraw-Hill, 1954), p. 110. It is sometimes claimed that D. Ewen Cameron pioneered insulin-coma therapy in the United States at the Worcester State Hospital. Yet Cameron and coworkers began their insulin work only in March 1936. See Cameron and R. G. Hoskins, "Some Observations on Sakel's Insulin-Hypoglycemia Treatment of Schizophrenia," *Schweizer Archiv für Neurologie und Psychiatrie*, 39, suppl. (1937), pp. 180–182.

85. Joseph Wortis, "On the Response of Schizophrenic Subjects to Hypoglycemic Insulin Shock," report given at the meeting of the New York Society of Clinical Psychiatry, Nov. 12, 1936, *JNMD*, 85 (Apr. 1937), pp. 446–456.

86. Joseph Wortis, "Early Experiences with Sakel's Hypoglycemic Insulin Treatment of the Psychoses in America," *Schweizer Archiv für Neurologie und Psychiatrie,* 39, suppl. (1937), p. 208.

87. Manfred Sakel, "The Origin and Nature of the Hypoglycemic Therapy of the Psychoses," *Bulletin of the New York Academy of Medicine*, ser. 2, 13 (1937), pp. 97–109.

88. As recorded by Michael Shepherd, *Journal of Psychopharmacology* 1990, p. 131. Cameron had published his own experiences with insulin therapy at the Münsingen conference in 1937. See Cameron and R. G. Hoskins, "Some Observations . . . ," *Schweiz. Arch. Neurol.* (1937), pp. 180–182; the paper was sent in, not delivered.

89. William L. Laurence, "Tribute to Manfred Sakel," in Max Rinkel, ed., *Biological Treatment of Mental Illness* (New York: Page, 1966), p. 38. Uwe Henrik Peters points out that it was Ruth Wilmanns (later Wilmanns-Lidz), a young Jewish émigré psychiatrist from Heidelberg, who introduced insulin shock treatment at the Phipps Clinic. Peters, *Fortschritte der Neurologie und Psychiatrie* 1992, p. 359.

90. Walter Freeman, *Psychiatrist*, p. 35.

91. Slater, *Contemporary Review* 1975, p. 74.

92. Roberts, "Myths and Truths," pp. 17–18.

93. On the same results as barbiturate-narcosis, see Brian Ackner et al., "Insulin Treatment of Schizophrenia: A Controlled Study," *Lancet*, 2 (Mar. 23, 1957), pp. 607–611. For a not unfavorable historical evaluation of insulin coma therapy, see W. A. Cramond, "Lessons from the Insulin Story in Psychiatry," *Australian and New Zealand Journal of Psychiatry*, 21 (1987), pp. 320–326.

94. For an account of Meduna's life and work, see Max Fink, ed., "Autobiography of L. J. Meduna," *Convulsive Therapy*, 1 (1985), pp. 43–57, 121–135. See also Fink, "Meduna and the Origins of Convulsive Therapy," *AJP*, 141 (1984), pp. 1034–41, esp. pp. 1034–36.

95. A. Glaus, "Über Kombinationen von Schizophrenie und Epilepsie," *Zeitschrift für die gesamte Neurologie und Psychiatrie*, 135 (1931), pp. 450–500.

96. Meduna autobiography, *Convulsive Therapy* 1985, p. 54.

97. On camphor's long history in the treatment of psychosis, see Linde, *Pharmakopsychiatrie*, pp. 106–107; Walter Sneader, "The Prehistory of Psychotherapeutic Agents," *Journal of Psychopharmacology*, 4 (1990), pp. 115–119, esp. pp. 117–118.

98. Laszlo Joseph [sic] Meduna, "The Convulsive Treatment: A Reappraisal," in Arthur M. Sackler et al., eds., *The Great Physiodynamic Therapies in Psychiatry: An Historical Reappraisal* (New York: Hoeber, 1956), pp. 76–90; for exact date, see p. 79n.

99. Ladislaus von Meduna, "Versuche über die biologische Beeinflussung des Ablaufes der Schizophrenie," *Zeitschrift für die gesamte Neurologie und Psychiatrie*, 152 (1935), pp. 235–262, L. Z.'s case pp. 237–238. The author gives "1933" as the year of admission but internal evidence suggests it was probably 1930.

100. Meduna autobiography, *Convulsive Therapy* 1985, p. 122.

101. Meduna, *Zeitschrift für die gesamte Neurologie* 1935, p. 237. Meduna's definitive report on his therapy appeared as *Die Konvulsionstherapie der Schizophrenie* (Halle/S.: Marhold, 1937).

102. Linde, *Pharmakopsychiatrie*, p. 107.

103. Müller, *Erinnerungen*, p. 244. "Qualvolle Todesangst und Vernichtungsgefühl."

104. Müller, *Erinnerungen*, pp. 73–74.

105. Henry R. Rollin, *Festina Lente: A Psychiatric Odyssey* (London: British Medical Journal, 1990), p. 69.

106. Freeman, *Psychiatrist*, pp. 41–42.

107. On Meduna's Chicago years, see Herbert L. Jackman, "Epilogue to the Autobiography of L. J. Meduna," *Convulsive Therapy*, 1 (1985), pp. 136–138.

108. Peter G. Cranford, *But for the Grace of God: The Inside Story of the World's Largest Insane Asylum, Milledgeville!* (Augusta: Great Pyramid Press,

1981), pp. 82–85; Bliss Forbush, *The Sheppard & Enoch Pratt Hospital, 1853–1970: A History* (Philadelphia: Lippincott, 1971), p. 123.

109. On previous uses of electricity in psychiatry, see for example, A. W. Beveridge and E. B. Renvoize, "Electricity: A History of Its Use in the Treatment of Mental Illness in Britain During the Second Half of the 19th Century," *BJP*, 153 (1988), pp. 157–162; Norman Endler, "The History of ECT," in Endler and Emmanuel Persad, eds., *Electroconvulsive Therapy: The Myths and the Realities* (Toronto: Huber, 1988), pp. 3–30, esp. p. 6.

110. Of the various obituaries of Cerletti, that by Henri Baruk does most to place his life in context. See Baruk, "Nécrologie, Le professeur Ugo Cerletti (1877–1963)," *Bulletin de l'académie nationale de médecine*, 150 (Nov. 1966), pp. 574–579.

111. Quote from Ferdinando Accornero, "Testimonianza Oculare sulla Scoperta dell'Elletroshock," *Pagine di Storia della Medicina*, 14 (1970), pp. 38–52, quote p. 38. On Cerletti's life, see A. Novelletto, "Cerletti, Ugo," in *Dizionario biografico degli italiani*, vol. 23 (Rome: Istituto della Enciclopedia Italiana, 1979), pp. 759–763.

112. See Ugo Cerletti, "Electroshock Therapy," *Journal of Clinical and Experimental Psychopathology*, 15 (1954), pp. 191–217, esp. p. 191.

113. Some information I owe to a personal communication from Prof. Lamberto Longhi.

114. This narrative is drawn from Accornero, *Pagine di Storia della Medicina* 1970, p. 39ff.

115. Müller, *Erinnerungen*, p. 170. For the congress papers, see "Bericht über die wissenschaftlichen Verhandlungen auf der 89. Versammlung der Schweizerischen Gesellschaft für Psychiatrie in Münsingen b. Bern am 29-31. Mai 1937: Die Therapie der Schizophrenie, Insulinschock, Cardiazol, Dauerschlaf," *Schweizer Archiv für Neurologie und Psychiatrie*, 39, suppl. [Ergänzungsheft] (1937), pp. 1–238. Bini's "Ricerche sperimentali sull'accesso epilettico da corrente elettrica" appeared on pp. 121–122. Bini concluded by saying that the group at the Rome clinic would indeed progress to human experimentation.

116. Accornero, *Pagine di Storia della Medicina* 1970, p. 43.

117. Accornero, *Pagine di Storia della Medicina* 1970, p. 43.

118. This account is based on Accornero, *Pagine di Storia della Medicina* 1970, pp. 43–48; Cerletti, *J. Clin. Exper.* 1954, pp. 193–194. See also Cerletti, "Old and New Information about Electroshock," *AJP*, 107 (1950), pp. 87–94. Kalinowsky believed he was present at the first trial of ECT, but it was in fact the second he attended. Kalinowsky, *Comprehensive Psychiatry* 1980, pp. 430–431. For a historical account, see Endler, "The History of ECT."

119. Ugo Cerletti and Lucio Bini, "L'Elettroshock," *Archivio generale di neurologia*, 19 (1938), pp. 266–268. On May 28, 1938, the authors made a preliminary communication to the Academy of Medicine of Rome.

120. Cerletti, *J. Clin. Exper.* 1954, p. 194.

121. W. H. Shepley and J. S. McGregor, "The Clinical Applications of Electrically Induced Convulsions," *Proceedings of the Royal Society of Medicine*, 33 (1940), pp. 267–274. Kalinowsky introduced ECT to British audiences in his article, "Electric-Convulsion Therapy in Schizophrenia," *Lancet*, 2 (Dec. 9, 1939), pp. 1232–33. Almost simultaneously, another group of researchers at Bristol's Burden Neurological Institute were beginning ECT at the nearby Barnwood House Mental Hospital in Gloucester: They had a London firm make their apparatus. See G. W. T. H. Fleming, F. L. Golla, and W. Grey Walter, "Electric-Convulsion Therapy of Schizophrenia," *Lancet*, 2 (Dec. 30, 1939), pp. 1353–55. For Kalinowsky's recollections of these events, see Richard Abrams, "Interview with Lothar Kalinowsky, M.D.," *Convulsive Therapy*, 4 (1988), pp. 25–39, esp. pp. 32–33.

122. E. B. Strauss and Angus MacPhail, "Treatment of Out-Patients by Electrical Convulsant Therapy with a Portable Apparatus," *BMJ*, 2 (Dec. 7, 1940), pp. 779–782.

123. Kalinowsky, in Pongratz, ed., *Psychiatrie in Selbsdarstellungen*, pp. 155–157. Endler, *ECT*, p. 21.

124. Norton, *BMJ* 1979, p. 430.

125. Felix Post, "Then and Now," *BJP*, 133 (1978), pp. 83–86, quote p. 83.

126. Sargant and Slater, *Physical Methods*, p. 64.

127. David J. Impastato and Renato Almansi, "The Electrofit in the Treatment of Mental Disease," *JNMD*, 96 (1942), pp. 395–409; see also Impastato, "The Story of the First Electroshock Treatment," *AJP*, 116 (1960), pp. 1113–14, which is basically about an interview Impastato had with Cerletti. Douglas Goldman at Longview Hospital coclaims priority. "History of Psychopharmacology in North America," *Psychiatry Journal of the University of Ottawa*, 14 (1989), pp. 266–267. For another early application (from March 1940 on), see Victor E. Gonda, "Treatment of Mental Disorders with Electrically Induced Convulsions," *Diseases of the Nervous System*, 2 (1941), pp. 84–92.

128. See Endler, *ECT*, p. 22.

129. An influential U.S. textbook on the three shock therapies thought little of ECT and preferred insulin-shock for schizophrenia. Lucie Jessner and V. Gerard Ryan, *Shock Treatment in Psychiatry: A Manual* (New York: Grune and Stratton, 1941), pp. 101, 122.

130. Harry Stack Sullivan, *Conceptions of Modern Psychiatry* (Washington, DC: W. A. White Foundation, 1947), p. 73 n. 51. The first edition was published in 1940.

131. Group for the Advancement of Psychiatry, *Shock Therapy*, report no. 1, Sept. 15, 1947, quote p. 1.

132. Group for the Advancement of Psychiatry, *Revised Electro-Shock Therapy Report*, report no. 15, Aug. 1950.

133. For a review, see L. Bruce Boyer, "Fantasies Concerning Convulsive Therapy," *Psychoanalytic Review*, 39 (1952), pp. 252–270.

134. Robert P. Knight deplored this state of affairs in his presidential address to the American Psychoanalytic Association in December 1952, claiming that the inability of asylum-trained residents to do psychotherapy, and the inability of residents trained in psychoanalytic institutes and psychoanalytically oriented departments to do ECT, was driving "an ever greater cleavage between practitioners of the so-called physiological therapies on the one hand and practitioners of the psychological therapies on the other." Knight, "The Present Status of Organized Psychoanalysis in the United States," *American Psychoanalytic Association Journal*, 1 (1953), pp. 197–221, quote p. 217.

135. Arnold A. Rogow, *The Psychiatrists* (New York: Putnam, 1970), p. 79.

136. Rollin, *Journal of Psychopharmacology* 1990, pp. 111–112.

137. On this story, see Walter Sneader, *Drug Discovery: The Evolution of Modern Medicines* (Chichester: Wiley, 1985), p. 128.

138. Abram E. Bennett, "Preventing Traumatic Complications in Convulsive Shock Therapy by Curare," *JAMA*, 114 (Jan. 27, 1940), pp. 332–324.

139. G. Holmberg and S. Thesleff, "Succinyl-Choline-Iodide as a Muscular Relaxant in Electroshock Therapy," *AJP*, 108 (1952), pp. 842–846. The researchers were at the Karolinska Institutet in Stockholm.

140. Lothar B. Kalinowsky, "Convulsive Shock Treatment," in Silvano Arieti, *American Handbook of Psychiatry*, vol. 2 (New York: Basic, 1959), pp. 1499–1520, quote p. 1510.

141. Louis Casamajor, "Notes for an Intimate History of Neurology and Psychiatry in America," *JNMD*, 98 (1943), pp. 600–608, quote p. 607. Casamajor had trained with Kraepelin and had a thoroughly organic orientation to psychiatry.

142. O. Lindvall, "Transplants in Parkinson's Disease," *European Neurology*, 31 (suppl. 1) (1991), pp. 17–27.

143. Michael A. Jenike et al., "Cingulotomy for Refractory Obsessive-Compulsive Disorder," *Archives of General Psychiatry*, 48 (1991), pp. 548–555; Lee Baer et al., "Cingulotomy in a Case of Concomitant Obsessive-Compulsive Disorder and Tourette's Syndrome, ibid., 51 (1994), pp. 73–74.

144. On Burckhardt's life, see Marco Mumenthaler, "Medizingeschichtliches zur Entwicklung der Neurologie in der Schweiz," *Schweizer Archiv für Neurologie und Psychiatrie*, 138 (1987), pp. 15–30, esp. pp. 15–16; Christian Müller, "Gottlieb Burckhardt, the Father of Topectomy," *AJP*, 117 (1960), pp. 461–463. Christian Müller, himself a psychiatrist, was Max Müller's son.

145. See "Application de l'hypnotisme au traitement des maladies mentales," a summary of seven of Burckhardt's cases apparently taken from the annual report of Préfargier. *Revue de l'hypnotisme*, 3 (1889), pp. 56–59.

146. Gottlieb Burckhardt, "Über Rindenexcisionen, als Beitrag zur operativen Therapie der Psychosen," *Allgemeine Zeitschrift für Psychiatrie*, 47 (1891), pp. 463–548. For a tidy summary of Burckhardt's work and data, see German E. Berrios, "Psychosurgery in Britain and Elsewhere: A Conceptual History,"

in Berrios and Hugh Freeman, eds., *150 Years of British Psychiatry, 1841–1991* (London: Gaskell, 1991), pp. 180–196.

147. See Albert Moll's letter to August Forel of Aug. 11, 1890, in Hans H. Walser, ed., *August Forel, Briefe/Correspondance, 1864–1927* (Berne: Huber, 1968), pp. 242–243.

148. See, for example, William Ireland, "German Retrospect," in *Journal of Mental Science*, 37 (1891), pp. 606–618; the section summarizing Burckhardt's work begins on p. 613.

149. See Berrios, "Psychosurgery," pp. 182–185.

150. Karl Bonhoeffer alludes to these operations in his autobiography, written around 1940 and published in J. Zutt et al., eds., *Karl Bonhoeffer zum hundertsten Geburtstag* (Berlin: Springer, 1969), p. 57. The *Index-Medicus* for these years includes no article by Mikulicz on this subject.

151. Valentin Magnan, *Les Dégénérés* (Paris: Rueff, 1895), p. 219.

152. Quoted in Elliot S. Valenstein, *Great and Desperate Cures: The Rise and Decline of Psychosurgery and Other Radical Treatments for Mental Illness* (New York: Basic, 1986), p. 78. For my account of Moniz, I rely on Valenstein's study, on Berrios, and on Stanley Finger, *Origins of Neuroscience: A History of Explorations into Brain Function* (New York: Oxford U. P., 1994), pp. 290–296.

153. In an early English-language presentation of findings, Moniz gave details on only 3 patients in a series of 18, the second such series he had done. "Prefrontal Leucotomy in the Treatment of Mental Disorders," *AJP*, 93 (1937), pp. 1379–85; Moniz's account of the development of his procedure contained no data and was filled with windy speculation about hypothetical mechanisms. Moniz, "How I Came to Perform Prefrontal Leucotomy," in *Psychosurgery, First International Conference* (Aug. 4–7, 1948) (Lisbon: no publ. given, 1949), pp. 15–21; see also Valenstein, *Great and Desperate Cures*, p. 113.

154. For a concise and well-informed overview of the history of psychosurgical procedures, see Victor W. Swayze, II, "Frontal Leukotomy and Related Psychosurgical Procedures in the Era before Antipsychotics (1935–1954): A Historical Overview," *AJP*, 152 (1995), pp. 505–515, esp. tab. 1, p. 509.

155. Valenstein, *Great and Desperate Cures*, p. 229.

156. Sargant and Slater, *Physical Methods*, p. 145.

157. Joseph W. Friedlander and Ralph S. Banay, "Psychosis Following Lobotomy in a Case of Sexual Psychopathy," *Archives of Neurology and Psychiatry*, 59 (1948), pp. 302–321, quote p. 319.

158. Cranford, *Milledgeville*, p. 157.

159. Gerald N. Grob, *From Asylum to Community: Mental Health Policy in Modern America* (Princeton: Princeton U. P., 1991), p. 130.

160. David Crossley, "The Introduction of Leucotomy: A British Case History," *History of Psychiatry*, 4 (1993), pp. 553–564, esp. p. 562.

161. Although the number of lobotomies declined sharply after the early 1950s, the procedure continued to be performed for another decade at least. In

1961, 58 lobotomies were conducted in the psychiatric hospitals of Ontario, down from 157 in 1953. See Roger Baskett, "The Life of the Toronto Psychiatric Hospital," in Edward Shorter, ed., *TPH: History and Memories of the Toronto Psychiatric Hospital* (Toronto: Wall & Emerson, 1996), pp. 96–153, see p. 152, fn. 239.

162. Eben Alexander, "A Perspective of the 1940s," *Surgery and Neurology*, 28 (1987), pp. 319–320, quote p. 320.

163. Grob, *Asylum to Community*, p. 131.

164. Finger, *Origins of Neuroscience*, p. 294.

165. See Edward Shorter, "Private Clinics in Central Europe, 1850–1933," *Social History of Medicine*, 3 (1990), pp. 159–195, esp. pp. 177, 181.

166. See David Kennedy Henderson, *The Evolution of Psychiatry in Scotland* (Edinburgh: Livingstone, 1964), pp. 95–100.

167. Caspar Max Brosius, *Aus meiner psychiatrischen Wirksamkeit* (Berlin: Hirschwald, 1878), pp. 23–27.

168. Theodor Kirchhoff, *Deutsche Irrenärzte*, vol. 2 (Berlin: Springer, 1924), p. 71.

169. Grob, *Asylum to Community*, pp. 239–240.

170. Johannes Bresler gives the founding dates of German hospital psychiatry departments in "Eine oberschlesische Nervenklinik," *PNW*, 26 (Aug. 9, 1924), pp. 104–106, esp. p. 104.

171. For an overview of English mental-health legislation, see Kathleen Jones, *Asylums and After: A Revised History of the Mental Health Services: From the Early 18th Century to the 1990s* (London: Athlone, 1993).

172. Jones, *Asylums and After*, pp. 137–138.

173. On Thomas Percy Rees's life, see *Munk's Roll*, vol. 5, pp. 344–345; interview with Edward Hare in Wilkinson, *Talking about Psychiatry*, pp. 62–63.

174. Joshua Bierer, "Psychotherapy in Mental Hospital Practice (Being the Preliminary Report of a Full-Time Psychotherapist in a Public Mental Hospital)," *Journal of Mental Science*, 86 (1940), pp. 928–952. For details of Bierer's life, see Raghu Gaind, "Bierer Obituary," *International Journal of Social Psychiatry*, 31 (1985), pp. 82–83.

175. Joshua Bierer, "From Psychiatry to Social and Community Psychiatry," *International Journal of Social Psychiatry*, 26 (1980), pp. 77–79.

176. Joshua Bierer, "Group Psychotherapy," *BMJ*, 1 (Feb. 14, 1942), pp. 214–217, quote p. 216.

177. These details from Bierer, *J. Ment. Sci.* 1940, pp. 933–934; Bierer, "A Self-Governed Patients' Social Club in a Public Mental Hospital," *Journal of Mental Science*, 87 (1941), pp. 419–424, quote p. 419. The historians of social psychiatry and the therapeutic community have not done well by Bierer. N. P. Manning's brief history of the movement does not even mention him. "Innovation in Social Policy—the Case of the Therapeutic Community," *Journal of Social Policy*, 5 (1976), pp. 265–279.

178. Bierer, *J. Ment. Sci.* 1940, p. 934. Owing to the pressures of war, Bierer abandoned the experiment at Runwell after two years. See Bierer, "Introduction to the Second Volume," *International Journal of Social Psychiatry,* 2 (1956), pp. 5–11, esp. p. 5.

179. For these details, see Maxwell Jones, *Social Psychiatry: A Study of Therapeutic Communities* (London: Tavistock, 1952), pp. 1–15, quotes pp. 2, 13.

180. Maxwell Jones interview, in Wilkinson, *Talking about Psychiatry,* pp. 53–54.

181. See Sargant, *The Unquiet Mind,* pp. 77–78.

182. See Sargant, *The Unquiet Mind,* p. 29.

183. See Sargant, *The Unquiet Mind,* p. 30.

184. On the treatment of psychoneuroses at the Northfield Military Hospital, see Robert H. Ahrenfeldt, *Psychiatry in the British Army in the Second World War* (London: Routledge, 1958), pp. 149–153; see also Main's obituary in the *Times,* June 5, 1990, p. 14.

185. Thomas F. Main, "The Hospital as a Therapeutic Institution," *Menninger Clinic Bulletin,* 10 (1946), pp. 66–70, quote p. 67.

186. Thomas F. Main, "The Ailment," *Medical Psychology,* 30 (1957), pp. 129–145, quote p. 144.

187. Main, *Medical Psychology,* 1957, p. 139.

188. H. V. Dicks, *Fifty Years of the Tavistock Clinic* (London: Routledge, 1970), p. 111.

189. This is the gist of Bierer's philosophy, although he did not use such terms as empowerment and normalization. See his "Theory and Practice of Psychiatric Day Hospitals," *Lancet,* 2 (Nov. 21, 1959), pp. 901–902: "The assumption that faulty relationships are the *result* of mental illness is probably onesided. We assume more and more that faulty or inadequate relationships are one of the *causes* of mental illness" (p. 901).

190. D. Ewen Cameron, "The Day Hospital: An Experimental Form of Hospitalization for Psychiatric Patients," *Modern Hospital,* 69 (1947), pp. 60–62. For reports of the Day Centre's activities (as it was called after 1950), see D. Ewen Cameron, "The Day Hospital," in A. E. Bennett et al., eds., *The Practice of Psychiatry in General Hospitals* (Berkeley: University of California Press, 1956), pp. 134–150; and A. E. Moll, "Psychiatric Service in a General Hospital with Special Reference to a Day Treatment Unit," *AJP,* 109 (1953), pp. 774–776.

191. Joshua Bierer, *The Day Hospital: An Experiment in Social Psychiatry* (London: Lewis, 1951), p. 10.

192. James Farndale, *The Day Hospital Movement in Great Britain* (Oxford: Pergamon, 1961), pp. 2, 5.

193. Bierer, *Lancet* 1959, p. 901.

194. Elmer E. Southard, "Alienists and Psychiatrists: Notes on Divisions and Nomenclature of Mental Hygiene," *Mental Hygiene,* 1 (1917), pp. 567–571, quote p. 569. On Southard, see David Henderson [letter], in

"Introduction to the Second Volume," *International Journal of Social Psychiatry*, 2 (1956), pp. 8–9.

195. John B. MacDonald, "Social Service and Out-Patient Relations," *AJP*, 1 (1921), pp. 141–157; Owen Copp, "Some Problems Confronting the Association," ibid., 1 (1921), pp. 1–13; Albert M. Barrett, "The Broadened Interests of Psychiatry," ibid., 2 (1922), pp. 1–13; the latter two papers were presidential addresses.

196. See, for example, Arthur J. Viseltear, "Milton C. Winternitz and the Yale Institute of Human Relations: A Brief Chapter in the History of Social Medicine," *Yale Journal of Biology and Medicine*, 57 (1984), pp. 869–889.

197. Paul Schilder, "Results and Problems of Group Psychotherapy in Severe Neuroses," *Mental Hygiene*, 23 (1939), pp. 87–98, quotes pp. 87–88, 90.

198. Leo Srole et al., *The Midtown Manhattan Study, vol. 1: Mental Health in the Metropolis* (New York: McGraw-Hill, 1962), and Thomas S. Langner and Stanley T. Michael, *The Midtown Manhattan Study: vol 2: Life Stress and Mental Health* (Glencoe: Free Press, 1963). See also Grob, *Asylum to Community*, pp. 100–102. On the community study of New Haven, see August B. Hollingshead and Frederick C. Redlich, *Social Class and Mental Illness: A Community Study* (New York: Wiley, 1958).

199. Marvin I. Herz, "The Therapeutic Community: A Critique," *Hospital and Community Psychiatry*, 23 (1972), pp. 69–72, quote p. 69.

200. Farndale, *Day Hospital Movement*, p. 1. Lawrence Friedman's study of the Menninger Clinic mentions a Patients' Council and other dimensions of a therapeutic community. The outpatients' club must have been the functional equivalent of a day hospital. *Menninger: The Family and the Clinic* (Lawrence: University of Kansas Press, 1990), p. 275.

201. On the genesis of the Mental Retardation and Community Mental Health Centers Construction Act of 1963, see Grob, *From Asylum to Community* 1991, pp. 216–234.

202. For evidence of the continuing resilience of communitarian thinking in British mental-health circles, see Lindsay Prior, *The Social Organization of Mental Illness* (London: Sage, 1993), who sees "community centred services" as the summit of twentieth-century psychiatry (p. 1).

Chapter 7: The Second Biological Psychiatry

1. Richard von Krafft-Ebing, "Untersuchungen über Irresein zur Zeit der Menstruation: ein klinischer Beitrag zur Lehre vom periodischen Irresein," *Archiv für Psychiatrie*, 8 (1878), pp. 65–107; quote p. 93; see the synoptic table of the 19 cases on pp. 94–97.

2. Emil Kraepelin, *Psychiatrie*, 8th ed., vol. 3, pt. 2 (Leipzig: Barth, 1913), p. 918.

3. Thomas Clouston, "The Neuroses of Development, Lecture III," *Edinburgh Medical Journal*, 37 (1891), pp. 104–124, see p. 108.

4. Clouston, "The Neuroses of Development [Lecture 1]," *Edinburgh Medical Journal*, 36 (1891), pp. 593–602, quote pp. 600–601.

5. Quote from the "Preface" by the Medical Research Council in Eliot Slater's, *Psychotic and Neurotic Illnesses in Twins* (London: HMSO, 1953), p. iii.

6. See Peter McGuffin et al., *Seminars in Psychiatric Genetics* (London: Gaskell, 1994), pp. 88–89.

7. Francis Galton, "The History of Twins, as a Criterion of the Relative Powers of Nature and Nurture," *Fraser's Magazine*, NS, 12 (Nov. 1875), pp. 556–576, quote p. 566. See also, C. G. Nicholas Mascie-Taylor, "Galton and the Use of Twin Studies," in Milo Keynes, ed., *Sir Francis Galton, FRS: The Legacy of His Ideas* (London: Macmillan, 1993), pp. 119–218.

8. Hans Luxenburger, "Vorläufiger Bericht über psychiatrische Serienuntersuchungen an Zwillingen," *Zeitschrift für die gesamte Neurologie und Psychiatrie*, 116 (1928), pp. 297–326, see tab. 4, p. 313.

9. On Luxenburger's life, see Thomas Haenel, *Zur Geschichte der Psychiatrie: Gedanken zur allgemeinen und Basler Psychiatriegeschichte* (Basel: Birkhäuser, 1982), pp. 167–168.

10. Kenneth S. Kendler and Scott R. Diehl, "The Genetics of Schizophrenia: A Current Genetic-Epidemiologic Perspective," *Schizophrenia Bulletin*, 19 (1993), pp. 261–285, anecdote p. 262.

11. On Rosanoff's life, see the obituaries in *AJP*, 99 (1943), pp. 616–617 and 773–774.

12. Aaron J. Rosanoff et al., "The Etiology of So-Called Schizophrenic Psychoses," *AJP*, 91 (1934), pp. 247–286, see esp. p. 252.

13. Rosanoff, "The Etiology of Manic-Depressive Syndromes with Special Reference to Their Occurrence in Twins," *AJP*, 91 (1935), pp. 725–762, see esp. p. 726, quote p. 758.

14. Robert N. Proctor writes scornfully of the psychiatric geneticists following Galton, "Twin studies purportedly demonstrated the heritability of everything from epilepsy, criminality, memory, and hernias to tuberculosis, cancer, schizophrenia, and divorce." *Racial Hygiene: Medicine under the Nazis* (Cambridge: Harvard U. P., 1988), p. 42. Weindling, without mentioning twin studies as such, airily dismisses this whole approach: "A range of diseases such as epilepsy, cretinism and hysteria, as well as deviant behaviors, were ascribed to the mysterious power of heredity." *Health, Race and German Politics*, p. 82. In fact, all items on this list save cretinism have significant genetic components (if one understands hysteria to mean chronic psychosomatic illness). It goes without saying that the Nazis abused twin research to fortify their doctrines of racial hygiene, just as they abused physics to manufacture missiles. Yet neither physics nor psychiatric genetics may be swept from the table simply because they are capable of misuse.

15. Henry A. Bunker's overview of U.S. contributions gives Rosanoff a passing nod midst hundreds of other references. "American Psychiatric Literature

during the Past One Hundred Years," in American Psychiatric Association, *One Hundred Years of American Psychiatry* (New York: Columbia U. P., 1944), p. 257. Rosanoff's name does not appear in the index of Walter E. Barton's *The History and Influence of the American Psychiatric Association* (Washington: APA, 1987), which contains 15 references to himself and 12 to William Menninger.

16. Franz J. Kallmann, *The Genetics of Schizophrenia: A Study of Heredity and Reproduction in the Families of 1,087 Schizophrenics* (New York: Augustin, 1938).

17. Kallmann, "The Genetic Theory of Schizophrenia: An Analysis of 691 Schizophrenic Twin Index Families," *AJP*, 103 (1946), pp. 309–322, esp. fig. 7, p. 313. Kallmann's life work came together in his book *Heredity in Health and Mental Disorder: Principles of Psychiatric Genetics in the Light of Comparative Twin Studies* (New York: Norton, 1953).

18. Franz J. Kallmann, "The Genetics of Psychoses," in *Premier Congrès Mondial de Psychiatrie Paris 1950* (Paris: Hermann, 1952), vol. 6, pp. 12–20; for the discussion see pp. 57–74.

19. A notable example was Slater's *Psychotic and Neurotic Illnesses in Twins.*

20. See McGuffin, *Seminars Psychiatric Genetics*, fig. 5.1, p. 88.

21. Seymour S. Kety et al., "The Types and Prevalence of Mental Illness in the Biological and Adoptive Families of Adopted Schizophrenics," *Journal of Psychiatric Research*, 6, suppl. 1 (Nov. 1968), pp. 345–362, quote p. 361.

22. Seymour S. Kety and Loring J. Ingraham, "Genetic Transmission and Improved Diagnosis of Schizophrenia from Pedigrees of Adoptees," *Journal of Psychiatric Research*, 26 (1992), pp. 247–255, esp. p. 250.

23. Kety et al., "Mental Illness in the Biological and Adoptive Relatives of Schizophrenic Adoptees: Replication of the Copenhagen Study in the Rest of Denmark," *Archives of General Psychiatry*, 51 (1994), pp. 442–455, see p. 449.

24. A. Bertelsen et al., "A Danish Twin Study of Manic-Depressive Disorders," *BJP*, 130 (1977), pp. 330–351.

25. Svenn Torgersen, "Genetic Factors in Anxiety Disorders," *Archives of General Psychiatry*, 40 (1983), pp. 1085–89.

26. Michael Bohman et al., "An Adoption Study of Somatoform Disorders, III. Cross-Fostering Analysis and Genetic Relationship to Alcoholism and Criminality," *Archives of General Psychiatry*, 41 (1984), pp. 872–878; C. Robert Cloninger et al., "Symptom Patterns and Causes of Somatization in Men: II. Genetic and Environmental Independence from Somatization in Women," *Genetic Epidemiology*, 3 (1986), pp. 171–185.

27. Oguz Arkonac and Samuel B. Guze, "A Family Study of Hysteria," *NEJM*, 268 (Jan. 31, 1963), pp. 239–242; C. Robert Cloninger and Samuel B. Guze, "Hysteria and Parental Psychiatric Illness," *Psychological Medicine*, 5 (1975), pp. 27–31.

28. For a summary, see Robert Plomin, "Genetic Risk and Psychosocial Disorders: Links Between the Normal and Abnormal," in Michael Rutter and

Paul Casaer, eds., *Biological Risk Factors for Psychosocial Disorders* (Cambridge: Cambridge U. P., 1991), pp. 101–138, tab. 5.1, p. 107.

29. Robert Plomin and Denise Daniels, "Why Are Children in the Same Family So Different from One Another?" *Behavioral and Brain Sciences,* 10 (1987), pp. 1–59, quote p. 1.

30. Shengbiao Wang et al., "Evidence for a Susceptibility Locus for Schizophrenia on Chromosome 6pter-p22," *Nature Genetics,* 10 (1995), pp. 41–46.

31. Wade H. Berrettini et al., "Chromosome 18 DNA Markers and Manic-Depressive Illness: Evidence for a Susceptibility Gene," *Proceedings of the National Academy of Science USA,* 91 (1994), pp. 5918–21; Richard E. Straub, "Possible Vulnerability Locus for Bipolar Affective Disorder on Chromosome 21q22.3," *Nature Genetics,* 8 (1994), pp. 291–294.

32. Arturas Petronis and James L. Kennedy, "Unstable Genes—Unstable Mind," *AJP,* 152 (1995), pp. 164–172.

33. Otto Loewi and E. Navratil, "Über humorale Übertragbarkeit der Herznervenwirkung. X. Mitteilung. Über das Schicksal des Vagusstoffs," *Pflügers Archiv für die gesamte Physiologie,* 214 (1926), pp. 678–688.

34. See A. M. Fiamberti, "L'Acétylcholine dans la physio-pathogénèse et dans la thérapie de la schizophrénie," *Premier Congrès Mondial de Psychiatrie Paris 1950,* vol. 4, pp. 16–22; also Fiamberti, "Sul meccanismo d'azione terapeutica della 'burrasca vascolare' provocate con derivati della colina," *Giornale di psichiatria e di neuropatologia,* 67 (1939), pp. 270–280. The author speculated that vascular shock might be the mechanism of action.

35. Heinz Lehmann, "The Introduction of Chlorpromazine to North America," *Psychiatric Journal of the University of Ottawa,* 14 (1989), pp. 263–265, quote p. 263.

36. On the introduction of chlorpromazine, see the monograph by Judith P. Swazey, *Chlorpromazine in Psychiatry: A Study of Therapeutic Innovation* (Cambridge: MIT Press, 1974), which builds on Anne E. Caldwell's pioneering study, *Origins of Psychopharmacology from CPZ to LSD* (Springfield: Thomas, 1970); see also Caldwell, "History of Psychopharmacology," in William G. Clark and Joseph del Giudice, eds., *Principles of Psychopharmacology,* 2nd ed. (New York: Academic, 1978), pp. 9–40, esp. 23–30.

37. Swazey, *Chlorpromazine,* p. 79, quote from Swazey's interview with Laborit.

38. Swazey, *Chlorpromazine,* pp. 100–103.

39. This story is told in Henri Laborit, *La Vie antèrieure* (Paris: Grasset, 1989), pp. 91–92. The maverick hypnotherapist and quasi-psychoanalyst Léon Chertok, at the time a staff psychiatrist at Villejuif, was present at the experiment. At its conclusion, Chertok asked permission to try chlorpromazine on patients at Villejuif but was refused. Chertok later said, "Thus I failed to become one of the pioneers [of psychopharmacology]." Léon Chertok, "30 Ans Après: La petite histoire de la découverte des neuroleptiques," *Annales médico-psychologiques,* 140 (1982), pp. 971–976, quote p. 974.

40. Details on lunch and lack of enthusiasm from Swazey, *Chlorpromazine,* p. 117.

41. Henri Laborit et al., "Un nouveau stabilisateur végétatif (le 4560 RP)," *Presse médicale,* 60 (Feb. 13, 1952), pp. 206–208, quote p. 208.

42. Joseph Hamon, Jean Paraire, and Jean Velluz, "Remarques sur l'action du 4560 R.P. sur l'agitation maniaque," *Annales médico-psychologiques,* 110 (March 1952), pp. 332–335, reporting the meeting of the Parisian Medico-Psychological Society of Feb. 25, 1952.

43. First to undertake a major clinical trial using only chlorpromazine were Parisian psychiatrists J. Sigwald and D. Bouttier, who, starting on Feb. 18, 1952, ultimately gave the compound to 48 patients. However, the authors published only in 1953, demonstrating the importance of rushing into print to ascertain medical priority. "Le Chlorhydrate de chloro-3. . . . ," *Annales de médecine,* 54 (1953), pp. 150–182.

44. Jean Delay, Pierre Deniker, and J. -M. Harl, "Utilisation en thérapeutique psychiatrique d'une phénothiazine d'action centrale élective (4560 RP)," *Annales médico-psychologiques,* 110 (2) (1952), pp. 112–120. Harl was an intern.

45. Jean Delay, Pierre Deniker, and J. -M. Harl, "Traitement des états d'excitation par une méthode médicamenteuse dérivée de l'hibernothérapie," *Annales médico-psychologiques,* 110 (2) (1952), pp. 267–273. Simultaneously, in June 1952 Andrée Deschamps, an asylum psychiatrist at Fleury-les-Aubrais who was directly inspired by Laborit, reported the results of a deep-sleep cure of eight days that she had successfully attempted with RP 4560 and barbiturates on four patients. "Hibernation artificielle en psychiatrie," *Presse médicale,* 60 (June 21, 1952), pp. 944–946. It is clear that numerous physicians were giving the compound at the same time as Delay and Deniker.

46. As one puff piece on Delay said, "In 1952, in a survey of the therapeutic shock methods, Professor Delay and his co-worker, Pierre Deniker, described a different and new method of treatment, by means of a simple medicament, called chlorpromazine. . . . Thanks to the discovery of this first neuroleptic . . . there was a radical transformation from the lunatic asylums of those days to the psychiatric clinics as they are known today throughout the world." "Leading Men of Science: Jean Delay," in *Triangle,* 6 (1964), pp. 306–307. Laborit received proper credit for his role in 1957 when he shared a Lasker Prize with Delay, Deniker, and Heinz Lehmann, among others. Deniker later gave Laborit (almost) full marks in "Introduction of Neuroleptic Chemotherapy into Psychiatry," in Frank J. Ayd, Jr., and Barry Blackwell, eds., *Discoveries in Biological Psychiatry* (Baltimore: Ayd Medical Communications, 1984), pp. 155–164, esp. p. 157.

47. Delay, *Ann. med.-psych.,* June 1952, case 1, pp. 268–269 Medico-Psychological Society, meeting of June 23, 1952. This paper did mention Laborit, but only his tangential work on the deep-cooling of surgical patients.

48. Caldwell, "History of Psychopharmacology," p. 30. I have singled out the chlorpromazine story as the most important narrative strand in the history

of the antipsychotics but the reader should be aware there are other strands, such as the reserpine story, that figure in the beginning but ultimately peter out. On reserpine, see Frances R. Frankenburg, "History of the Development of Antipsychotic Medication," *Psychiatric Clinics of North America*, 17 (1994), pp. 531–540, esp. p. 532. Psychiatrist Nathan Kline was a major actor in the reserpine story, as he was in the development of the monoamine oxidase inhibitors for depression, another story this book slides over in silence because the MAOIs ultimately declined in importance. On Kline see Heinz Lehmann, "Nathan Kline," in Thomas A. Ban and Hanns Hippius, eds., *Psychopharmacology in Perspective* (New York: Springer, n.d. [1992]), pp. 26–28. David Healy's forthcoming *History of the Antidepressants* (Cambridge: Harvard U. P., 1996) reviews all of these narratives.

49. See Simone Courvoisier et al., "Propriétés pharmacodynamiques du . . . 4.560 R.P.," *Archives internationales de pharmacodynamie*, 92 (1953), pp. 305–361.

50. John D. M. Griffin, "An Historic Oversight," *Canadian Psychiatric Association Bulletin*, 26 (2) (April 1994), p. 5. Kajander never published her work, and ended up practicing in Thunder Bay, Ontario.

51. Interview of Heinz Lehmann by David Healy, p. 2. Dr. Healy kindly made a copy of the interview available to me.

52. Heinz E. Lehmann and Gorman E. Hanrahan, "Chlorpromazine: New Inhibiting Agent for Psychomotor Excitement and Manic States," [American Medical Association] *Archives of Neurology and Psychiatry*, 71 (1954), pp. 227–237.

53. Heinz Lehmann, "Introduction of Chlorpromazine to North America," p. 264.

54. Healy interview, p. 9.

55. Lehmann, "Introduction of Chlorpromazine to North America," p. 265.

56. Lehmann, *Archives of Neurology*, p. 231.

57. John R. Young, personal communication. On Smith Kline & French's involvement with chlorpromazine, see Swazey, *Chlorpromazine*, pp. 159–190; for a few added details, see Shorter, *The Health Century* (New York: Doubleday, 1987), pp. 120–126.

58. Willis H. Bower, "Chlorpromazine in Psychiatric Illness," *NEJM*, 251 (Oct. 21, 1954), pp. 689–692. Swazey's monograph makes no mention of Bower's work. N. William Winkelman's earlier study was done primarily on psychoneurotic patients. "Chlorpromazine in the Treatment of Neuropsychiatric Disorders," *JAMA*, 155 (May 1, 1954), pp. 8–21. Winkelman allowed that chlorpromazine had some benefits but that it "should never be given as a substitute for analytically oriented psychotherapy" (p. 21).

59. See on this Swazey, *Chlorpromazine*, pp. 201–207.

60. *Time*, Mar. 7, 1955, p. 56.

61. Bliss Forbush, *The Sheppard & Enoch Pratt Hospital, 1853–1970: A History* (Philadelphia: Lippincott, 1971), pp. 124–125.

62. See Pierre Deniker, "From Chlorpromazine to Tardive Dyskinesia (Brief History of the Neuroleptics)," *Psychiatry Journal of the University of Ottawa*, 14 (1989), pp. 253–259, esp. p. 254.

63. Henry R. Rollin, "The Dark before the Dawn," *Journal of Psychopharmacology*, 4 (1990), pp. 109–114, quote p. 113.

64. John F. J. Cade, "Lithium Salts in the Treatment of Psychotic Excitement," *Medical Journal of Australia*, 2 (Sept. 3, 1949), pp. 349–352, quote p. 351. See also Cade's recounting of his discovery in *Discoveries in Biological Psychiatry*, pp. 218–225.

65. Cade in *Discoveries in Biological Psychiatry*, p. 219.

66. Mogens Schou et al., "The Treatment of Manic Psychoses by the Administration of Lithium Salts," *Journal of Neurology, Neurosurgery and Psychiatry*, 17 (1954), pp. 250–260. The psychiatric hospital of Aarhus University is in fact at Risskov.

67. Mogens Schou, "Lithium: Personal Reminiscences," *Psychiatric Journal of the University of Ottawa*, 14 (1989), pp. 260–262, quote p. 261.

68. Eddie Kingstone, "The Lithium Treatment of Hypomanic and Manic States," *Comprehensive Psychiatry*, 1 (1960), pp. 317–320; Kingstone was Cameron's chief resident. See also Samuel Gershon and Arthur Yuwiler, "Lithium Ion: A Specific Psychopharmacological Approach to the Treatment of Mania," *Journal of Neuropsychiatry*, 1 (1960), pp. 229–241. On the complexities of the introduction of lithium to North America, see F. Neil Johnson, *The History of Lithium Therapy* (London: Macmillan, 1984), pp. 94–104.

69. See Frank J. Ayd., Jr., "The Early History of Modern Psychopharmacology," *Neuropsychopharmacology*, 5 (1991), pp. 71–84, details p. 82.

70. On Lewis and Shepherd, see Felix Post interview in Greg Wilkinson, ed., *Talking about Psychiatry* (London: Gaskell, 1993), p. 167.

71. It suits the logic of the exposition to describe psychosis and depression as entirely separate disorders. Yet it is not entirely clear that schizophrenia is a different disorder from psychotic depression. Depression, for example, often responds well to chlorpromazine, a drug supposedly for schizophrenia. (See Donald F. Klein and Max Fink, "Behavioral Reaction Patterns with Phenothiazines, *Archives of General Psychiatry*, 7 [1962], pp. 449–459, especially category E.) What has tended to maintain the airtight distinction between the two disorders is more the marketing strategies of the pharmaceutical companies than scientific findings.

72. Of the various accounts Kuhn has given of the "imipramine story," most complete is that in Ludwig J. Pongratz, ed., *Psychiatrie in Selbstdarstellungen* (Berne: Huber, 1977), pp. 219–257, esp. pp. 235–239. The accounts of Geigy insiders differ somewhat from his own, and I thank David Healy for sharing some of this material with me.

73. Roland Kuhn, "Über die Behandlung depressiver Zustände mit einem Iminodibenzylderivat (G22355)," *Schweizerische Medizinische Wochenschrift*, 87 (Aug. 31, 1957), pp. 1135–40.

74. Kuhn, *Schweiz. Med. Wochenschrift* 1957. The first international notice was Kuhn's article in the main American psychiatry journal in 1958: "The Treatment of Depressive States with G22355 (Imipramine Hydrochloride)," *AJP*, 115 (1958), pp. 459–464. This article incorrectly identified Kuhn as "chief medical officer"; he was in fact a ward chief (Oberarzt). Heinz Lehmann did the first North American trials. See his, "Tricyclic Antidepressants: Recollections," in M. J. Parnham and J. Bruinvels, eds., *Psycho- and Neuro-Pharmacology*, vol. 1 (Amsterdam: Elsevier, 1983), pp. 211–216.

75. National Center for Health Statistics, H. Koch, "Drug Utilization in Office-Based Practice, A Summary of Findings. National Ambulatory Medical Care Survey, United States, 1980," *Vital and Health Statistics*, ser. 13, no. 65, DHHS Pub. No. (PHS) 83-1726. Public Health Service, Washington, DC, U.S. Government Printing Office, Mar., 1983, tab. 1, p. 15; tab. 2, p. 17.

76. Felix Post, "Then and Now," *BJP*, 133 (1978), pp. 83–86, quotes pp. 84, 85.

77. Heinrich Laehr, *Über Irrsein und Irrenanstalten* (Halle: Pfeffer, 1852), pp. ix, 16.

78. Clouston, *Edinburgh Medical Journal* 1891, p. 595.

79. Mention should be made of the pioneering but largely ignored work on neurochemistry of John William Thudichum, a lecturer at St. Thomas's Hospital in London. He was interested in the biochemistry of psychiatric illness. See David L. Drabkin, ed., J. L. W. Thudichum, *A Treatise on the Chemical Constitution of the Brain* (1884) (reprint ed. Hamden, CT: Archon, 1962).

80. C. Grabow and Felix Plaut, "Experimentelle Untersuchungen zur Frage der Antikörperbildung im Liquorraum," *Zeitschrift für Immunitätsforschung und experimentelle Therapie*, 54 (1927), pp. 335–354. On these early stirrings at the Deutsche Forschungsanstalt, see Matthias M. Weber, " 'Ein Forschungsinstitut für Psychiatrie . . .': Die Entwicklung der Deutschen Forschungsanstalt für Psychiatrie in München zwischen 1917 und 1945," *Sudhoffs Archiv*, 75 (1991), pp. 74–89, esp. pp. 82–83.

81. On Plaut's end, see David Krasner, "Smith Ely Jelliffe and the Immigration of European Physicians to the United States in the 1930s," *Transactions and Studies of the College of Physicians of Philadelphia*, ser. 5, 12 (1990), pp. 49–67, p. 57.

82. Denis Hill, "Electroencephalography as an Instrument of Research in Psychiatry," *Premier Congrès Mondial de Psychiatrie*, vol. 3, pp. 163–177, quote p. 164.

83. See W. C. Corning, "Bootstrapping toward a Classification System," in Theodore Millon and Gerald L. Klerman, eds., *Contemporary Directions in Psychopathology* (New York: Guilford, 1986), pp. 279–306, esp. pp. 296–299.

84. Summary of paper by R. E. Hemphill and M. Reiss, "The Isotopes in Psychiatry," *Premier Congrès Mondial de Psychiatrie*, vol. 3, pp. 290–291.

85. Summary of paper by Richter, "Biochemical Changes in the Brain in Functional Activity," *Premier Congrès Mondial de Psychiatrie*, vol. 3, p. 296.

86. See Wilder Penfield, *The Difficult Art of Giving: The Epic of Alan Gregg* (Boston: Little Brown, 1967), pp. 273, 282–283, quote p. 282.

87. For this story see Tracy J. Putnam, "The Demonstration of the Specific Anticonvulsant Action of Diphenylhydantoin and Related Compounds," in *Discoveries Biological Psychiatry*, pp. 85–90. This work was done while the group were still at the Boston City Hospital, where in 1934 Putnam replaced Cobb as head of neurology.

88. Johannes M. Nielsen and George N. Thompson, *The Engrammes of Psychiatry* (Springfield: Thomas, 1947). The book was dedicated "to the scientists interested in the neuronal basis of human behavior."

89. On the founding, see Jules H. Masserman, "Preface and Dedication," *Biological Psychiatry: Proceedings of the Scientific Sessions of the Society of Biological Psychiatry, San Francisco, May, 1958* (New York: Grune and Stratton, 1959), p. xv.

90. "The Society of Biological Psychiatry," *AJP*, 111 (1954), pp. 389–391, quotes p. 390.

91. The main title, "Psychopharmakon," appeared in Greek, the subtitle in Latin. Edited by Reinhard Lorich, the work was theological in nature and not medical. It was translated into English by H. Thorne as *Physicke for the Soule* (London: Denham, c. 1568). Rhegius, a Lutheran preacher, died in 1541.

92. Jacques-Joseph Moreau de Tours, *Du hachisch et de l'aliénation mentale: Études psychologiques* (1845) (reprint Paris: Ressources, 1980), pp. 29–30.

93. Claude Bernard, "Des effets physiologiques de la morphine et leur combinaison avec ceux de chloroform," *Bulletin thérapeutique*, 77 (1869), pp. 241–256.

94. Emil Kraepelin, *Über die Beeinflussung einfacher psychischer Vorgänge durch einige Arzneimittel* (Jena: Fischer, 1892), p. 227.

95. David I. Macht, "Contributions to Psychopharmacology," *Johns Hopkins Hospital Bulletin*, 31 (1920), pp. 167–173, quotes p. 167. Contemporary usage of the term psychopharmacology, however, dates not from Macht's article but from Jean Delay and Jean Thuillier who used the word in an article they wrote in 1956 (against the protests of Delay who disliked the neologism). Delay and Thuillier, "Psychiatrie expérimentale et psychopharmacologie," *Semaine des hôpitaux de Paris*, 32 (Oct. 22, 1956), pp. 3187–93. Thuillier, Delay's assistant, was in charge of the experimental-psychiatry lab at Ste-Anne. The term "psychopharmacology" was sanctified at a conference in Milan the following year. See Jean Thuillier, note, in Ban and Hippius, *Psychopharmacology in Perspective*, pp. 88–89.

96. On LSD, see Abraham Wikler, *The Relation of Psychiatry to Pharmacology* (Baltimore: Williams & Wilkins, 1957), pp. 20–22 and passim. The book was the first American textbook of psychopharmacology.

97. Wolfgang de Boor, *Pharmakopsychologie und Psychopathologie* (Berlin: Springer, 1956).

98. Ban, *Psychopharmacology in Perspective*, pp. xii–xiii.

99. Betty M. Twarog, "Serotonin: History of a Discovery," *Comparative Biochemistry and Physiology*, 91C (1988), pp. 21–24. Betty M. Twarog and Irvine H. Page, "Serotonin Content of Some Mammalian Tissues and Urine and a Method for Its Determination," *American Journal of Physiology*, 175 (1953), pp. 157–161. Her original paper on serotonin as a neurotransmitter, submitted in 1952, was not published until 1954 because the editor of the journal had initially dismissed it as unimportant without bothering to notify her.

100. Arvid Carlsson et al., "On the Presence of 3-Hydroxytyramine in Brain," *Science*, 127 (Feb. 28, 1958), p. 471. 3-hydroxytyramine is dopamine. The paper was submitted in 1957. The advent of spectrofluorimetry in the mid-1950s greatly aided Carlsson's work and made possible technically the coming push in studying the monoamines.

101. Arvid Carlsson and Margit Lindqvist, "Effect of Chlorpromazine or Haloperidol on Formation of 3-Methoxytyramine and Normetanephrine in Mouse Brain," *Acta Pharmacol. et Toxicol.*, 20 (1963), pp. 140–144.

102. Solomon H. Snyder, "The Dopamine Hypothesis of Schizophrenia: Focus on the Dopamine Receptor," *AJP*, 133 (1976), pp. 197–202. See also Snyder's 1974 paper cited earlier.

103. The first in this series of papers was Alfred Pletscher, Parkhurst A. Shore, and Bernard B. Brodie, "Serotonin Release as a Possible Mechanism of Reserpine Action," *Science*, 122 (Aug. 26, 1955), pp. 374–375.

104. I owe some of this perspective to an interview of Arvid Carlsson by David Healy, pp. 2–3. I am grateful to Dr. Healy for making a copy of the transcript available to me.

105. Elizabeth F. Marshall et al., "The Effect of Iproniazid and Imipramine on the Blood Platelet 5-Hydroxytryptamine Level in Man," *British Journal of Pharmacology*, 15 (1960), pp. 35–41.

106. Arvid Carlsson et al., "The Effect of Imipramine of [sic] Central 5-Hydroxytryptamine Neurons," *Journal of Pharmacy and Pharmacology*, 20 (1968), pp. 150–151. See also Carlsson et al., "Effects of Some Antidepressant Drugs on the Depletion of Intraneuronal Brain Catecholamine Stores . . . ," *European Journal of Pharmacology*, 5 (1969), pp. 367–373.

107. Solomon Snyder et al., "Drugs, Neurotransmitters, and Schizophrenia," *Science*, 184 (1974), pp. 1243–53.

108. David Healy, "The Structure of Psychopharmacological Revolutions," *Psychiatric Developments*, 4 (1987), pp. 349–376, quote p. 351. I have also benefited from Healy's "The History of British Psychopharmacology," in Hugh

Freeman and German E. Berrios, eds., *150 Years of British Psychiatry. Volume II: the Aftermath* (London: Athlone, 1996), pp. 61–88.

109. See David T. Healy, "The Psychopharmacologic Era: Notes toward a History," *Journal of Psychopharmacology*, 4 (1990), pp. 152–167, esp. p. 164. On clozapine's role in challenging the dopamine hypothesis, see Alfred Goodman Gilman et al., eds., *Goodman and Gilman's The Pharmacological Basis of Therapeutics*, 8th ed. (New York: McGraw-Hill, 1990), p. 391.

110. See Floyd E. Bloom, "Advancing a Neurodevelopmental Origin for Schizophrenia," *Archives of General Psychiatry*, 50 (1993), pp. 224–227, quote p. 224.

111. Joyce A. Kovelman and Arnold B. Scheibel, "A Neurohistological Correlate of Schizophrenia," *Biological Psychiatry*, 19 (1984), pp. 1601–1621, quote p. 1616.

112. Francine M. Benes et al., "Increased Vertical Axon Numbers in Cingulate Cortex of Schizophrenics," *Archives of General Psychiatry*, 44 (1987), pp. 1017–21.

113. Sarnoff A. Mednick et al., "Adult Schizophrenia Following Prenatal Exposure to an Influenza Epidemic," *Archives of General Psychiatry*, 45 (1988), pp. 189–192. See also Mednick and Tyrone D. Cannon, "Fetal Development, Birth and the Syndromes of Adult Schizophrenia," in Mednick et al., eds., *Fetal Neural Development and Adult Schizophrenia* (Cambridge: Cambridge U. P., 1991), pp. 3–13, also pp. 227–237.

114. Christopher E. Barr et al., "Exposure to Influenza Epidemics during Gestation and Adult Schizophrenia: A 40-Year Study," *Archives of General Psychiatry*, 47 (1990), pp. 869–874.

115. Janice R. Stevens, "Neuropathology of Schizophrenia," *Archives of General Psychiatry*, 39 (1982), pp. 1131–39.

116. Eve C. Johnstone et al., "Cerebral Ventricular Size and Cognitive Impairment in Chronic Schizophrenia," *Lancet*, 2 (Oct. 30, 1976), pp. 924–926. For an overview, see Herbert Y. Meltzer, "Biological Studies in Schizophrenia," *Schizophrenia Bulletin*, 13 (1987), pp. 77–111, esp. 78–81.

117. See Mary Seeman, "Schizophrenia: D4 Receptor Elevation: What Does It Mean?" *Journal of Psychiatry and Neuroscience*, 19 (1994), pp. 171–176, esp. 172.

118. Bloom, *Archives of General Psychiatry* 1993, p. 224.

119. Mednick and Cannon, *Fetal Neural Development*, pp. 6–9. See also Barbara Fish et al., "Infants at Risk for Schizophrenia: Sequelae of a Genetic Neurointegrative Defect: A Review and Replication Analysis of Pandysmaturation in the Jerusalem Infant Development Study," *Archives of General Psychiatry*, 49 (1992), pp. 221–235.

120. As Thomas Clouston put it, in the language of the day, "All sorts of postponements of developmental processes, all forms of asymmetry about the head and face, should be danger signals taken along with neurotic heredity." Clouston, *Edinburgh Medical Journal* 1891, pp. 119–120.

121. Bloom, *Archives of General Psychiatry* 1993, p. 226.

122. Godfrey D. Pearlson and Amy E. Veroff, "Computerised Tomographic Scan Changes in Manic-Depressive Illness," *Lancet*, 2 (Aug. 29, 1981), p. 470.

123. Otto Fenichel, *Outline of Clinical Psychoanalysis* (New York: Norton, 1934), p. 146.

124. Lewis R. Baxter, Jr., et al., "Local Cerebral Glucose Metabolic Rates in Obsessive-Compulsive Disorder," *Archives of General Psychiatry*, 44 (1987), pp. 211–218.

125. See P. K. McGuire et al., "Functional Anatomy of Obsessive-Compulsive Phenomena," *BJP*, 164 (1994), pp. 459–468; Scott L. Rauch et al., "Regional Cerebral Blood Flow Measured during Symptom Provocation in Obsessive-Compulsive Disorder using Oxygen 15-Labeled Carbon Dioxide and Positron Emission Tomography," *Archives of General Psychiatry*, 51 (1994), pp. 62–70.

126. Rudolf Hoehn-Saric et al., "Effects of Fluoxetine on Regional Cerebral Blood Flow in Obsessive-Compulsive Patients," *AJP*, 148 (1991), pp. 1243–45.

127. National Advisory Mental Health Council, *Approaching the 21st Century: Opportunities for NIMH Neuroscience Research. Report to Congress on the Decade of the Brain* (Rockville: National Institute of Mental Health, 1988), p. 2.

128. For this argument, see Edward Shorter, *Bedside Manners: The Troubled History of the Doctor-Patient Relationship* (New York: Simon and Schuster, 1985); reprinted with a new preface as *Doctors and Their Patients: A Social History* (New Brunswick: Transaction, 1991).

129. For these examples, see Sherry Hirsch et al., eds., *Madness Network News Reader* (San Francisco: Glide, 1974), pp. 81, 91.

130. On the history of the antipsychiatry movement, see Norman Dain, "Psychiatry and Anti-Psychiatry in the United States," in Mark S. Micale and Roy Porter, *Discovering the History of Psychiatry* (New York: Oxford U. P., 1994), pp. 415–444; Gerald N. Grob, *From Asylum to Community: Mental Health Policy in Modern America* (Princeton: Princeton U. P., 1991), pp. 262–268, 279–287; and Digby Tantam, "The Anti-Psychiatric Movement," in German E. Berrios and Hugh Freeman, *150 Years of British Psychiatry, 1841–1991* (London: Gaskell, 1991), pp. 333–347.

131. For a succinct overview, see Mitchell Wilson, "*DSM-III* and the Transformation of American Psychiatry: A History," *AJP*, 150 (1993), pp. 399–410, esp. p. 402.

132. Thomas S. Szasz, *The Myth of Mental Illness*, rev. ed. (New York: Harper and Row, 1974; first ed. 1960), quote p. xiii.

133. Erving Goffman, *Asylums: Essays on the Social Situation of Mental Patients and Other Inmates* (New York: Doubleday, 1961), pp. 14, 67–68, 111. According to Goffman, "The perception of losing one's mind is based on culturally derived and socially engrained stereotypes . . . ." (p. 132).

134. Ken Kesey, *One Flew Over the Cuckoo's Nest* (New York: Viking, 1962), p. 20.

135. Thomas J. Scheff, *Being Mentally Ill: A Sociological Theory* (Chicago: Aldine, 1966), pp. 28, 92–93, 96.

136. Samuel B. Guze, *Why Psychiatry Is a Branch of Medicine* (New York: Oxford U. P., 1992), p. 14.

137. Ronald D. Laing, *The Divided Self: A Study of Sanity and Madness* (London: Tavistock, 1960), p. 179.

138. Ronald D. Laing, *The Politics of Experience* (New York: Random House, 1967), pp. 127, 129. This essay was initially published in 1964.

139. Ronald D. Laing, "The Invention of Madness," *New Statesman*, 73 (June 16, 1967), p. 843. Michel Foucault's work was a doctoral thesis, initially appearing as *Folie et déraison: Histoire de la folie à l'âge classique* (Paris: Plon, 1961).

140. Laurice L. McAfee, "Interview with Joanne Greenberg," in Ann-Louise S. Silver, ed., *Psychoanalysis and Psychosis* (Madison: International Universities Press, 1989), pp. 513–531, quotes pp. 527–528.

141. William A. White, "Presidential Address," *AJP*, 5 (1925), pp. 1–20, esp. p. 3.

142. Albert Deutsch, *The Shame of the States* (New York: Harcourt, 1948), quotes pp. 28, 42–43, 49.

143. *Time*, Dec. 20, 1948, quote p. 41.

144. Morton Kramer et al., *A Historical Study of the Disposition of First Admissions to a State Hospital: Experience of the Warren State Hospital during the Period 1916–50* (Public Health Service, Public Health Monograph no. 32; Washington, DC: Department of Health, Education and Welfare, 1955), see fig. 3, p. 13, for all mental disorders, under 65 years, both sexes, cohort of 1946–50. Release rates had been climbing steadily, but even for the earliest cohort of patients admitted in 1916–25, 55 percent were released within five years.

145. See P. John Mathai and P. S. Gopinath, "Deficits of Chronic Schizophrenia in Relation to Long-Term Hospitalization," *BJP*, 148 (1985), pp. 509–516.

146. The following chronology reflects primarily American events. In Germany, it was not until the student revolt of the 1970s and the rise of antipsychiatry that deinstitutionalization began. See K. Heinrich, "Psychopharmakologie seit 1952," *Fortschritte der Neurologie und Psychiatrie*, 62 (1994), pp. 31–39, esp. p. 36.

147. See Frank J. Ayd, Jr., "Henry Brill," in Ban, *Psychopharmacology in Perspective*, pp. 2–3.

148. See U.S. Bureau of the Census, *Historical Statistics of the United States, Colonial Times to 1970, Bicentennial Edition*, part 2 (Washington, DC: GPO, 1975), tab. B-426, p. 84; Center for Mental Health Services and National Institute of Mental Health, R. W. Manderscheid and M. A. Sonnenschein, eds., *Mental Health, United States, 1992*. DHHS Pub. No. (SMA) 92–1942

(Washington, DC: GPO, 1992), tab. 1.2, p. 24. The figures for 1955 and 1970 refer to the mental-hospital census on July 1 of a given year, that for 1988 to the number of beds. Yet the figures should be closely comparable.

149. DHHS, Center for Mental Health Services, Richard W. Redick et al., "The Evolution and Expansion of Mental Health Care in the United States Between 1955 and 1990," *Data Highlights, Mental Health Statistical Note*, no. 210, May 1994, p. 1.

150. See E. Fuller Torrey, *Nowhere to Go: The Tragic Odyssey of the Homeless Mentally Ill* (New York: Harper and Row, 1988), pp. 25–29, 126–128 passim.

151. See Torrey, *Nowhere to Go*, pp. 7–9, 11.

152. See H. Richard Lamb and Victor Goertzel, "Discharged Mental Patients: Are They Really in the Community?" *Archives of General Psychiatry*, 24 (1971), pp. 29–34.

153. For an early *prise de conscience* of this problem, see George E. Crane, "Clinical Psychopharmacology in Its 20th Year: Late, Unanticipated Effects of Neuroleptics May Limit Their Use in Psychiatry," *Science*, 181 (1973), pp. 124–128.

154. A 1984 newspaper account, quoted in Torrey, *Nowhere to Go*, p. 33.

155. Henry R. Rollin, *Festina Lente: A Psychiatric Odyssey* (London: British Medical Journal Memoir Club, 1990), p. 92.

156. *United States Mental Health 1992*, p. 21.

157. *United States Mental Health 1994*, p. 38.

158. Lucy Freeman, "We're Overdoing Shock Treatments," *Science Digest*, 34 (Sept. 1953), pp. 26–29. This was condensed from her book *Hope for the Troubled*.

159. Peter G. Cranford, *But for the Grace of God: The Inside Story of the World's Largest Insane Asylum, Milledgeville!* (Augusta: Great Pyramid Press, 1981), pp. 86–87, 108, 149.

160. Goffman, *Asylums*, p. 81.

161. Kesey, *One Flew*, pp. 14, 15.

162. L. Ron Hubbard, *Dianetics: The Modern Science of Mental Health* (Los Angeles: American Saint Hill Org., 1950), pp. 97–98, 151, 193–194, 318, 367–369, 383. "Dianetics" first appeared as an article, "Dianetics, The Evolution of a Science," *Astounding Science Fiction*, May 1950, pp. 43f.

163. Church of Scientology of California, *What Is Scientology?* (Los Angeles: CSC, 1978), p. 98.

164. William J. Winslade et al., "Medical, Judicial, and Statutory Regulation of ECT in the United States," *AJP*, 141 (1984), pp. 1349–55, see p. 1350.

165. See "Attack on Electroshock," *Newsweek*, Mar. 17, 1975, p. 86. "Court Stays Curb on Shock Therapy," *New York Times*, Jan. 3, 1975, p. 20; "Curb on Therapy Stirs a Dispute," *New York Times*, April 6, 1975, p. 18.

166. "Berkeley Voters Ban ECT," *Science News*, 122 (Nov. 13, 1982), p. 309; "Electroshock Therapy on Trial," *Science Digest*, 92 (Oct. 1984), p. 14.

167. "Bill Would Ban ECT in Texas," *Psychiatric News*, Apr. 21, 1995, pp. 1, 34.

168. Haroutun M. Babigian and Laurence B. Guttmacher, "Epidemiologic Considerations in Electroconvulsive Therapy," *Archives of General Psychiatry*, 41 (1984), pp. 246–253, see tab. 2, p. 247.

169. On these events, see Max Fink, "Die Geschichte der EKT in den Vereinigten Staaten in den letzten Jahrzehnten," *Nervenarzt*, 64 (1993), pp. 689–695, esp. p. 690.

170. Fred H. Frankel, "Electro-Convulsive Therapy in Massachusetts: A Task Force Report," *Massachusetts Journal of Mental Health*, 3 (1973), pp. 3–29, quotes pp. 18, 19.

171. American Psychiatric Association, *Report of the Task Force on Electroconvulsive Therapy* (Washington, DC: APA, May, 1978), pp. 3, 11, 12, 161–162.

172. Max Fink, "Convulsive and Drug Therapies of Depression," *Annual Review of Medicine*, 32 (1981), pp. 405–412; Fink's paradoxical conclusion was, "While ECT is clearly more effective than tricyclic antidepressants and monoamine oxidase inhibitors, the additional difficulty in administering ECT, the public image of its special hazards, and the ease of administering the drug therapies make their use generally preferred" (p. 410).

173. National Institutes of Health, Office of Medical Applications of Research, "Electroconvulsive Therapy," *Consensus Development Conference Statement*, 5 (11) [1985], quotes pp. 2, 3. The report was reprinted, together with abstracts of presentations made to the panel, in *Psychopharmacology Bulletin*, 22 (1986), pp. 445–502. See also "Electroconvulsive Therapy," *JAMA*, 254 (Oct. 18, 1985), pp. 2103–08.

174. See John Pippard and Les Ellam, *Electroconvulsive Treatment in Great Britain, 1980* (London: Gaskell, 1981); the authors summarized their report in *Lancet*, 2 (Nov. 21, 1981), pp. 1160–61. The techniques and equipment used in Britain, however, were said to be sadly out of date. See editorial: "ECT in Britain: a Shameful State of Affairs," ibid., Nov. 28, 1981, pp. 1207–08.

175. American Psychiatric Association, *The Practice of Electroconvulsive Therapy: Recommendations for Treatment, Training, and Privileging: A Task Force Report* (Washington, DC: APA, 1990), pp. 7–8.

176. Laurence B. Guttmacher, *Concise Guide to Psychopharmacology and Electroconvulsive Therapy* (Washington, DC: American Psychiatric Press, 1994), tab. 5–1, p. 122.

177. Robert A. Dorwart et al., "A National Study of Psychiatrists' Professional Activities," *AJP*, 149 (1992), pp. 1499–1505, see p. 1503.

178. Norman S. Endler, *Holiday of Darkness: A Psychologist's Personal Journey out of His Depression* (New York: Wiley, 1982), pp. 50–51, 72–73, 81–83.

179. On these terms, see Hagop S. Akiskal and William T. McKinney, Jr., "Psychiatry and Pseudopsychiatry," *Archives of General Psychiatry*, 28 (1973), pp. 367–373, esp. p. 370.

180. Samuel B. Guze, "Biological Psychiatry: Is There Any Other Kind?" *Psychological Medicine*, 19 (1989), pp. 315–323, quote p. 315. Guze contrasted "toughmindedness vs. tendermindedness." See his "The Need for Toughmindedness in Psychiatric Thinking," *Southern Medical Journal*, 63 (1970), pp. 662–671, esp. p. 670.

181. Ross J. Baldessarini, "Drugs and the Treatment of Psychiatric Disorders," in *Goodman and Gilman*, 8th ed., pp. 383–435, quote p. 385.

Chapter 8: From Freud to Prozac

1. William E. Narrow et al., "Use of Services by Persons with Mental and Addictive Disorders: Findings from the National Institute of Mental Health Epidemiologic Catchment Area Program," *Archives of General Psychiatry*, 50 (1993), pp. 95–107, statistics p. 95.

2. Mark Olfson and Harold Alan Pincus, "Outpatient Psychotherapy in the United States, I: Volume, Costs, and User Characteristics," *AJP*, 151 (1994), pp. 1281–88, see tab. 2, p. 1285.

3. See Joseph Veroff et al., *Mental Health in America: Patterns of Help-Seeking from 1957 to 1976* (New York: Basic, 1981), p. 79. The proportion of the population that had "used help" almost doubled from 14 percent in 1957 to 26 percent in 1976.

4. See, for example, Ronald Mac Keith and Martin Bax, eds., *Minimal Cerebral Dysfunction* (London: Heinemann Medical, 1963). The symposium, after much agonizing, finally determined the diagnosis was inadvisable in the absence of concrete indications of brain damage.

5. American Psychiatric Association, *DSM-II: Diagnostic and Statistical Manual of Mental Disorders*, 2nd ed. (Washington, DC: APA, 1968), p. 50.

6. American Psychiatric Association, *DSM-III: Diagnostic and Statistical Manual of Mental Disorders*, 3d ed. (Washington, DC: APA, 1980), p. 41. Within the highly heterogeneous group of children, mainly boys, diagnosed as having ADHD, there exists a core with some kind of apparently genetically based cerebral organicity. See Joseph Biederman et al., "Family-Genetic and Psychosocial Risk Factors in *DSM-III* Attention Deficit Disorder," *Journal of the American Academy of Child and Adolescent Psychiatry*, 29 (1990), pp. 526–533; Hans C. Lou et al., "Focal Cerebral Dysfunction in Developmental Learning Disabilities," *Lancet*, 335 (Jan. 6, 1990), pp. 8–11. On the history of such diagnoses, see Russell J. Schachar, "Hyperkinetic Syndrome: Historical Development of the Concept," in Eric A. Taylor, ed., *The Overactive Child* (Oxford: Blackwell, 1986), pp. 19–40.

7. *New York Times*, Jan. 13, 1996, p. A9. Synthesized in 1955, Ritalin was first recommended for "hyperkinetic behavior syndrome" in children two years later. See Maurice W. Laufer and Eric Denhoff (at the Emma Pendleton Bradley Home in Providence, RI), "Hyperkinetic Behavior Syndrome in Children," *Journal of Pediatrics*, 50 (1957), pp. 463–474. The authors, however,

preferred amphetamines. First to come out emphatically for Ritalin in the control of hyperactive children who made trouble ("disturbed" children) were C. Keith Conners and Leon Eisenberg (both psychiatrists at Johns Hopkins University), "The Effects of Methylphenidate on Symptomatology and Learning in Disturbed Children," *AJP*, 120 (1963), pp. 458–464.

8. "Media Coverage Can Trigger Stress Disorder in Kids," *Medical Post*, June 13, 1995, p. 34.

9. Cross-National Collaborative Group, "The Changing Rate of Major Depression: Cross-National Comparisons," *JAMA*, 268 (Dec. 2, 1992), pp. 3098–3104. On long-term trends in the presentation of depression, see Edward Shorter, "The Cultural Face of Melancholy," in Shorter, *From the Mind into the Body: The Cultural Origins of Psychosomatic Symptoms* (New York: Free Press, 1994), pp. 118–148.

10. "National Depression Screening Day Set Records in 1993," *Psychiatric News*, April 1, 1994, p. 11.

11. S. M. Schappert, "Office Visits to Psychiatrists: United States, 1989–1990," *Advance Data from Vital and Health Statistics*, no. 237 (Hyattsville, MD: National Center for Health Statistics, 1993), see tab. 6, p. 6.

12. Narrow, *Arch. Gen. Psych.* 1993, p. 101.

13. For critiques of this entity, see Harold Merskey, "The Manufacture of Personalities: The Production of Multiple Personality Disorder," *BJP*, 160 (1992), pp. 327–340; Herman M. van Praag, *"Make-Believes" in Psychiatry, or The Perils of Progress* (New York: Brunner/Mazel, 1993), pp. 203–209.

14. Allen J. Frances et al., "An A to Z Guide to DSM-IV Conundrums," *Journal of Abnormal Psychology*, 100 (1991), pp. 407–412, quote p. 410.

15. Robert S. Wallerstein, "The Future of Psychotherapy," *Bulletin of the Menninger Clinic*, 55 (1991), pp. 421–443, quote pp. 430–431.

16. See Edward Shorter, *From Paralysis to Fatigue: A History of Psychosomatic Illness in the Modern Era* (New York: Free Press, 1992), pp. 51–64.

17. Hagop S. Akiskal and William T. McKinney, Jr., "Psychiatry and Pseudopsychiatry," *Archives of General Psychiatry*, 28 (1973), pp. 367–373, quotes p. 372.

18. Adolf Meyer, "Historical Sketch and Outlook of Psychiatric Social Work" (1922), in Eunice E. Winters, ed., *Collected Papers of Adolf Meyer*, vol. 4 (Baltimore: Hopkins, 1952), pp. 237–240.

19. National Conference of Social Work, *Proceedings of the National Conference of Social Work, 47th session, 1920* (Chicago: University of Chicago Press [1920], quotes pp. 256, 378.

20. E. Fuller Torrey, *Nowhere to Go: The Tragic Odyssey of the Homeless Mentally Ill* (New York: Harper and Row, 1989), p. 164.

21. Stuart A. Kirk and Herb Kutchins, *The Selling of DSM: The Rhetoric of Science in Psychiatry* (New York: Aldine, 1992), p. 8.

22. See Harry Specht, "Social Work and the Popular Psychotherapies," *Social Service Review*, 64 (1990), pp. 345–357, quote p. 345.

23. Specht, *Soc. Serv. Review* 1990, p. 346.

24. Carl R. Rogers, *Client-Centered Therapy: Its Current Practice, Implications, and Theory* (Boston: Houghton Mifflin, 1951), p. 23.

25. Carl R. Rogers, "In Retrospect: Forty-Six Years," *American Psychologist*, 29 (1974), pp. 115–123, quotes pp. 115, 116.

26. The quotation is Specht's summary of Rogers, *Soc. Serv. Review* 1990, p. 351.

27. Rogers, *American Psychologist* 1974, p. 117.

28. American Psychological Association, personal communication, 6,574 members as of Jan. 1996.

29. Group for the Advancement of Psychiatry, *Psychotherapy in the Future* (Washington, DC: APA, 1992; report no. 133), p. 1.

30. Ronald C. Kessler et al., "Lifetime and 12-Month Prevalence of DSM-III-R Psychiatric Disorders in the United States," *Archives of General Psychiatry*, 51 (1994), pp. 8–19. Americans 15 to 54 were interviewed. See tab. 2, p. 12.

31. Kessler, *Archives of General Psychiatry*, tab. 4, p. 14.

32. Province of Ontario, Premier's Council on Health, Well-Being and Social Justice, *Mental Health in Ontario: Selected Findings from the Mental Health Supplement to the Ontario Health Survey* (Toronto: Ministry of Health, n.d. [1994]), p. 40.

33. Daniel Freedman, "Foreword," in Lee N. Robins and Darrel A. Regier, eds., *Psychiatric Disorders in America*, (New York: Free Press, 1991), p. xxiii.

34. See, for example, "Congress Takes First Step . . . ," *Psychiatric News*, July 7, 1995, p. 1.

35. Henri Ellenberger, "A Comparison of European and American Psychiatry," *Bulletin of the Menninger Clinic*, 19 (1955), pp. 43–52, quote p. 48.

36. R. E. Kendell et al., "Diagnostic Criteria of American and British Psychiatrists," *Archives of General Psychiatry*, 25 (1971), pp. 123–130, see p. 128.

37. Mitchell Wilson, "*DSM-III* and the Transformation of American Psychiatry: A History," *AJP*, 150 (1993), pp. 399–410, quote p. 403; Wilson interviewed Spitzer and paraphrased his remarks.

38. On Stengel's life, see F. A. Jenner, "Erwin Stengel: A Personal Memoir," in German E. Berrios and Hugh Freeman, eds., *150 Years of British Psychiatry, 1841–1991* (London: Gaskell, 1991), pp. 436–444. Felix Post interview in Greg Wilkinson, ed., *Talking about Psychiatry* (London: Gaskell, 1993), p. 169.

39. Erwin Stengel, "Classification of Mental Disorders," *Bulletin of the World Health Organization*, 21 (1959), pp. 601–663, quote p. 603.

40. Morton Kramer, "Cross-National Study of Diagnosis of the Mental Disorders: Origin of the Problem," *AJP*, 125 (suppl. 10) (1969), pp. 1–11; Heinz Lehmann in ibid., "Discussion: A Renaissance of Psychiatric Diagnosis?" pp. 43–46, quote p. 46.

41. Donald W. Goodwin and Samuel B. Guze, *Psychiatric Diagnosis* (1974), 4th ed. (New York: Oxford U.P., 1989), p. vii.

42. American Medico-Psychological Association and National Committee for Mental Hygiene, *Statistical Manual for the Use of Institutions for the Insane* (New York: no publ. given, 1918). See also Gerald N. Grob, "Origins of *DSM-I*: A Study in Appearance and Reality," *AJP*, 148 (1991), pp. 421–431, esp. p. 426; Theodore Millon, "On the Past and Future of the *DSM-III*: Personal Recollections and Projections," in Millon and Gerald L. Klerman, eds., *Contemporary Directions in Psychopathology: Toward the DSM-IV* (New York: Guilford, 1986), pp. 29–70, esp. pp. 30–34.

43. National Conference on Nomenclature of Disease, H. B. Logie, ed., *A Standard Classified Nomenclature of Disease* (New York: Commonwealth, 1933); of the three-page section on "mental diseases," two are given over to psychoses. The American Neurological Association approved the brief list of "psychoneuroses, neuroses, maladjustment . . ." and so on (pp. 88–90). On these events, see the Foreword of American Psychiatric Association, *Diagnostic and Statistical Manual, Mental Disorders* (Washington, DC: APA, 1952), pp. v–vi. "*DSM-I.*"

44. *DSM-I*, p. vii.

45. *DSM-I*, p. xii.

46. *DSM-I*, p. 31.

47. Also at issue in drafting *DSM-II* was harmonizing the American nosology with the international ICD nosology, see Millon, *Contemporary Directions*, pp. 34–36. Millon's claim, however, that the drafters of *DSM-II* "eschew[ed] theory-based positions" seems improbable (p. 35).

48. *DSM-II*, p. 39.

49. On the "Neo-Kraepelinians," see Gerald Klerman, "The Contemporary American Scene: Diagnosis and Classification of Mental Disorders, Alcoholism and Drug Abuse," in Norman Sartorius et al., eds., *Sources and Traditions of Classification in Psychiatry* (Toronto: Hogrefe, 1990), pp. 93–138, quote, p. 109.

50. George Winokur and Paula Clayton, *The Medical Basis of Psychiatry* (Philadelphia: Saunders, 1986).

51. John P. Feighner et al., "Diagnostic Criteria for Use in Psychiatric Research," *Archives of General Psychiatry*, 26 (1972), pp. 57–63; see p. 58 for the criteria for depression.

52. Robert Spitzer et al., "Research Diagnostic Criteria," *Archives of General Psychiatry*, 35 (1978), pp. 773–782. Spitzer and colleagues took the RDC criteria for an initial promenade in a discussion of how schizophrenia and other psychoses should be diagnosed. See Spitzer et al., "Schizophrenia and Other Psychotic Disorders in *DSM-III*," *Schizophrenia Bulletin*, 4 (1978), pp. 489–509, esp. p. 500f.

53. See Ronald Bayer, *Homosexuality and American Psychiatry: The Politics of Diagnosis* (New York: Basic, 1981), pp. 101f.

54. On these events, see Kirk and Kutchins, *Selling of DSM*, p. 79.

55. See Millon, *Contemporary Directions*, pp. 36–38. As early as 1970, Millon had been urging Sabshin to undertake a more radical revision of *DSM-II* (p. 36).

56. Ronald Bayer and Robert L. Spitzer, "Neurosis, Psychodynamics, and *DSM-III*," *Archives of General Psychiatry*, 42 (1985), pp. 187–196, quote p. 188.

57. *DSM-III*, quote p. 3, field-testing p. 5.

58. Kenneth S. Kendler et al., "Independent Diagnoses of Adoptees and Relatives as Defined by *DSM-III* in the Provincial and National Samples of the Danish Adoption Study of Schizophrenia," *Archives of General Psychiatry*, 51 (1994), pp. 456–468, see especially p. 464.

59. Gerald L. Klerman, "The Advantages of *DSM-III*," *AJP*, 141 (1984), pp. 539–542, quote p. 542. See also Klerman, "Is the Reliability of *DSM-III* a Scientific or a Political Question?" *Social Work Research*, 23 (1987), p. 3.

60. Wilson, *AJP* 1993, p. 399.

61. M. Bourgeois, "Connaissance et usage du *DSM-III*," in Pierre Pichot, ed., *DSM-III et psychiatrie française* (Paris: Masson, 1985), pp. 51–59; the attitudes of typical psychiatry residents in France are described on pp. 51–52.

62. *Diagnostisches und Statistisches Manual psychischer Störungen: DSM-III-R*, H.-U. Wittchen et al., eds. and trans. (Weinheim: Beltz, 1989), see the translators' introduction, p. x.

63. Kirk, *Selling of DSM*, pp. 118, 199. American Psychiatric Association, *Diagnostic and Statistical Manual of Mental Disorders*, 4th ed: *DSM-IV* (Washington, DC: APA, 1994). The actual number of numerical codes in *DSM-IV*, minus the "V" codes, is 374. Herb Kutchins and Stuart Kirk assert that the net gain is 5 and I accept their mathematics. "*DSM-IV*: Does Bigger and Newer Mean Better?" *Harvard Mental Health Letter*, May, 1995, pp. 4–6, see especially p. 5.

64. See Herman van Praag's critique of this "new-disorder-rush" in his "*Make-Believes*" *in Psychiatry*, p. 250 and passim.

65. Philippe Pinel, *Traité médico-philosophique sur l'aliénation mentale*, 2nd ed. (Paris: Brosson, 1809), pp. xx–xxi, 138–139.

66. Millon, *Contemporary Directions*, p. 39.

67. I am grateful to Mitchell Weiss for this notion.

68. George E. Vaillant, "The Disadvantages of *DSM-III* Outweigh Its Advantages," *AJP*, 141 (1984), pp. 542–545, quote p. 543.

69. *DSM-II*, p. 44.

70. Millon, *Contemporary Directions*, pp. 50–51.

71. See Wilson, *AJP* (1993), pp. 406–407; Bayer and Spitzer, *Arch. Gen. Psych.* 1985.

72. *DSM-III*, p. 9; for example, phobic disorders also become "phobic neuroses" (p. 225).

73. Wilbur J. Scott, "PTSD in *DSM-III*: A Case in the Politics of Diagnosis and Disease," *Social Problems*, 37 (1990), pp. 294–310, quote p. 308.

74. American Psychiatric Association, *Diagnostic and Statistical Manual of Mental Disorders*, 3d. rev. ed.: *DSM-III-R* (Washington, DC: APA, 1987), pp. 371–374, 367–369.

75. *DSM-IV*, 1994, pp. 715–718. For an exchange on the scientific usefulness of *DSM-IV*, see Kutchins and Kirk, *Harvard Mental Health Letter*, May, 1995, pp. 4–6; and the response by Allen Frances et al., "*DSM-IV*: Its Value and Limitations," *Harvard Mental Health Letter*, June, 1995, pp. 4–6.

76. Wilson, *AJP* 1993, p. 407.

77. Nathan G. Hale, Jr., *The Rise and Crisis of Psychoanalysis in the United States: Freud and the Americans, 1917–1985* (New York: Oxford, 1995), p. 355.

78. For an account of the therapeutic effectiveness of the main psychotherapies, see American Psychiatric Association, Commission on Psychiatric Therapies, vol. 2: *The Psychosocial Therapies* (Washington, DC: APA, 1984).

79. Hans J. Eysenck, "The Effects of Psychotherapy: An Evaluation," *Journal of Consulting Psychology*, 16 (1952), pp. 319–324. On the increasing dubiety about the effectiveness of formal systems of psychotherapy, contrasted with spontaneous recovery and placebo psychotherapy, see Leslie Prioleau et al., "An Analysis of Psychotherapy versus Placebo Studies," *Behavioral and Brain Sciences*, 6 (1983), pp. 275–310. The authors write, "Thirty years after Eysenck (1952) first raised the issue of the effectiveness of psychotherapy . . . we are still not aware of a single convincing demonstration that the benefits of psychotherapy exceed those of placebos for real patients" (p. 284).

80. Wallerstein, *Bull. Menninger Clin.* 1991, pp. 423, 425, 430, 433.

81. Bertram S. Brown, "The Life of Psychiatry," *AJP*, 133 (1976), pp. 489–495, quote p. 492.

82. Kenneth Z. Altshuler, "Whatever Happened to Intensive Psychotherapy?" *AJP*, 147 (1990), pp. 428–430, quote p. 430.

83. Hoch is quoted indirectly in Milton Greenblatt and Myron R. Sharaf, "Poverty and Mental Health: Implications for Training," in Nolan D. C. Lewis and Margaret O. Strahl, eds., *The Complete Psychiatrist: The Achievements of Paul H. Hoch* (Albany: SUNY Press, 1968), pp. 688–697, quote p. 688.

84. *Complete Psychiatrist Hoch*, p. 692.

85. A 1988–1989 poll found that "only 2.7 percent of psychiatrists' outpatients were engaged in psychoanalysis." See Robert A. Dorwart et al., "A National Study of Psychiatrists' Professional Activities," *AJP*, 149 (1992), pp. 1499–1505, statistic p. 1503. The exact percentage of practicing analysts is unknown because many psychiatrists who were trained as analysts later abandoned it.

86. Fritz Redlich and Stephen R. Kellert, "Trends in American Mental Health," *AJP*, 135 (1978), pp. 22–28, quotes p. 26.

87. Linda Hilles, "Changing Trends in the Application of Psychoanalytic Principles to a Psychiatric Hospital," *Bulletin of the Menninger Clinic*, 32 (1968), pp. 203–218, statistics pp. 210–211. The Menningers, unfortunately, misjudged the *Zeitgeist* and shifted from psychoanalysis to social psychiatry rather than biological. See Lawrence J. Friedman, *Menninger: The Family and the Clinic* (Lawrence: University Press of Kansas, 1990), pp. 264–265.

88. Turan Itil, "Fritz Flügel," in T. A. Ban and Hanns Hippius, eds., *Psychopharmacology in Perspective* (New York: Springer, n.d. [1992]), pp. 17–19, quote p. 18.

89. Daniel S. Jaffe et al., "Survey of Psychoanalytic Practice 1976," *American Psychoanalytic Association Journal*, 26 (1978), pp. 615–631, quotes pp. 619, 620.

90. Jaffe, *J. Am. Pa. Assn.*, 1978, p. 618.

91. Bruce Cohen, "Watch the Clock . . . ," *Psychiatric News*, Feb. 4, 1994, p. 14.

92. Paul Gray, "The Assault on Freud," *Time*, Nov. 29, 1993, pp. 47–50.

93. On this philosophy at Chestnut Lodge, see Sandra G. Boodman, "The Mystery of Chestnut Lodge," *Washington Post Magazine*, Oct. 8, 1989, pp. 18f, esp. pp. 23, 41.

94. For details of the Osheroff case, see Gerald L. Klerman, "The Psychiatric Patient's Right to Effective Treatment: Implications of *Osheroff v. Chestnut Lodge*," AJP, 147 (1990), pp. 409–418; see also Klerman, "The *Osheroff* Debate: Finale," AJP, 148 (1991), pp. 387–388.

95. See Robert Pear, "M.D.s Are Making Room for Others among the Ranks of Psychoanalysts," *New York Times*, Aug. 19, 1992, p. C12. The figure for 1989 was 17 percent. See James Morris, "Psychoanalytic Training Today," *American Psychoanalytic Association Journal*, 40 (1992), pp. 1185–1210, esp. pp. 1191–92.

96. Robert Michels, "Psychoanalysis and Psychiatry—The End of the Affair," [New York Academy of Psychoanalysis] *Academy Forum*, 25 (1981), quote p. 9.

97. Adolf Grünbaum, "Does Psychoanalysis Have a Future? Doubtful," *Harvard Mental Health Letter*, 11 (4) (Oct. 1994), pp. 3–6, quote p. 4.

98. "Centre Offers Course," *Medical Post*, Oct. 11, 1994, p. 27.

99. Amer. Pa. Assoc., meeting of Dec. 1952, "Scientific Committees: Evaluation of Psychoanalytic Therapy," *American Psychoanalytic Association Bulletin*, 9 (Apr. 1953), p. 331. Committee chair Jean G. N. Cushing formally recommended that the committee's work be held "in abeyance" at the May 1953 meeting. Ibid. (Oct. 1953), p. 730.

100. Robert P. Knight, "The Present Status of Organized Psychoanalysis in the United States," *American Psychoanalytic Association Journal*, 1 (1953), pp. 197–220, quotes pp. 219–220.

101. Dec. 1954 meeting, "Committee Reports," *Amer. Pa. Assoc. Bull.*, 11 (1) (Apr. 1955), p. 327.

102. Meeting of Apr. 1956. "Central Fact-Gathering Committee," *Amer. Pa. Assoc. Bull.* 12 (2) (Oct. 1956), pp. 712–713.

103. Dec. 1957 meeting, "Central Fact-Gathering Committee," *Amer. Pa. Assoc. Bull.*, 14 (1) (Apr. 1958), p. 362.

104. David A. Hamburg et al., "Report of Ad Hoc Committee on Central Fact-Gathering Data of the American Psychoanalytic Association," *Amer. Pa. Assoc. Journal*, 15 (1967), pp. 841–861.

105. Eysenck, *Journal of Consulting Psychology*, 1952, see tab. 1, p. 321. ". . . Two-thirds of a group of neurotic patients will recover or improve to a marked extent within about two years of the onset of their illness, whether they are treated by means of psychotherapy or not" (p. 322).

106. William Mayer-Gross, Eliot Slater, and Martin Roth, *Clinical Psychiatry* (London: Cassell, 1954), p. 17.

107. Donald F. Klein, "Anxiety Reconceptualized," in Klein and Judith G. Rabkin, eds., *Anxiety: New Research and Changing Concepts* (New York: Raven, 1981), pp. 235–263, quote p. 239. Klein's skepticism about psychoanalysis was further strengthened when the panic patients responded to imipramine but not to chlorpromazine.

108. Philip R. A. May and A. Hussain Tuma, "The Effect of Psychotherapy and Stelazine on Length of Hospital Stay . . . ," *JNMD*, 139 (1964), pp. 362–369. Statistically, only the drug therapy had any significant effect in reducing length of stay. The psychotherapy patients were indistinguishable from the untreated controls. The combination of drugs and therapy was not statistically significant.

109. Seymour Fisher and Roger P. Greenberg, *The Scientific Credibility of Freud's Theories and Therapy* (1977) (reprint New York: Columbia U. P., 1985), p. 395. Although the authors' assessment of research done since 1977 turned out more favorably toward psychoanalysis than in previous work, they still found that Freud's basic conception of insight-oriented psychotherapy was deficient: "Patients' awareness of their own motivations or dynamics has proven to be of more limited value in directly promoting change than Freud initially postulated." Fisher and Greenberg, *Freud Scientifically Reappraised: Testing the Theories and Therapy* (New York: Wiley, 1996), p. 282.

110. Adolf Grünbaum, *The Foundations of Psychoanalysis: A Philosophical Critique* (Berkeley: University of California Press, 1984); Grünbaum, *Validation in the Clinical Theory of Psychoanalysis: A Study in the Philosophy of Psychoanalysis* (Madison, CT: International Universities Press, 1993).

111. Richard Webster, *Why Freud Was Wrong: Sin, Science and Psychoanalysis* (New York: Basic, 1995).

112. Grünbaum, *Harvard Mental Health Letter* 1994, p. 5.

113. Hans J. Eysenck, *Decline and Fall of the Freudian Empire* (1985) (London: Penguin, 1991), p. 207.

114. Peter D. Kramer, "The New You," *Psychiatric Times*, Mar. 1990, pp. 45–46.

115. Peter D. Kramer, *Listening to Prozac* (New York: Penguin, 1993), pp. xvi and passim.

116. Kessler, *Archives of General Psychiatry* 1994, p. 12.

117. On this argument, see Shorter, *Bedside Manners: The Troubled History of Doctors and Patients* (New York: Simon and Schuster, 1985), chs. 3, 8.

118. This account of meprobamate's development depends mainly on Berger's recollections. See Frank M. Berger [an interview with], "The

'Social-Chemistry' of Pharmacological Discovery: The Miltown Story," *Social Pharmacology*, 2 (1988), pp. 189–204, quote p. 191; see also Berger, "Anxiety and the Discovery of the Tranquilizers," in Frank J. Ayd, Jr., and Barry Blackwell, eds., *Discoveries in Biological Psychiatry* (Baltimore: Ayd Medical Communications, 1984), pp. 115–129.

119. Berger, *Social Pharmacology* 1988, pp. 192–193.

120. These details are from Ayd, "The Early History of Modern Psychopharmacology," *Neuropsychopharmacology*, 5 (1991), pp. 71–84, esp. pp. 73–74.

121. S. J. Perelman, *The Road to Miltown or, Under the Spreading Atrophy* (New York: Simon and Schuster, 1957). The volume of humorous essays is not about Miltown.

122. Mickey C. Smith, *Small Comfort: A History of the Minor Tranquilizers* (New York: Praeger Scientific, 1985), tab. 5.1, p. 67.

123. "'Ideal' in Tranquility," *Newsweek*, Oct. 29, 1956, p. 63.

124. The following account is based on Willy Haefely, "Alleviation of Anxiety: The Benzodiazepine Saga," in M. J. Parnham and J. Bruinvels, eds., *Psycho- and Neuro-Pharmacology*, vol. 1 (Amsterdam: Elsevier, 1983), pp. 270–306, esp. pp. 272–277; Leo H. Sternbach, *The Benzodiazepine Story* (Basel: Eds. Roche, 1980; this is a revised version of Sternbach, "The Benzodiazepine Story," *Progress in Drug Research*, 22 (1978), pp. 229–266; Sternbach's "The Discovery of Librium," *Agents and Actions*, 2 (1972), pp. 193–196; also on a personal communication from Sternbach.

125. Irvin M. Cohen, "The Benzodiazepines," in Ayd, *Discoveries in Biological Psychiatry*, pp. 130–141, quote p. 130.

126. Haefely, *Psycho- and Neuro-Pharmacology*, p. 274.

127. Lowell O. Randall, "Pharmacology of Methaminodiazepoxide," *Diseases of the Nervous System*, 21 (suppl. no. 3) (1960), pp. 7–10, quote p. 7.

128. See Joseph M. Tobin et al., "Preliminary Evaluation of Librium (Ro-5-0690) in the Treatment of Anxiety Reactions," *Diseases of the Nervous System*, 21 (suppl. no. 3) (1960), pp. 11–19, as well as the other papers on Librium offered at a "Symposium on Newer Antidepressant and Other Psychotherapeutic Drugs" at the University of Texas in Galveston in Nov. 1959. See also Cohen, in *Discoveries Biological Psychiatry*. Both Tobin and Cohen share the priority for introducing chlordiazepoxide clinically.

129. Sternbach, *Benzodiazepine Story*, p. 43.

130. On side effects from stopping Librium, see Leo H. Hollister et al., "Withdrawal Reactions from Chlordiazepoxide ('Librium')," *Psychopharmacologia*, 2 (1961), pp. 63–68.

131. Sternbach, *Benzodiazepine Story*, p. 7.

132. Hugh J. Parry et al., "National Patterns of Psychotherapeutic Drug Use," *Archives of General Psychiatry*, 28 (1973), pp. 769–783, tab. 6, p. 775.

133. National Center for Health Statistics, "Office Visits to Psychiatrists: National Ambulatory Medical Care Survey, United States, 1975–1976," *Vital and Health Statistics, Advance Data*, no. 38 (Aug. 25, 1978), tab. 4, p. 4.

Shappert, *Vital and Health Statistics, Advance Data,* 1993, p. 11, tab. 10. The figure for 1980 was 36.0 percent. National Center for Health Statistics, H. Koch, "Drug Utilization in Office-Based Practice . . . 1980," *Vital and Health Statistics,* ser. 13, no. 65, DHHS pub. no. (PHS) 83-1726 (Public Health Service, Washington, DC: GPO, March 1983), p. 28, tab. 10.

134. Smith, *Small Comfort,* p. 217.

135. NCHS, "Drug Utilization" 1980, p. 15.

136. David Healy, "The History of British Psychopharmacology," in Hugh Freeman and German E. Berrios, eds., *150 Years of British Psychiatry, Volume II: The Aftermath* (London: Athlone, 1996), pp. 61–68, quote p. 74.

137. *DSM-II,* p. 39.

138. Donald F. Klein, "Delineation of Two Drug-Responsive Anxiety Syndromes," *Psychopharmacologia,* 5 (1964), pp. 397–408.

139. *DSM-III,* pp. 230–231.

140. Gerald L. Klerman, "Overview of the Cross-National Collaborative Panic Study," *Archives of General Psychiatry,* 45 (1988), pp. 407–412. On Upjohn and alprazolam, see David Healy, *Images of Trauma: From Hysteria to Post-Traumatic Stress Disorder* (London: Faber, 1993), pp. 230–231; also Healy, "The Psychopharmacological Era: Notes toward a History," *Journal of Psychopharmacology,* 4 (1990), pp. 152–167, esp. pp. 158–159. Healy and others have argued that Ciba-Geigy performed a similar feat in repositioning its antidepressant clomipramine as a drug specific for obsessive-compulsive disorder.

141. See the exchange between the doubters of alprazolam and the supporters: Isaac M. Marks et al. [the doubters], "Alprazolam and Exposure Alone and Combined in Panic Disorder with Agoraphobia," *BJP,* 162 (1993), pp. 776–787; for the supporters' reply, see David A. Spiegel et al., "Comment on the London/Toronto Study of Alprazolam and Exposure in Panic Disorder with Agoraphobia," ibid., pp. 788–789; Marks et al. replied to this on pp. 790–794; for an earlier exchange, see Marks, letter: "The 'Efficacy' of Alprazolam in Panic Disorder and Agoraphobia: A Critique of Recent Reports," *Archives of General Psychiatry,* 46 (1989), pp. 668–670; the original investigators answered on pp. 670–672.

142. "The Promise of Prozac," *Newsweek,* Mar. 26, 1990, p. 39.

143. John H. Gaddum, "Drugs Antagonistic to 5-Hydroxytryptamine," in G. E. W. Wolstenholme and Margaret P. Cameron, eds., *Ciba Foundation Symposium on Hypertension* (London: Churchill, 1954), pp. 75–77, quote p. 77.

144. Merton Sandler and David Healy, "The Place of Chemical Pathology in the Development of Psychopharmacology," *Journal of Psychopharmacology,* 8 (1994), pp. 124–133, quote p. 124.

145. See, however, D. W. Woolley and E. Shaw, researchers at the Rockefeller Institute for Medical Research in New York, "A Biochemical and Pharmacological Suggestion about Certain Mental Disorders," *Proceedings, National Academy of Sciences,* 40 (1954), pp. 228–231, in which the authors argued that "serotonin has an important role to play in mental processes and that the

suppression of its action results in a mental disorder" (p. 230). See Woolley's reconstruction of this story in his *The Biochemical Bases of Psychoses, or the Serotonin Hypothesis about Mental Diseases* (New York: Wiley, 1962), pp. 189–192.

146. Bernard B. Brodie and Parkhurst A. Shore, "A Concept for a Role of Serotonin and Norepinephrine as Chemical Mediators in the Brain," *Annals of the New York Academy of Sciences*, 66 (1957), pp. 631–642; for some context, see Robert Kanigel, *Apprentice to Genius: The Making of a Scientific Dynasty* (New York: Macmillan, 1986), pp. 97–101, quote p. 101.

147. Alec Coppen et al., "Potentiation of the Antidepressive Effect of a Monoamine-Oxidase Inhibitor by Tryptophan," *Lancet*, 1 (Jan. 12, 1963), pp. 79–81. Tryptophan is a precursor of serotonin. The following year, Coppen went to West Park Hospital, where he remained for the rest of his career.

148. Undated transcript of an interview David Healy did with Coppen, p. 7. I am grateful to Dr. Healy for making a copy available to me.

149. Arvid Carlsson et al., "Effects of Some Antidepressant Drugs on the Depletion of Intraneuronal Brain Catecholamine Stores . . . ," *European Journal of Pharmacology*, 5 (1969), pp. 367–373.

150. See Alec Coppen et al., "Zimelidine: A Therapeutic and Pharmacokinetic Study in Depression," *Psychopharmacology*, 63 (1979), pp. 199–202; Arvid Carlsson et al., eds., *Recent Advances in the Treatment of Depression; Proceedings of an International Symposium, Corfu, Greece, April 16–18, 1980* (Copenhagen: Munksgaard, 1981; *Acta Psychiatrica Scandinavica*, suppl. 290, vol. 63 [1981]). On Carlsson's defense of his priority see his abstract, "A Historical Note on the Development of Zimelidine, the First Selective Serotonin Reuptake Inhibitor," *European Psychiatry*, 11 suppl. 4 (1996), pp. 235s–236s.

151. See Steven E. Hyman and Eric J. Nestler, *Molecular Foundations of Psychiatry* (Washington, DC: APA, 1993), p. 127.

152. David T. Wong et al., "A Selective Inhibitor of Serotonin Uptake: Lilly 110140 . . . ," *Life Sciences*, 15 (1974), pp. 471–479. The story of fluoxetine's development at Lilly is told in Pharmaceutical Manufacturers Association, *The Discoverers Awards, 1993* (Washington, DC: PMA, 1993). See also Bryan B. Molloy et al., "The Discovery of Fluoxetine," *Pharmaceutical News*, 1 (June 1994), pp. 6–10. Further information was obtained in interview with Joachim F. Wernicke, a psychiatrist on Lilly's staff between 1984 and 1988. I have compressed some of the detail in a quite complex story.

153. Louis Lemberger et al., "The Effect of Nisoxetine (Lilly Compound 94939), a Potential Antidepressant, on Biogenic Uptake in Man," *British Journal of Clinical Pharmacology*, 3 (1976), pp. 215–220. See also M. J. Schmidt and J. F. Thornberry, "Norepinephrine-Stimulated Cyclic AMP Accumulation . . . ," *Archives internationales de pharmacodynamie et de thérapie*, 229 (1977), pp. 42–51.

154. The acronym SSRI became current with the publication of John P. Feighner and William F. Boyer, eds., *Selective Serotonin Re-uptake Inhibitors* (Chichester: Wiley, 1991).

155. Louis Lemberger et al., "Pharmacologic Effects in Man of a Specific Serotonin-Reuptake Inhibitor," *Science*, 199 (1978), pp. 436–437. With this research, Lilly verified that fluoxetine inhibited serotonin reuptake in humans, without side effects on blood pressure.

156. The first published clinical report was so negative, it is a wonder Lilly did not kill the drug. None of the three patients responded and one developed a severe dystonia. Herbert Y. Meltzer et al., "Extrapyramidal Side Effects and Increased Serum Prolactin Following Fluoxetine, a New Antidepressant," *Journal of Neural Transmission*, 45 (1979), pp. 165–175.

157. John P. Feighner, "The New Generation of Antidepressants," *Journal of Clinical Psychiatry*, 44 (1983), pp. 49–55, see tab. 2, p. 51.

158. "Gilding Lilly," *Barron's*, May 12, 1986, pp. 15, 63. Lilly scientist David Wong told the author in an interview that the company never lost interest in depression, despite the enthusiasm about weight-loss.

159. On the field trials, see William Boyer and John P. Feighner, "An Overview of Fluoxetine, A New Serotonin-Specific Antidepressant," *Mount Sinai Journal of Medicine*, 56 (1989), pp. 136–140.

160. In 1986, Prozac had been approved in Belgium.

161. James L. Hudson and Harrison G. Pope, Jr., "Affective Spectrum Disorder: Does Antidepressant Response Identify a Family of Disorders with a Common Pathophysiology?" *AJP*, 147 (1990), pp. 552–564, quote p. 558.

162. Quoted in Colette Dowling, *You Mean I Don't Have to Feel This Way? New Help for Depression, Anxiety and Addiction* (1991) (New York: Bantam, 1993), p. 20.

163. Schappert, *Advance Data* 1993, tab. 7, p. 7; 43.1 percent of all visits were for mood disorders: 48.8 percent for women, 34.9 percent for men.

164. "The Personality Pill," *Time*, Oct. 1, 1993, p. 53.

165. Schappert, *Advance Data* 1993, tab. 14, p. 13.

166. *New York Times*, Dec. 13, 1993, p. 1.

167. "The Culture of Prozac," *Newsweek*, Feb. 7, 1994, p. 41.

168. "Listening to Eli Lilly," *Wall Street Journal*, Mar. 31, 1994, p. B1. By 1993, Prozac ranked among the top 20 brand-name drugs prescribed by American doctors, though it was not among the top 2 (Amoxicillin and Tylenol). D. A. Woodwell and S. M. Schappert, "National Ambulatory Medical Care Survey: 1993 Summary," *Advance Data from Vital and Health Statistics*, no. 270 (Hyattsville, MD: National Center for Health Statistics, 1995), tab. 21, p. 14.

169. *Newsweek* 1990, p. 41.

170. Healy, *Journal of Psychopharmacology* 1990, p. 159.

171. *Encyclopedia of Associations*, 1996, pp. 1794, 1795.

172. Pierre Deniker, "The Neuroleptics: A Historical Survey," *Acta Psychiatrica Scandinavica*, 82 (suppl. 358) (1990), pp. 83–87, quote p. 87.

173. Association of American Medical Colleges, *AAMC Data Book* (Washington, DC: AAMC, 1995), unpaginated, tabs. B13, F1; data on PGY-1

residencies; the remainder of the 1,327 available first-year positions were filled mainly with foreign medical graduates.

174. An editorial in the *Lancet* also asked this question. "Molecules and Minds," *Lancet*, 343 (Mar. 19, 1994), pp. 681–682.

175. Mark F. Longhurst, "Angry Patient, Angry Doctor," *Canadian Medical Association Journal*, 123 (1980), pp. 597–598, quote p. 598.

176. Kelly Kelleher et al., "Major Recent Trends in Mental Health in Primary Care," in *Mental Health, United States*, 1994, pp. 149–164, see fig. 9.6, "Mean Duration of Physician-Patient Contact, by Specialty, 1989," p. 155.

177. Robert Wood Johnson Foundation, *Special Report: Medical Practice in the United States* (Princeton: Robert Wood Johnson Foundation, 1981), fig. 2.4, p. 25.

178. Lester Luborsky et al., "Comparative Studies of Psychotherapies: Is it True That 'Everyone Has Won and All Must Have Prizes'?" *Archives of General Psychiatry*, 32 (1975), pp. 995–1008, quote p. 1004.

179. This is the argument of Shorter, *Bedside Manners*.

180. Kenneth S. Bowers, *Hypnosis for the Seriously Curious* (Monterey: Brooks, 1976), p. 152.

Index

Index

423

Index

429